Binary Data Analysis of Randomized Clinical Trials with Noncompliance

Statistics in Practice

Series Advisors

Human and Biological Sciences
Stephen Senn
University of Glasgow, UK

Earth and Environmental Sciences
Marian Scott
University of Glasgow, UK

Industry, Commerce and Finance
Wolfgang Jank
University of Maryland, USA

Statistics in Practice is an important international series of texts which provide detailed coverage of statistical concepts, methods and worked case studies in specific fields of investigation and study.

With sound motivation and many worked practical examples, the books show in down-to-earth terms how to select and use an appropriate range of statistical techniques in a particular practical field within each title's special topic area.

The books provide statistical support for professionals and research workers across a range of employment fields and research environments. Subject areas covered include medicine and pharmaceutics; industry, finance and commerce; public services; the earth and environmental sciences, and so on.

The books also provide support to students studying statistical courses applied to the above areas. The demand for graduates to be equipped for the work environment has led to such courses becoming increasingly prevalent at universities and colleges. It is our aim to present judiciously chosen and well-written workbooks to meet everyday practical needs. Feedback of views from readers will be most valuable to monitor the success of this aim.

A complete list of titles in this series appears at the end of the volume.

Binary Data Analysis of Randomized Clinical Trials with Noncompliance

Kung-Jong Lui

Department of Mathematics and Statistics
San Diego State University, USA

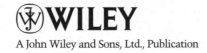

A John Wiley and Sons, Ltd., Publication

Registered office
John Wiley & Sons Ltd, The Atrium, Southern Gate, Chichester, West Sussex, PO19 8SQ, United Kingdom

For details of our global editorial offices, for customer services and for information about how to apply for permission to reuse the copyright material in this book please see our website at www.wiley.com.

Library of Congress Cataloging-in-Publication Data

Lui, Kung-Jong, author.
  Binary data analysis of randomized clinical trials with noncompliance/Kung-Jong Lui, Department of Mathematics and Statistics, San Diego State University, USA.
    p. ; cm.
  Includes bibliographical references and index.
  ISBN 978-0-470-66095-9 (cloth) – ISBN 978-1-119-99160-1 (epdf) – ISBN 978-1-119-99161-8 (obook) – ISBN 978-1-119-99390-2 (epub) – ISBN 978-1-119-99391-9 (mobi)
1. Clinical trials–Statistical methods.   2. Drugs–Testing–Statistical methods.   I. Title.
  [DNLM: 1. Randomized Controlled Trials as Topic–methods. 2. Medication Adherence. 3. Statistics as Topic–methods. QV 771]
  RM301.27.L85 2011
  615.5072′4–dc22

                                                                                          2010051072

A catalogue record for this book is available from the British Library.

Print ISBN: 978-0-470-66095-9
ePDF ISBN: 978-1-119-99160-1
oBook ISBN: 978-1-119-99161-8
ePub ISBN: 978-1-119-99390-2
Mobi ISBN: : 978-1-119-99391-9

Typeset in 11.75/14pt Times by Aptara Inc., New Delhi, India
Printed and bound in Great Britain by TJ International Ltd, Padstow, Cornwall

Dedicated to

*Professors William G. Cumberland and Abdelmonem A. Afifi
at UCLA, as well as
Professor Daniel McGee at Florida State University*

Contents

Preface

In a randomized clinical trial (RCT), it is quite common to encounter patients who do not comply with their assigned treatment due to ethical reasons, patient's decision or the feature of a study design (such as pre-randomized consent designs). Since noncompliance often occurs non-randomly, the commonly-used subgroup analyses, including as-treated (AT) analysis and as-protocol (AP) analysis, are well known to produce a possibly biased inference of treatment efficacy due to the incomparability of the underlying prognostic conditions for patients between two comparison groups. To alleviate this concern, the intent-to-treat (ITT) (or as-randomized (AR)) analysis has been often suggested for a RCT with noncompliance. However, the ITT analysis estimates the programmatic effectiveness rather than the treatment efficacy. Although ITT analysis may provide us with unbiased test for assessing the superiority of an experimental treatment to a standard treatment, the ITT analysis tends to underestimate the relative treatment effect in the presence of noncompliance under certain commonly-assumed conditions. Thus, how to assess the treatment efficacy in a RCT with noncompliance becomes practically useful and important.

The analysis of data for a RCT with noncompliance is generally quite complicated even for the simplest case of a simple noncompliance RCT, in which only patients assigned to the experimental treatment can have access to the experimental treatment. Furthermore, the frequent involvement of sophisticated numerical iterative procedures based on likelihoods to obtain parameter estimates makes this topic even more challenging and difficult for many clinicians and data analysts to appreciate. This book is to focus attention on the level which clinicians with one year of solid training in biostatistics can comprehend, and provides readers with a simple, systematic, and organized approach to study treatment effect for a RCT with noncompliance when the patient response is dichotomous and the noncompliance status is all-or-none in a variety of situations. This book adopts an instructive and easily-understood approach by using contingency tables to explicitly lay down the latent probability structure of observed data so that readers can easily visualize the logics and the ideas behind the development of the proposed test procedures and estimators in a one unified model frame. By contrast, when using the proportion difference (PD) to measure the relative treatment effect, we assume the structural risk additive model based on the model-based approach. While using the proportion ratio (PR) to measure the relative treatment effect, we assume the structural risk multiplicative model. Furthermore, this book presents all test procedures, estimators and sample size calculation procedures in closed forms. Readers may simply use a hand calculator to calculate all the test statistics, interval estimators or sample size calculation formulae without the need of employing any iterative numerical procedures in the situations considered here. For the easy access of the particular topic of reader's interest, this book is written in such a constructive structure that the underlying assumptions, notation, test procedures and formulae in each chapter are self-contained. Readers may directly refer to the particular chapter without the need of reading the details in all the preceding chapters, although I must admit that some assumptions, definitions in notation, and important notes are repeated to avoid confusions in narrative or ambiguities in formulae and findings. Through some real-life examples and computer-simulated data, readers can appreciate the practical usefulness of the test procedures and estimators discussed in this book. The exercises given at the end of each chapter can further help readers better understand the underlying assumptions, the theory and limitations of the proposed test procedures and estimators, as well as other relevant issues and extensions. To facilitate the use of sample size determination presented here, we include in Appendix SAS programs that can be easily modified by readers to accommodate the situations in which they are interested. Despite the book generally adopting the principal stratification approach to account for the effect due to noncompliance, this book also briefly addresses use of the model-based approach (which is related to a quite general class of the structural mean models (SMMs) proposed elsewhere) and notes the relations of parameters and estimators between these two approaches. Because the discussion on the SMM is truly beyond the modest scope of this book, the SMM is not discussed in the book. Readers who are interested in this area may begin with reading a few key references regarding the SMMs cited here.

This book is intended for postgraduates, clinicians, biostatisticians and data analysts. This book can be used as supplemental material for an introductory-level course focusing on clinical statistics or experimental trials in Epidemiology, Psychology and Sociology. This book may also be used as a desk reference for clinicians or biostatisticians when they come across binary data in the presence of noncompliance. To clarify the main issues raised by noncompliance and strengthen the narrative, we explicitly define and discuss some common assumptions and terms encountered in a RCT with noncompliance, as well as include numerical examples to illustrate the bias of most commonly-used subgroup analyses in Chapter 1. Because testing superiority, non-inferiority and equivalence, interval estimation and sample size calculation are all the most fundamental statistical topics for analyzing clinical data, this book concentrates discussions on these when we use the PD, the PR and the odds ratio (OR) to measure treatment efficacy under various frequently-encountered situations. These include parallel groups design (Chapter 2), stratified sampling (Chapter 3), cluster sampling (Chapter 4), parallel sampling with subsequent missing outcomes (Chapter 5) and data in repeated binary measurements (Chapter 6). Clinicians and biostatisticians should find that this book is useful and handy.

I wish to express my indebtedness to my colleagues Drs. Richard Levine, Barbara Bailey and Kristin Duncan at San Diego State University and the five anonymous reviewers who generously provided valuable comments and suggestions on an early draft and outlines of contents of the manuscript. I also wish to thank my wife Jen-Mei, whose continued patience and understanding have endured throughout so many years and made the work much more pleasant than it otherwise would have been. I want to thank my brothers Dan-Yang, Kung-Yi and Kung-Jen for their encouragements in many years. Finally I want to express my deepest appreciation to my parents, Shung-Wu and Li-Ching for their endless love, spiritual support and guidance, which continue to last in my memory.

Kung-Jong Lui
San Diego

About the Author

Kung-Jong Lui is a professor in the Department of Mathematics and Statistics at San Diego State University. He obtained his Ph.D. in biostatistics in 1982, M.S. in biostatistics in 1979, M.A. in Mathematics in 1977, all from UCLA, and B.S. in Mathematics in 1975 at Fu-Jen Catholic University at Taipei, Taiwan. He has had 150 publications in peer-reviewed journals, including *Biometrics, Statistics in Medicine, Biometrical Journal, Computational Statistics and Data Analysis, Psychometrika, Journal of Biopharmaceutical Statistics, Drug Information Journal, Contemporary Clinical Trials, Journal of Applied Statistics, Statistical Methodology, Communications in Statistics, Theory and Methods, Science, Nature, Proceedings of National Academy of Sciences, Journal of Official Statistics, IEEE Transactions on Reliability, Environmetrics, Test, American Journal of Epidemiology, American Journal of Public Health, New England Journal of Medicine, Journal of the American Medical Association,* etc. He is the author of the book *Statistical Estimation of Epidemiological Risk* published by Wiley in 2004. He is an Associate Editor for *Biometrical Journal.* He is a Fellow of the American Statistical Association, a Fellow of the American College of Epidemiology, and a life member of International Chinese Statistical Association.

1

Randomized clinical trials with noncompliance: issues, definitions and problems of commonly used analyses

When comparing an experimental treatment with a standard treatment (or placebo), we often employ a randomized clinical trial (RCT), in which eligible patients (after obtaining their informed consents) are randomized to one of the two treatments under comparison. One of the most fundamental ideas behind use of the RCT is, as shown in Figure 1.1, that all (known or unknown) covariates affecting patients' responses are expected to balance through randomization. Thus, when there is a difference in the distribution of patient responses between two treatments under perfect compliance, we may attribute this to different treatments they receive between the two randomized groups.

However, noncompliance can often occur in a RCT. When a patient feels that the burden of taking his/her assigned treatment is not worth its perceived benefits, the patient may decide not to comply with his/her assigned treatment (Heitjan, 1999). Noncompliance can also occur as a result of a negative experience of taking a treatment, drug sharing among participated patients, an error in treatment administration by study staff,

Binary Data Analysis of Randomized Clinical Trials with Noncompliance, First Edition. Kung-Jong Lui.
© 2011 John Wiley & Sons, Ltd. Published 2011 by John Wiley & Sons, Ltd.

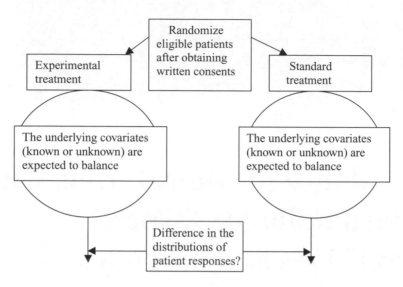

Figure 1.1   Schema for a RCT.

or even the feature of a pre-randomized study design (Zelen, 1979, 1982, 1986, 1990). Because noncompliance often occurs nonrandomly, simply excluding patients who do not comply with their assigned treatment from data analysis may produce a misleading inference. For convenience in the following discussion, we call the RCT with noncompliance, in which only patients assigned to an experimental treatment group can have access to the experimental treatment, the simple noncompliance RCT.

Example 1.1   Consider the simple noncompliance RCT, in which children who resided in 225 villages randomly selected out of 450 villages were assigned to the intervention group of receiving two large oral doses of vitamin A supplementation, while children who resided in the remaining 225 villages were assigned to the control group of receiving no vitamin A supplementation (Sommer and Zeger, 1991; Sommer, Tarwotjo and Djunaedi *et al.*, 1986). Approximately 20 % of children assigned to the intervention group did not receive vitamin A supplementation, but children assigned to the control group were all assumed to receive no vitamin A supplementation. To investigate whether there was a self-selection bias due to noncompliance, we might compare the mortality rate of children who were assigned to the intervention group but received no vitamin A supplementation with the mortality rate of children who were assigned to the control group. We summarize these data in Table 1.1 (Sommer and Zeger, 1991). For the purpose of illustration, we ignore the intraclass correlation (which will be discussed in Chapter 4) of survival outcomes between children within villages here. When employing the commonly used two independent sample-proportion statistics to test the equality of mortality rates (Fleiss, 1981), we find strong statistical significance (p-value < 0.001) based on the data in Table 1.1. In other words, there is strong evidence that children who declined receiving vitamin A supplementation tended to be in poorer health or at a higher risk of mortality. To help readers easily appreciate the schema of this simple noncompliance RCT, we may use the schema as shown in Figure 1.2.

Table 1.1   The observed cell frequency and the corresponding cell proportion (in parenthesis) in preschool children who were assigned to the intervention group but did not receive the vitamin A supplementation versus those in preschool children who were assigned to the control group and assumed to all receive no vitamin A supplementation.

	Patients assigned to the intervention group but received no vitamin A supplementation	Patients assigned to the control group
Death	34 (1.4 %)	74 (0.6 %)
Survival	2385 (98.6 %)	11514 (99.4 %)
Total	2419 (100 %)	11588 (100 %)

Because noncompliance does not, as shown in Figure 1.2, occur randomly, we cannot directly compare the mortality in preschool children between the two randomized arms by simply excluding those children who did not comply with taking vitamin A supplementation from the experimental arm. This is because the underlying prognostic conditions on children between the two arms would not balance; the experimental arm would consist of children at the low risk of mortality and the control arm would consist of children at both low and high risks of mortality. Thus, if we included only children who complied with their assigned treatment in our analysis and found a reduction in the mortality rate of

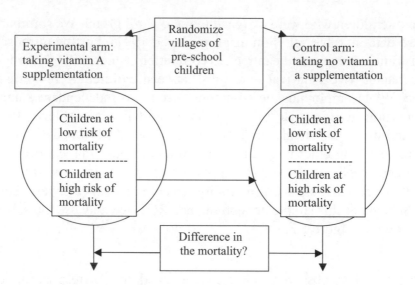

Figure 1.2   Schema for the simple noncompliance RCT of studying vitamin A supplementation to reduce mortality among pre-school children.

the experimental arm as compared with the control arm, this could be due to the reason that the children at a high risk of mortality were excluded from the experimental arm.

1.1   Randomized encouragement design (RED)

For certain treatments, such as flu vaccine or quitting smoking, it is not ethical to randomly assign high-risk patients to receive either the treatment or the placebo. Thus, to alleviate the ethical concern in application of the traditional RCT, the randomized encouragement design (RED) is often suggested (Multiple Risk Factor Intervention Trial Research Group, 1982; McDonald, Hui and Tierney, 1992; Zhou and Li, 2006; Jo, 2002).

RED – Patients are randomly assigned to either the intervention group of receiving an encouragement to accept the experimental treatment or the control group of receiving no such encouragement.

Because of randomization, the underlying prognostic conditions between the intervention and control groups are expected to balance in a RED. Since we do not interfere with patients assigned to the control group to receive their usual medical treatment in a RED, there are no ethical issues involved. Note that the rate of taking the experimental treatment in the intervention group of receiving an encouragement is expected to be higher than that in the control group through the encouragement. Thus, when there is a difference in the proportion of patient responses between the two randomized groups, we may attribute this to the difference in the two treatments under comparison. Note that because patients may decide to take or decline the experimental treatment despite whether they receive an encouragement or not, the extent of noncompliance is generally large in a RED. Thus, the RED can be relatively inefficient to the traditional RCT for detecting a difference between two treatments, especially when the extent of noncompliance is not small. How to achieve a high compliance rate becomes a very important and critical issue in designing a good RED.

Example 1.2   If we employed the traditional RCT to randomly assign high-risk patients to receive either the flu vaccine or the placebo, we would withhold vaccination from some high-risk patients. This would raise the ethical concern. The RED has been employed to study the influenza vaccine efficacy in reducing morbidity by using computer-generated reminder for flu shots (McDonald, Hui and Tierney, 1992). Physicians were randomly assigned to either the intervention group of receiving a computer-generated reminder when a patient with a scheduled appointment was eligible for a flu shot or the control group of receiving no such reminders. Each physician at the clinic cared for a fixed group of patients and his/her patients were then similarly classified. Since the study did not keep information on the clustering of patients by doctor, we ignore clustering for the purpose of illustration (Zhou and Li, 2006). We summarize these data in Table 5.1 (Chapter 5). Approximately 79 % of patients who were assigned to the intervention group of receiving reminders did not receive the flu vaccine, while approximately 14 % of patients who were assigned to the control group of receiving no reminders received the flu vaccine. There were also many patients with subsequent missing outcomes. How to obtain a consistent estimator of the flu vaccine effect on morbidity in the presence of a large percentage of noncompliance and a nonnegligible percentage of missing outcomes is likely to be of practical interest. We will discuss hypothesis testing and estimation of the treatment effect for a RCT with both noncompliance and subsequent missing outcomes in Chapter 5.

1.2   Randomized consent designs

When we implement a traditional RCT, the assignment of patients to a treatment completely depends on a chance mechanism after obtaining patients' informed consent. At the time of consent, neither physicians nor patients know exactly which treatment a patient will receive. This may compromise the relationship between physicians and patients (Zelen, 1990). Since physicians need to provide patients with all the relevant information on treatments, including the fact that they are not even sure which treatment can be the best to the patient, physicians may feel hesitated to enroll patients into a traditional RCT. This can cause the practical difficulty in recruiting patients into a RCT (Zelen, 1990). Furthermore, patients may originally agree to participate in a traditional RCT, but have reservation about continuing to participate or even decline the treatment once when the treatment is known. To account for these concerns, Zelen (1979, 1990) proposed the randomized consent design (or pre-randomized design), in which patients are randomly assigned to the treatments even before their consents are sought. After assigning an eligible patient to a treatment, physicians approach patients for consents and discuss potential risks, benefits, and treatment opinions. Patients will be given the assigned treatment if he/she is willing to accept the assigned one, and otherwise, the other. One important advantage of the randomized consent design over the traditional RCT is that the patient, at the time of consent, knows exactly which treatment he/she is going to receive (Zelen, 1990). By contrast, patients do not generally know exactly which treatment will be received in a traditional RCT. Based on whether noncompliance can occur in only one or both of the two randomized groups, the randomized consent designs can be classified as a single-consent randomized design (SCRD) and a double-consent randomized design (DCRD).

1.2.1   Single-consent randomized design (SCRD)

SCRD – Patients assigned to an experimental treatment are asked for consents, while patients assigned to a standard treatment are not.

If a patient in the assigned experimental treatment group agrees to receive the assigned treatment, he/she will be given the experimental treatment and otherwise, the patient will be given the standard treatment. However, all patients in the assigned standard treatment group are assumed to all receive the standard treatment. We may use the diagram in Figure 1.3 to illustrate the schema of the SCRD.

When comparing an experimental treatment with the best available standard treatment, Zelen (1979, 1990) contended that the SCRD could be a useful alternative design to the traditional RCT. This is because patients assigned to the standard treatment receive the best available treatment to them and hence it should not involve ethical issues if we did not seek their consents. On the other hand, patients assigned to the experimental treatment could be allowed to switch the best standard

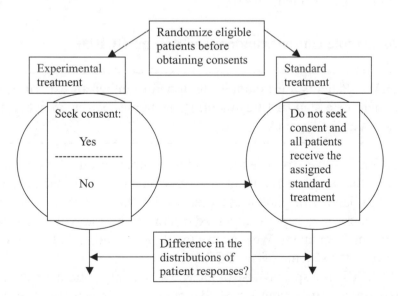

Figure 1.3   Schema for the single-consent randomized design.

treatment if they were not willing to accept the assigned (experimental) treatment. Thus, patients and physicians know exactly which treatment the patient will be given. Zelen (1990) provided an excellent discussion on when the randomized consent design can be more efficient than the traditional RCT through an increase of the enrollment rate of patients into a trial. Anbar (1983), Matts and McHugh (1993) as well as Brunner and Neumann (1985) also discussed estimation and testing hypothesis under the randomized consent design.

Example 1.3   The SCRD has been employed to study the extracorporeal membrane oxygenation (ECMO) on new infants having a diagnosis of persistent pulmonary hypertension (PPH) (Zelen, 1990). When infants were diagnosed with PPH, using the traditional RCT would require that the parents of an infant near death provide informed consent for an invasive surgical procedure (ECMO) which might not be even administered to their babies. This can raise an unnecessarily stressful burden to both parents and health administrators. The SCRD only required that parents whose infants were assigned ECMO be approached for giving consents because this was a deviation from the conventional therapy. Other practical applications of the randomized consent design can be found elsewhere (Zelen, 1990).

1.2.2   Double-consent randomized design (DCRD)

> **DCRD** – Patients are randomly assigned to either an experimental treatment or a standard treatment. Patients are then approached for consents in both groups.

If a patient assigned to the experimental treatment group does not agree to accept the assigned treatment, he/she will be given the standard treatment. Similarly, if a patient assigned to the standard treatment group does not agree to accept the assigned treatment, he/she will be given the experimental treatment. We may use the diagram shown in Figure 1.4 in to illustrate the schema of the DCRD.

The SCRD is a special case of DCRD when only patients assigned to the experimental treatment are asked for consents. Because noncompliers in the assigned experimental treatment group do not necessarily represent the same subpopulation as noncompliers in the assigned standard

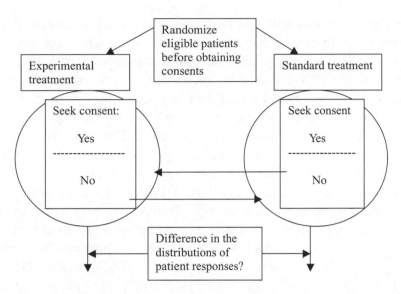

Figure 1.4   Schema for double consent randomized design.

treatment group, a direct comparison of patient responses by excluding those noncompliers from data analysis can be misleading due to the underlying prognostic conditions are no longer comparable between the two comparison groups. Some discussions on hypothesis testing and interval estimation under the DCRD appeared elsewhere (Anbar, 1983; Brunner and Neumann, 1985; Lui and Lin, 2003).

1.3   Treatment efficacy versus programmatic effectiveness

Before discussing the bias of an estimator for treatment efficacy, it is essential to clarify the definition of treatment efficacy in the presence of noncompliance to avoid the confusion noted elsewhere (Lui, 2009). Following Last (1988), we define the treatment efficacy as the treatment effect relative to a control (or placebo) among compliers who would fully comply with whatever their assigned treatment regimen. The treatment efficacy provides us with the useful information on the biological action of a treatment and is most interesting to clinicians. By contrast, we define the programmatic effectiveness as the treatment assignment effect relative to a control (or placebo) in a population consisting of both compliers and noncompliers. On the basis of the programmatic effectiveness, a drug with low treatment efficacy but an extremely high compliance rate can be more useful than a drug with high treatment efficacy but an extremely low compliance rate (Nagelkerke, Fidler and Bernsen *et al.*, 2000). This is because a drug can be beneficial to only those patients who would accept the drug, and using the former with a very high compliance rate may save more patients than the latter with an extremely low compliance rate in practice. Thus, the programmatic effectiveness can be of interest and importance to health policy administrators. When subjects in a population are all compliers, the treatment efficacy and the programmatic effectiveness are, by definition, identical. Note that the programmatic effectiveness can vary as compliance changes. A meta-analysis of empirical research showed an overall 26 % difference in response rates between patients with high and low compliance rates (Walter, Guyatt and Montori *et al.*, 2006; DiMatteo, Giordani and Lepper *et al.*, 2002). Unless the distribution of noncompliance for patients participated into a RCT is quite similar to that for patients of the targeted population, we may not be able to extrapolate the findings on the programmatic effectiveness from a particular RCT to the targeted population. Thus, we will focus our attention on the treatment efficacy, and use the terms treatment efficacy and treatment effect synonymously in this book.

1.4   Definitions of commonly used terms and assumptions

To estimate the efficacy of a treatment in the presence of noncompliance, we first make the stable unit treatment value assumption (SUTVA) (Rubin, 1978).

> **SUTVA** – There is no interference between patients; the treatment-received status of one patient does not influence the response or the treatment-received status of another patient (Sato, 2001; Matsuyama, 2002). Also, we often include consistency – the responses of patients remain identical regardless of possibly different forms or versions in administration of a treatment, as a part of the SUTVA as well (Ten Have, Elliott and Joffe *et al.*, 2004; Bellamy, Lin and Ten Have, 2007).

The SUTVA can sometimes be violated in practice. For example, consider the study of quitting smoking on the mortality of coronary heart disease (CHD) (Matsui, 2005; Multiple Risk Factor Intervention Trial Research Group, 1982). Smoking can have a direct effect on the outcome of a patient who smoked and an indirect effect on the outcome of a patient whose roommate smoked. An analysis without accounting for this indirect effect can lead us to a biased estimate of the effect due to smoking if both of these patients are included into the trial. Other examples about the violation of SUTVA can be found elsewhere (Cox, 1958; Bellamy, Lin and Ten Have, 2007). Also, for simplicity, we focus our attention on the situation in which there is only a single one form or version of administrating treatments and hence consistency is implicitly assumed to be satisfied throughout this book.

Say, we compare an experimental treatment with a standard treatment. Following Angrist, Imbens and Rubin (1996), we define for each patient the vector $(d(1), d(0))$ of his/her potential treatment-received status: $d(g) = 1$ if the patient assigned to treatment g $(= 1$ for experimental, and $= 0$ for standard) actually receives the experimental treatment, and $d(g) = 0$ otherwise. Therefore, we can divide our sampling population into four subpopulations, including compliers $(d(1) = 1$ and $d(0) = 0)$, never-takers $(d(1) = d(0) = 0)$, always-takers $(d(1) = d(0) = 1)$, and defiers $(d(1) = 0$ and $d(0) = 1)$. To allow the parameter representing the treatment efficacy to be identifiable, we commonly make the monotonicity assumption as well as the exclusion restriction assumption for always-takers and never-takers.

The Monotonicity Assumption – We assume $d(1) \geq d(0)$ for all patients; or equivalently, there are no defiers.

The Exclusion Restriction Assumption – The treatment affects a patient response only through the treatment which the patient actually receives and the treatment assignment itself does not affect the patient response.

Brunner and Neumann (1985) contended that a patient who refused a proffered treatment should only stay in the trial if he/she preferred the other treatment. In fact, it is very likely that a patient who is a defier may not even provide his/her written consent and enter into a RCT in practice. Thus, the monotonicity assumption should be plausible in most encountered RCTs, although one may find situations in which the assumption of no defiers does not hold (Bellamy, Lin and Ten Have, 2007; Ten Have, Elliott and Joffe et $al.$, 2004). Based on the monotonicity assumption, if a patient assigned to an experimental treatment ($g = 1$) receives a standard treatment ($g = 0$), he/she must be a never-taker (i.e. a patient with $d(1) = 0$ must have $d(0) = 0$). Similarly, if a patient assigned to a standard treatment receives an experimental treatment, he/she must be an always-taker (i.e. a patient with $d(0) = 1$ must have $d(1) = 1$). However, if a patient assigned to an experimental treatment receives his/her assigned (experimental) treatment, he/she can be either a complier or an always-taker. Also, if a patient assigned to a standard treatment receives his/her assigned (standard) treatment, he/she can be either a complier or a never-taker. Because we cannot distinguish compliers from always-takers in the assigned experimental treatment or compliers from never-takers in the assigned standard treatment, the difference in the probabilities of response among compliers between the experimental and standard treatments is not directly estimatible from data without making some assumptions. This is actually the fundamental issue in estimation of treatment effect (among compliers) under a RCT with noncompliance.

The exclusion restriction assumption is likely to be reasonable in a double-blind study. Frangakis and Baker (2001) contended that the exclusion restriction assumption for always-takers and never-takers is probably to hold when noncompliance occurs soon after assignment. This is because, within the defined groups of always-takers and never-takers, different assignment results in the same extent of actual exposure to the experimental treatment (for always-takers) and the standard treatment (for never-takers). On the other hand, for example, in the RED studying the flu vaccine, the exclusion restriction assumption for always-takers might not necessarily hold (Hirano, Imbens and Rubin et $al.$, 2000; Zhou and Li, 2006). This is because always-takers who received the flu shot regardless of their assigned group tended to be patients who were most likely at high risk for getting flu. If the flu reminder prompted the physician to take other medical treatments beyond the flu shot to improve the health outcomes on such patients, the exclusion restriction assumption for always-takers could be violated. Note that the exclusion restriction assumption is generally not testable without having the additional auxiliary information. Hirano, Imbens and Rubin *et al.* (2000) proposed a Bayesian approach and discussed sensitivity analysis to violation of the exclusion restriction assumption. Their results can depend, however, on their assumed specific form of the likelihood function and prior distribution. Note also that there is a subtle difference in the definition of compliers between the traditional RCT and RED. A complier in the former represents a patient who receives whatever treatment he/she is assigned to, while a complier in the latter represents a patient who will accept a treatment if he/she is assigned to an intervention group of receiving an encouragement and who will decline a treatment if he/she is assigned to a control of group of receiving no encouragement. Thus, the treatment efficacy defined in compliers between the traditional RCT and RED can be nonidentical. The compliers in a RED can be trial specific and hence the extrapolation of findings from a RED to the targeted population should also be treated with caution.

1.5   Most commonly used analyses for a RCT with noncompliance

To analyze data in a RCT with noncompliance, the most commonly used approaches include as-protocol (AP) analysis, as-treated (AT) analysis, and intent-to-treat (ITT) analysis.

AP Analysis – Patients are compared between those who comply with their assigned treatments. Patients who do not comply with their assigned treatments are excluded from data analysis.

AT Analysis – Patients are compared according to the treatment they actually receive regardless of what their originally assigned treatment.

Because noncompliance often does not occur randomly, both the AT and AP analyses generally produce a biased inference of treatment efficacy. To clarify this point, we consider the following numerical examples.

Example 1.4   Consider comparing an experimental treatment with a standard treatment in a simple noncompliance RCT. Suppose that our population consist of two subpopulations: 70 % compliers (who fully accept whatever their assigned treatment) and 30 % never-takers (who always take the standard treatment regardless of whatever their assigned treatment). Suppose further that we randomly assign patients to either an experimental treatment ($g = 1$) or a standard treatment ($g = 0$). First, consider the case of equal treatment efficacy between the two treatments. Say, the conditional probabilities of death, given a complier for both the experimental and standard treatments, are given by: $P(death|complier, g = 1) = P(death|complier, g = 0) = 0.30$. Furthermore, because never-takers, who are randomly assigned to the two treatments under comparison, will take the same (standard) treatment, the conditional probabilities of death, given a never-taker, can be reasonably assumed to equal to each other between the two assigned treatment groups. This is actually the exclusion restriction assumption defined in the above for never-takers. We arbitrarily assume that these conditional probabilities are given by $P(death|never-takers, g = 1) = P(death|never-takers, g = 0) = 0.60$. If we randomly assigned 500 patients to each of the two treatments, we would obtain the expected frequencies as given in Table 1.2 (Exercise 1.1). When using the AP analysis excluding those patients who do not comply with their assigned treatments from the experimental treatment group, we obtain the hypothetical mortality data in Table 1.2a.

Based on these data, there is strong evidence that the mortality rate in patients complying with the assigned experimental treatment is lower than the mortality rate in patients complying with the assigned standard treatment (Exercise 1.2), although the underlying mortality rates among compliers between these two treatments are actually equal, as assumed in the example. The estimated proportion difference (PD) in the mortality rate between the two comparison groups in the AP analysis is -0.09 ($= 105/350\text{-}195/500$). Also, when using the AT analysis by comparing

Table 1.2 The expected cell frequency and the corresponding cell proportion (in parenthesis) for the experimental and standard treatments under the simple noncompliance RCT as described in Example 1.4.

	Patients assigned to the experimental treatment		
	Compliers	Never-takers	Total
Death	105 (21 %)	90 (18 %)	195 (39 %)
Survival	245 (49 %)	60 (12 %)	305 (61 %)
Total	350 (70 %)	150 (30 %)	500 (100 %)
	Patients assigned to the standard treatment		
	Compliers	Never-takers	Total
Death	–	–	195 (39 %)
Survival	–	–	305 (61 %)
Total	–	–	500 (100 %)

– denotes that the cell frequency is unobservable.

patients according to the treatment they actually receive, we obtain the data in Table 1.2b.

Again, there is strong evidence that the mortality rate in the experimental treatment is lower that that in the standard treatment (Exercise 1.3). The estimated PD in the mortality rate between the two

Table 1.2a The expected cell frequency and the conditional cell proportion (in parenthesis), given the column total fixed, between patients complying with their assigned treatment for the AP analysis.

	Patients complying with the assigned experimental treatment	Patients complying with the assigned standard treatment
Death	105 (30 %)	195 (39 %)
Survival	245 (70 %)	305 (61 %)
Total	350 (100 %)	500 (100 %)

Table 1.2b   The expected frequency and the conditional cell proportion (in parenthesis), given the column total fixed, between patients according to their actually received treatment for the AT analysis.

	Patients actually received the experimental treatment	Patients actually received the standard treatment
Death	105 (30%)	285 (44%)
Survival	245 (70%)	365 (56%)
Total	350 (100%)	650 (100%)

comparison groups is -0.14. The above results illustrate the case in which the bias in inference can occur for both hypothesis testing and estimation when we employ the AP and AT analyses to study treatment efficacy. To alleviate this concern, the ITT analysis has been suggested.

> **ITT Analysis** – Patients are compared according to the treatment to which they are randomly assigned, despite what treatment they actually receive. Thus, the ITT analysis is also called as-randomized (AR) analysis (Heitjan, 1999).

When using the ITT analysis in the above example, we can easily see that the estimated PD is 0 ($= 195/500\text{-}195/500$) based on Table 1.2, and there is obviously no evidence against the underlying assumed condition that the two treatment effects are equal to one another. These illustrate that the ITT analysis is unbiased in both hypothesis testing and estimation when an experimental treatment effect is equal to a standard treatment effect. In Chapter 2, we will explicitly show why use of the ITT analysis is unbiased under the null relative treatment effect and certain assumptions. On the other hand, the ITT analysis can be biased in estimation of the relative treatment efficacy when the underlying two treatment effects are different. To illustrate this point, we consider the following numerical example.

Example 1.5 Consider the above simple noncompliance RCT in Example 1.4, in which the population consist of two subpopulations:

70 % compliers and 30 % never-takers. However, we now assume that the conditional probability of death $P(death|compliers, g = 1) = 0.30$ among compliers assigned to the experimental treatment is different from the conditional probability of death $P(death|compliers, g = 0) = 0.70$ among compliers assigned to the standard treatment. Thus, the assumed underlying PD among compliers in the mortality rate is -0.40. We assume that the conditional probability of death among never-takers remains the same as that given in the previous example. If we randomly assigned 500 patients to each of the two treatments, we would obtain the expected frequencies as given in Table 1.3 (Exercise 1.4).

Table 1.3 The expected cell frequency and the corresponding cell proportion (in parenthesis) for the experimental and standard treatments under the simple noncompliance RCT as described in Example 1.5.

	Patients assigned to the experimental treatment		
	Compliers	Never-takers	Total
Death	105 (21 %)	90 (18 %)	195 (39 %)
Survival	245 (49 %)	60 (12 %)	305 (61 %)
Total	350 (70 %)	150 (30 %)	500 (100 %)
	Patients assigned to the standard treatment		
	Compliers	Never-takers	Total
Death	–	–	335 (67 %)
Survival	–	–	165 (33 %)
Total	–	–	500 (100 %)

– denotes that the cell frequency is unobservable.

When using the AP analysis, we obtain the data in Table 1.3a. Again, there is strong evidence that the mortality rate in the experimental treatment is lower than that in the standard treatment using the data in Table 1.3a (Exercise 1.5). The estimated PD is -0.37 ($= 105/350-335/500$), which is slightly different from the underlying assumed PD $= -0.40$. On the other hand, when using the AT analysis, we obtain the

Table 1.3a The expected cell frequency and the conditional cell proportion (in parenthesis), given the column total fixed, between patients complying with their assigned treatment for the AP analysis.

	Patients complying with the assigned experimental treatment	Patients complying with the assigned standard treatment
Death	105 (30 %)	335 (67 %)
Survival	245 (70 %)	165 (33 %)
Total	350 (100 %)	500 (100 %)

data in Table 1.3b. There is also strong evidence that the mortality rate in the experimental treatment is lower that that in the standard treatment (Exercise 1.6). The estimated PD is -0.35 for the AT analysis. When using the ITT analysis in the above example, we can easily see that the estimated PD in the mortality rate is -0.28 (=195/500-335/500), which is larger than the underlying assumed PD= -0.40 by 30 % (= (|$-0.28+0.40$|/0.40). This illustrates that the ITT analysis can be biased in estimation of the relative treatment efficacy and the magnitude of this bias can be even larger than that using the AP or AT analysis.

Table 1.3b The expected frequency and the conditional cell proportion (in parenthesis), given the column total fixed, between patients according to their actually received treatment for the AT analysis.

	Patients actually received the experimental treatment	Patients actually received the standard treatment
Death	105 (30 %)	425 (65 %)
Survival	245 (70 %)	225 (35 %)
Total	350 (100 %)	650 (100 %)

Since the underlying conditions between the two randomized groups are comparable, as illustrated in Example 1.4, the ITT analysis can preserve Type I error under the null hypothesis of no difference between the two treatment effects. Lachin (2000) advocated that the ITT analysis should be preferable to the other 'subgroup analyses' for a RCT with noncompliance. This is mainly because using the latter cannot warrant the underlying prognostic conditions between two comparison groups to be comparable as noted in use of the AP or AT analysis, or one needs to make certain additional assumptions (such as the monotonicity and exclusion restriction assumptions), of which most are inherently not testable without having the auxiliary information. These concerns can detract from the credibility of our trials (Begg, 2000). As illustrated by the above example, however, using the ITT analysis typically tends to attenuate the treatment efficacy when it is our interest. Furthermore, counting an event occurrence of interest in someone who has never received a treatment but has been assigned to it, as a failure (or success) of that treatment, also raises questions of some investigators (Nagelkerke, Fidler and Bernsen *et al.*, 2000).

Although the additional assumptions for estimation of treatment efficacy are mostly nontestable, these assumptions can often be judged whether they are reasonable or not based on one's subjective knowledge for a given trial (Mealli and Rubin, 2002). In fact, the programmatic effectiveness and the treatment efficacy address distinct scientific questions, and are both important (Sommer and Zeger, 1991). If our interest is to demonstrate only whether there is a difference between two treatment effects, then the ITT analysis will be sufficient in most situations. However, in practice we may often want to quantify the magnitude of the relative treatment efficacy especially when there is statistically significant evidence of finding a difference in the treatment effects between two comparison groups. Furthermore, spurious heterogeneity can often occur in the programmatic effectiveness due to the variation of noncompliance extents between trials even if the underlying treatment efficacy is constant in meta-analysis. Therefore, the investigation in hypothesis testing, estimation and other relevant topics with respect to the treatment efficacy for a RCT with noncompliance under various situations becomes essentially useful and important, and will be the primary focus of this book.

Exercises

1.1 Show that the expected frequencies under the assumed conditions considered in Example 1.4 are given in Table 1.2.

1.2 What is the p-value for testing equality of the mortality rate between the assigned experimental and standard treatment groups based on the data in Table 1.2a for the AP analysis? (Answer: 0.007)

1.3 What is the p-value for testing equality of the mortality rate between the received experimental and received standard treatments based on the data in Table 1.2b for the AT analysis? (Answer: 0.00002)

1.4 Show that the expected frequencies under the assumed conditions considered in Example 1.5 are given in Table 1.3.

1.5 What is the p-value for testing equality of the mortality rate between the assigned experimental and standard treatment groups based on the data in Table 1.3a for the AP analysis?

1.6 What is the p-value for testing equality of the mortality rate between the received experimental and received standard treatments based on the data in Table 1.3b for the AT analysis?

1.7 Discuss and provide examples, in which the SUTVA, the monotonicity assumption, or the exclusion restriction assumption for always-takers or never-takers is violated (Bellamy, Lin and Ten Have, 2007; Ten Have, Elliott and Joffe *et al.*, 2004; Zhou and Li, 2006).

2

Randomized clinical trials with noncompliance under parallel groups design

The randomized clinical trial (RCT) is the most frequently used standard design to establish a new treatment effect, because randomization can provide a protection against obtaining a biased estimate of the treatment effect due to the difference in the underlying prognostic variables between two comparison groups. Because of patient refusal, ethical constraints, or side effects, however, it is not uncommon that we may encounter a RCT in which there are patients not complying with their assigned treatment. For example, consider the RCT studying vitamin A supplementation to reduce mortality among preschool children in rural Indonesia (Sommer and Zeger, 1991; Sommer, Tarwotjo and Djunaedi *et al.*, 1986). Children who resided in 225 randomly selected villages out of 450 were assigned to an experimental group of receiving a large oral dose of vitamin A supplementation two to three months following baseline enumeration and again six months later, and children who resided in the remaining 225 villages were assigned to a control group of receiving no vitamin A supplementation (Sommer and Zeger, 1991). Nearly 20 % of children assigned to the experimental group failed to receive vitamin A supplementation.

Binary Data Analysis of Randomized Clinical Trials with Noncompliance, First Edition. Kung-Jong Lui.
© 2011 John Wiley & Sons, Ltd. Published 2011 by John Wiley & Sons, Ltd.

Deaths were ascertained in a second population census 12 months following the baseline census. Mortality rates in children were then compared between these two groups. Because noncompliance often occurs nonrandomly, as noted in Chapter 1, analyzing data as-treated (AT) or as-protocol (AP) can often produce a misleading inference on a treatment effect. To avoid the potential selection bias due to noncompliance, the intent-to-treat (ITT) analysis is frequently recommended. However, the ITT analysis estimates the programmatic effectiveness (Sommer and Zeger, 1991) or the treatment assignment effect (O'Malley and Normand, 2005) rather than the treatment efficacy (Last, 1988) or the biological action (Sommer and Zeger, 1991). Because the former can vary as the extent of compliance changes irrespective of a given fixed biological efficacy, the latter is probably a more appealing index to clinicians (Sommer and Zeger, 1991; Walter, Guyatt and Montori *et al.*, 2006). Note that the data structure for the RCT with noncompliance is essentially parallel to that of the pre-randomized consent design proposed by Zelen (1979, 1982, 1986 and 1990) and hence the results and findings presented here are applicable to the latter (Anbar, 1983; Bernhard and Compagnone, 1989; Matts and McHugh, 1987, 1993; McHugh, 1984; Lui and Lin, 2003) as well.

In this chapter, we first use a contingency table summarizing the underlying latent probability structure of observed data and express the programmatic effectiveness and treatment efficacy explicitly in terms of a mathematical equation to clarify the relationship between these two important terms. We discuss how one can apply the ITT analysis to test the superiority of an experimental treatment to a standard treatment for a RCT with noncompliance in Section 2.1. We further discuss testing noninferiority and equivalence with respect to the treatment efficacy measured by the proportion difference (PD), the proportion ratio (PR), and the odds ratio (OR) in the presence of noncompliance under a RCT in Sections 2.2 and 2.3, respectively. To quantify the magnitude of the relative treatment effect, we include interval estimators accounting for noncompliance for the PD, PR, and OR in Section 2.4. We address sample size determination for testing superiority, noninferiority, and equivalence based on the proposed test procedures in Section 2.5. We outline the structural risk model-based approaches (Sato, 2000, 2001; Matsuyama, 2002; Robins, 1994) as well as show that the model parameters, including the PD and PR, and their corresponding estimators are actually identical to those based on the principal stratification approach (Frangakis and Rubin, 2002) adopted here under certain assumptions in Section 2.6.

Consider comparing an experimental treatment ($g = 1$) with a standard treatment (or placebo) ($g = 0$) in a RCT, in which there are patients who do not comply with their assigned treatment. To estimate the effect of a treatment, we make the stable unit treatment value assumption (SUTVA) – there is no interference between patients with respect to their treatment receipts and response outcomes (Rubin, 1978). Furthermore, we define for each patient the vector $(d(1), d(0))$ of his/her potential treatment-received status: $d(g) = 1$ if the patient assigned to treatment g actually receives the experimental treatment, and $d(g) = 0$ otherwise. Thus, we can divide our sampling population into four subpopulations, including compliers ($d(1) = 1$ and $d(0) = 0$), never-takers ($d(1) = d(0) = 0$), always-takers ($d(1) = d(0) = 1$), and defiers ($d(1) = 0$ and $d(0) = 1$). As commonly assumed for a RCT with noncompliance, we assume monotonicity (i.e. $d(1) \geq d(0)$ for all patients) or equivalently, no defiers (see Section 1.4 in Chapter 1). We let $\pi_{1S}^{(g)}$ denote the cell probability for a randomly selected patient assigned to treatment g ($g = 1, 0$) who has a positive response and falls in category S: $S = C$ for compliers, $= A$ for always-takers, and $= N$ for never-takers. We further let $\pi_{2S}^{(g)}$ denote the corresponding cell probability of a negative response and status S ($-C$, A and N) for a randomly selected patient assigned to treatment g. We use '+' notation to designate summation of cell probabilities over that particular subscript. For example, $\pi_{+S}^{(1)}$ represents $\pi_{1S}^{(1)} + \pi_{2S}^{(1)}$. Because of random assignment of patients to treatments, we may assume that $\pi_{+S}^{(1)} = \pi_{+S}^{(0)} = \pi_{+S}$, where π_{+S} denotes the proportion of subpopulation S (for $S = C, A, N$) in the sampling population. Define $\pi_{1|S}^{(g)} = \pi_{1S}^{(g)}/\pi_{+S}$, the conditional probability of a positive response among subpopulation S ($S = C, A, N$) in the assigned treatment g ($g = 1, 0$). Because patients are randomly assigned to one of the two treatments and always-takers take the same (experimental) treatment regardless of their assigned treatment, we may reasonably assume $\pi_{1|A}^{(1)} = \pi_{1|A}^{(0)}$. Following similar arguments, we assume $\pi_{1|N}^{(1)} = \pi_{1|N}^{(0)}$ for never-takers. This assumption that $\pi_{1|A}^{(1)} = \pi_{1|A}^{(0)}$ and $\pi_{1|N}^{(1)} = \pi_{1|N}^{(0)}$ is, in fact, called the exclusion restriction assumption for always-takers and never-takers (Angrist, Imbens and Rubin, 1996; Frangakis and Rubin, 1999). When there is no confusion in the following discussion, we denote the common values for $\pi_{1|A}^{(1)} = \pi_{1|A}^{(0)}$ and $\pi_{1|N}^{(1)} = \pi_{1|N}^{(0)}$ by $\pi_{1|A}$ and $\pi_{1|N}$, respectively. The above arguments imply that $\pi_{rA}^{(1)} = \pi_{rA}^{(0)}(=\pi_{rA})$ and $\pi_{rN}^{(1)} = \pi_{rN}^{(0)}(=\pi_{rN})$ for $r = 1, 2$.

For clarity, we may use the following table to summarize the underlying latent probability structure for the observed data of patients assigned to the experimental treatment based on the above assumptions:

Patients assigned to the experimental treatment (g = 1)

		Treatment actually received		
		Experimental treatment	Standard treatment	Total
Outcome	Positive	$\pi_{1CA}^{(1)} = \pi_{1C}^{(1)} + \pi_{1A}$	π_{1N}	$\pi_{1+}^{(1)}$
	Negative	$\pi_{2CA}^{(1)} = \pi_{2C}^{(1)} + \pi_{2A}$	π_{2N}	$\pi_{2+}^{(1)}$
	Total	$\pi_{+CA}^{(1)} = \pi_{+C} + \pi_{+A}$	π_{+N}	1.0

For example, the parameter $\pi_{1CA}^{(1)} = \pi_{1C}^{(1)} + \pi_{1A}$ represents the cell probability that a randomly selected patient assigned to the experimental treatment has a positive response and receives his/her assigned (experimental) treatment. The marginal probability $\pi_{+CA}^{(1)} = \pi_{+C} + \pi_{+A}$ represents the compliance probability that a patient assigned to the experimental treatment receives his/her assigned (experimental) treatment. Similarly, we may use the following table to summarize the underlying latent probability structure for the observed data of patients assigned to the standard treatment:

Patients assigned to the standard treatment (g = 0)

		Treatment actually received		
		Standard treatment	Experimental treatment	Total
Outcome	Positive	$\pi_{1CN}^{(0)} = \pi_{1C}^{(0)} + \pi_{1N}$	π_{1A}	$\pi_{1+}^{(0)}$
	Negative	$\pi_{2CN}^{(0)} = \pi_{2C}^{(0)} + \pi_{2N}$	π_{2A}	$\pi_{2+}^{(0)}$
	Total	$\pi_{+CN}^{(0)} = \pi_{+C} + \pi_{+N}$	π_{+A}	1.0

The parameter $\pi_{1CN}^{(0)} = \pi_{1C}^{(0)} + \pi_{1N}$, for example, represents the cell probability that a randomly selected patient assigned to the standard treatment has a positive response and receives his/her assigned (standard) treatment. Also, the marginal probability $\pi_{+CN}^{(0)} = \pi_{+C} + \pi_{+N}$ represents the compliance probability that a randomly selected patient assigned to the standard treatment receives his/her assigned (standard) treatment. Note that the probabilities of compliance for the assigned experimental $(g = 1)$ and standard $(g = 0)$ treatments are given by $\pi_{+CA}^{(1)}(= \pi_{+C} + \pi_{+A})$ and $\pi_{+CN}^{(0)}(= \pi_{+C} + \pi_{+N})$, which are different from the proportion of compliers π_{+C} in the population unless there is perfect compliance (i.e. $\pi_{+A} = \pi_{+N} = 0$) in a RCT. Note also that in the above model assumptions, the subpopulation of patients who comply with their assigned (experimental) treatment in the assigned experimental treatment is different from the subpopulation of patients who comply with their assigned (standard) treatment in the assigned standard treatment. The former consists of compliers and always-takers, while the latter consists of compliers and never-takers. Thus, a comparison of the response rates between only patients who comply with their originally assigned treatments as for the AP analysis can be misleading. Following similar reasons, we can see that the AT analysis, in which one compares patients according to the treatment they actually receive irrespective of the treatment to which they are originally assigned, can also produce a biased inference on treatment efficacy as a result of the incomparability of the underlying subpopulations between the two comparison groups. Furthermore, use of the stratified analysis with strata formed by whether the post-treatment variable 'compliance' or 'noncompliance' to the assigned treatment is also not appropriate due to the same reason that the stratum of 'compliance' or 'noncompliance' can consist of patients with possibly different characteristics between the assigned experimental and standard treatments.

Suppose that we randomly assign n_g patients to the experimental treatment $(g = 1)$ and the control treatment $(g = 0)$. Let $n_{rS}^{(g)}$ denote the observed frequency corresponding to the cell with probability $\pi_{rS}^{(g)}$ $(r = 1, 2, S = CA, N$ for $g = 1$, and $S = CN, A$ for $g = 0)$. The random vector $(n_{1CA}^{(1)}, n_{1N}^{(1)}, n_{2CA}^{(1)}, n_{2N}^{(1)})$ then follows a multinomial distribution with parameters n_1 and $(\pi_{1CA}^{(1)}, \pi_{1N}^{(1)}, \pi_{2CA}^{(1)}, \pi_{2N}^{(1)})$, while the random vector $(n_{1CN}^{(0)}, n_{1A}^{(0)}, n_{2CN}^{(0)}, n_{2A}^{(0)})$ follows a multinomial distribution with parameters n_0 and $(\pi_{1CN}^{(0)}, \pi_{1A}^{(0)}, \pi_{2CN}^{(0)}, \pi_{2A}^{(0)})$. Thus, the maximum likelihood estimator (MLE) for $\pi_{rS}^{(g)}$ is $\hat{\pi}_{rS}^{(g)} = n_{rS}^{(g)}/n_g (r = 1, 2, S = CA,$ N for $g = 1$; and $S = CN, A$ for $g = 0$). By the functional invariance properties of the MLE (Casella and Berger, 1990), the MLEs for the marginal probabilities are: $\hat{\pi}_{r+}^{(1)} = \hat{\pi}_{rCA}^{(1)} + \hat{\pi}_{rN}^{(1)}$, $\hat{\pi}_{r+}^{(0)} = \hat{\pi}_{rCN}^{(0)} + \hat{\pi}_{rA}^{(0)} (r = 1, 2)$, and $\hat{\pi}_{+S}^{(g)} = \hat{\pi}_{1S}^{(g)} + \hat{\pi}_{2S}^{(g)}$ ($S = CA, N$ for $g = 1$, and $S = CN, A$ for $g = 0$). Note that since $\pi_{+C} = \pi_{+CA}^{(1)} - \pi_{+A}$, the MLE for π_{+C} is given by $\hat{\pi}_{+C} = \hat{\pi}_{+CA}^{(1)} - \hat{\pi}_{+A}^{(0)} = \hat{\pi}_{+CA}^{(1)} + \hat{\pi}_{+CN}^{(0)} - 1$. Note also that a cell (or marginal) proportion is, by definition, always greater than or equal to 0. If the MLE for a given cell (or marginal) proportion should be negative (due to sampling variation), we will say that the MLE for this parameter does not exist and arbitrarily set the MLE estimate of a cell proportion to be the closest boundary value. Similarly, we will say that the MLE for a ratio does not exist if the estimate of its denominator is 0 as well. As long as we obtain an adequate number of patients in each cell, the chance for finding no MLE should be minimal.

2.1   Testing superiority

When comparing an experimental treatment with a standard treatment, we may wish to find out whether the treatment efficacy of the former is better than that of the latter. However, it is advisable that we do a two-sided test rather than a one-sided test for ethical and safety reasons (Fleiss, 1981, p. 29; Fleiss, Levin and Paik, 2003, pp. 59–60). This is because we want to have an opportunity to detect that if the efficacy of an experimental treatment is unexpectedly worse than that of the standard treatment. We define $\delta = \pi_{1+}^{(1)} - \pi_{1+}^{(0)}$, the PD of a positive response between the two randomized groups despite what treatment patients actually receive. We further define the PD among compliers between two treatments as

$$\Delta = \pi_{1|C}^{(1)} - \pi_{1|C}^{(0)}, \qquad (2.1)$$

where $\pi_{1|C}^{(g)} = \pi_{1C}^{(g)}/\pi_{+C}$ is the conditional probability of a positive response among compliers in the assigned treatment g ($g = 1, 0$). Note that δ can be shown to equal $\Delta\pi_{+C}$ (Exercise 2.1). When we use the PD to measure the relative treatment effect, the parameters $\delta(= \pi_{1+}^{(1)} - \pi_{1+}^{(0)})$ and $\Delta(= \pi_{1|C}^{(1)} - \pi_{1|C}^{(0)})$ actually represent the programmatic effectiveness and treatment efficacy, respectively. Given a fixed treatment efficacy Δ, we can easily see that the programmatic effectiveness δ ($= \Delta\pi_{+C}$) may change as the proportion of compliers π_{+C} varies between trials. Suppose that the proportion π_{+C} of compliers in the studied population is similar to that in the targeted populations. Given the treatment efficacy Δ fixed, the programmatic effectiveness can have a useful interpretation – when the drug is applied to the targeted population, the parameter δ represents the expected difference in the probabilities of a positive response between the two assigned treatments. However, because the extent of compliance usually varies between populations, the treatment efficacy Δ, representing the difference in the biological action between two treatments, is generally more interesting than the programmatic effectiveness δ in a RCT. Of course, if we can obtain an estimate of the treatment efficacy Δ, we will be able to draw an inference on the programmatic effectiveness δ in the population, of which the proportion of compliers π_{+C} is known or estimable.

In this section, we are interested in testing the null hypothesis $H_0 : \Delta = 0$ versus the alternative hypothesis $H_a : \Delta \neq 0$. Because $\delta = \Delta\pi_{+C}$ (where $\pi_{+C} > 0$), $\delta = 0$ if and only if $\Delta = 0$. Thus, when testing $H_0 : \Delta = 0$, we may apply the following statistic for the ITT analysis to test $H_0 : \delta = 0$,

$$\hat{\delta} = \hat{\pi}_{1+}^{(1)} - \hat{\pi}_{1+}^{(0)}. \tag{2.2}$$

This leads us to consider the following most commonly-used test statistic based on two independent sample proportions,

$$Z = \hat{\delta}/\sqrt{\hat{Var}(\hat{\delta}|H_0)}, \tag{2.3}$$

where $\hat{Var}(\hat{\delta}|H_0) = \hat{\pi}_{1+}^{(p)}(1 - \hat{\pi}_{1+}^{(p)})(1/n_1 + 1/n_0)$ and $\hat{\pi}_{1+}^{(p)} = (n_1\hat{\pi}_{1+}^{(1)} + n_0\hat{\pi}_{1+}^{(0)})/(n_1 + n_0)$. We will reject $H_0 : \Delta = 0$ at the α-level if the test statistic (2.3), $Z > Z_{\alpha/2}$ or $Z < -Z_{\alpha/2}$, where Z_α is the upper $100(\alpha)$th percentile of the standard normal distribution.

Furthermore, we will claim that the experimental treatment is superior to the standard treatment if $Z > Z_{\alpha/2}$. Note that because the transformation, $\tanh^{-1}(x)(=0.5\log((1+x)/(1-x)))$, has been successfully applied to improve power for test statistics relevant to the PD under other situations (Edwardes, 1995; Lui, 2002), we may also consider use of this transformation when applying $\hat{\delta} = \hat{\pi}_{1+}^{(1)} - \hat{\pi}_{1+}^{(0)}$(2.2) to test superiority. Using the delta method (Agresti, 1990; Lui, 2004), we obtain the asymptotic variance of $\tanh^{-1}(\hat{\delta})$ as given by $Var(\tanh^{-1}(\hat{\delta})) = Var(\hat{\delta})/(1-\delta^2)^2$ (Exercise 2.2). Thus, we have $Var(\tanh^{-1}(\hat{\delta})|H_0) = Var(\hat{\delta}|H_0)$ under the null hypothesis $H_0 : \Delta = 0$ (which implies $\delta = 0$). This leads us to obtain the following test statistic with the $\tanh^{-1}(\hat{\delta})$ transformation,

$$Z = \tanh^{-1}(\hat{\delta})/\sqrt{\hat{Var}(\hat{\delta}|H_0)}. \qquad (2.4)$$

If the test statistic (2.4), $Z > Z_{\alpha/2}$ or $Z < -Z_{\alpha/2}$, then we will reject $H_0 : \Delta = 0$ at the α- level. Furthermore, when the above rejection of $H_0 : \Delta = 0$ is due to the case $Z > Z_{\alpha/2}$, we claim that the experimental treatment is superior to the standard treatment. Note that the programmatic effectiveness δ would be small if π_{+C} was small. Thus, the tests based on statistics (2.3) or (2.4) for the ITT analysis may lack power when the extent of compliance is low. This may motivate us to consider a test procedure directly based on the following MLE for Δ(Exercise 2.3) to improve power in finite-sample cases:

$$\hat{\Delta} = \hat{\pi}_{1|C}^{(1)} - \hat{\pi}_{1|C}^{(0)},$$
$$= (\hat{\pi}_{1+}^{(1)} - \hat{\pi}_{1+}^{(0)})/(\hat{\pi}_{+CA}^{(1)} - \hat{\pi}_{+A}^{(0)}), \qquad (2.5)$$

where $\hat{\pi}_{1|C}^{(g)} = \hat{\pi}_{1C}^{(g)}/\hat{\pi}_{+C}$. Based on the likelihood kernel, Baker and Lindeman (1994) also obtained the MLE $\hat{\Delta}$ (2.5). Note that the MLE $\hat{\Delta}$(2.5) is actually identical to the instrumental variable (IV) estimator for treatment effect in binary data (Angrist, Imbens and Rubin, 1996).

Note that the simple noncompliance RCT or the single-consent randomized design (SCRD) (Zelen, 1979, 1986 and 1990), in which patients assigned to the experimental treatment can be allowed to switch to receive the standard treatment, while patients assigned to the standard treatment are all assumed to comply with their assigned (standard) treatment, will correspond to the above model with the assumption of no always-takers (i.e. $\pi_{+A} = 0$) (Frangakis and Rubin, 1999; Bellamy,

Lin and Ten Have, 2007). Note further that because of the assumption $\pi_{+A} = 0$ under the simple noncompliance RCT, the MLE $\hat{\Delta}(2.5)$ reduces to $\hat{\Delta}_{CA} = (\hat{\pi}_{1+}^{(1)} - \hat{\pi}_{1+}^{(0)})/\hat{\pi}_{+CA}^{(1)}$. On the other hand, the assumption that $\pi_{+A} = 0$ may not be necessarily true in reality. For example, we may encounter a simple noncompliance RCT with a placebo-controlled group. If noncompliers in the placebo group do not receive the experimental treatment due to the study feature of a trial, some of these noncompliers in the placebo group can be always-takers (but who are forced not to receive any treatment by study design). Suppose that the placebo effect is minimal so that the effect due to the placebo is approximately equal to that due to taking no treatment. The estimator $\hat{\Delta}_{CA} = (\hat{\pi}_{1+}^{(1)} - \hat{\pi}_{1+}^{(0)})/\hat{\pi}_{+CA}^{(1)}$ in this case actually estimates the PD $\Delta_{CA} = \pi_{1|CA}^{(1)} - \pi_{1|CA}^{(0)}$, where $\pi_{1|CA}^{(g)} = (\pi_{1C}^{(g)} + \pi_{1A}^{(g)})/\pi_{+CA}^{(1)}$ is the conditional probability of a positive response among patients who would accept the experimental treatment in the assigned treatment g ($g = 1, 0$) (Lui, 2006a and 2006b). Note that the PD $\Delta_{CA} = \pi_{1|CA}^{(1)} - \pi_{1|CA}^{(0)}$ is different from the PD $\Delta(= \pi_{1|C}^{(1)} - \pi_{1|C}^{(0)})$ as discussed here unless the equality $\pi_{1|C}^{(1)} - \pi_{1|C}^{(0)} = \pi_{1|A}^{(1)} - \pi_{1|A}^{(0)}$ holds (Exercise 2.4) or $\pi_{+A} = 0$. Although the parameter $\Delta_{CA} = \pi_{1|CA}^{(1)} - \pi_{1|CA}^{(0)}$ is generally not the same as Δ, the former representing the treatment effect on those patients who would accept the experimental treatment can be a parameter of interest itself. This is because an effective treatment can only be beneficial to those patients who would accept it. The asymptotic variance of $\hat{\Delta}_{CA} = (\hat{\pi}_{1+}^{(1)} - \hat{\pi}_{1+}^{(0)})/\hat{\pi}_{+CA}^{(1)}$ under the SCRD (Exercise 2.5) can be found elsewhere (Lui, 2006a). To improve the power of the test procedures in the ITT analysis, Lui (2006a) developed two simple test procedures directly based on $\hat{\Delta}_{CA}$ (Exercise 2.6) and demonstrated that his test procedures could outperform the test procedures for the ITT analysis in a variety of situations.

Note that the estimator $\hat{\Delta} = (\hat{\pi}_{1+}^{(1)} - \hat{\pi}_{1+}^{(0)})/(\hat{\pi}_{+CA}^{(1)} - \hat{\pi}_{+A}^{(0)})(2.5)$ may no longer be a consistent estimator of $\Delta(2.1)$ when noncompliers (who are supposed to be always-takers) in the standard treatment (or placebo) do not actually receive the experimental treatment so that the exclusion restriction assumption for always-takers is violated. Note also that we assume that each patient can be either a complier or a noncomplier (such as an always-takers or a never-taker), but not both. Because $\delta = \Delta\pi_{+C}$, the equality of treatment efficacy (i.e. $\Delta = 0$) among compliers between two treatments will imply, as noted previously, the equality of the corresponding programmatic effectiveness (i.e. $\delta = 0$), and vice versa. Thus, the case in which the equality of treatment efficacy does not necessarily imply the null programmatic effectiveness in the ITT analysis when compliers lately becomes noncompliant as noted elsewhere (Robins, 1998) under different structural assumptions cannot occur here under the above assumptions.

Example 2.1   Consider the data in Table 2.1 regarding the use of vitamin A supplementation to reduce the mortality among preschool children in rural Indonesia (Sommer and Zeger, 1991). These data were actually collected from a cluster randomized trial, in which randomized units are villages rather than children. For the purpose of illustration only, we ignore clusters here and assume that children were randomly assigned to either the experimental group of receiving doses of vitamin A supplementation or to the control group of receiving no vitamin A

Table 2.1   The data regarding use of vitamin A supplementation to reduce mortality among pre-school children.

Experimental group: receiving vitamin A supplementation ($g = 1$)

		Vitamin A actually	Supplementation received	
		Yes	No	Total
Outcome	Survival	9663 (79.90 %)	2385 (19.72 %)	12048 (99.62 %)
	Death	12 (0.10 %)	34 (0.28 %)	46 (0.38 %)
	Total	9675 (80.00 %)	2419 (20.00 %)	12094 (100 %)

Control group: receiving no vitamin A supplementation ($g = 0$)

		Vitamin A actually	Supplementation received	
		No	Yes	Total
Outcome	Survival	11514 (99.36 %)	0	11514 (99.36 %)
	Death	74 (0.64 %)	0	74 (0.64 %)
	Total	11588 (100 %)	0	11588 (100 %)

supplementation. The discussion about the cluster effect on hypothesis testing will be presented in Chapter 4. In the control group, because children were precluded from receiving a placebo for ethical reasons, we could observe only the total number of children surviving without the information on children who would decline to take vitamin A supplementation if they were actually assigned to the treatment group. As commonly assumed for a simple noncompliance trial, we assume that there are no always-takers (i.e. $\pi_{+A} = 0$) and all children assigned to the control group receive no vitamin A supplementation. Using the data in Table 2.1, we have $n_{1CA}^{(1)} = 9663$, $n_{1N}^{(1)} = 2385$, $n_{2CA}^{(1)} = 12$, and $n_{2N}^{(1)} = 34$ for a total number of 12 094 children assigned to the treatment of receiving vitamin A supplementation. Furthermore, we see that $(n_{1+}^{(0)} =)11\,514$ out of $(n_0 =)11\,588$ children survived in the control group. Thus, we obtain the MLE estimate for the PD in the survival rate between the experimental and control groups $\hat{\delta}(= \hat{\pi}_{1+}^{(1)} - \hat{\pi}_{1+}^{(0)}) = 0.0026$. Suppose that we are interested in finding out whether there is a difference in the survival rates between the group receiving vitamin A supplementation and the group without receiving any vitamin A among children who were compliers. When applying test statistics (2.3) and (2.4), we obtain p-values (two-sided test) of 0.005 in both cases. Given such a large sample size as considered in this example, it is not surprising to find such strong significant evidence that vitamin A supplementation has an effect on reducing mortality in preschool children, although the resulting estimate $\hat{\delta}$ is quite small.

Example 2.2   Consider the data taken from the Coronary Drug Project Research Group (1980) studying the cholesterol lowering drug Clofibrate to reduce mortality (Piantadosi, 1997; Nagelkerke, Fidler and Bernsen *et al.*, 2000). The Coronary Drug Project was a randomized, double-blind, placebo-controlled, multicenter clinical trial. The primary objective was to evaluate the efficacy and safety of several lipid-influencing drugs in the long-term therapy of coronary heart disease (CHD). Participants, who had to be a patient of 30–64 years old with electrocardiographic evidence of a myocardial infarction that had occurred not less than three months previously, were followed through clinic visits and examinations conducted every four months for a minimum of five and a maximum of 8.5 years. Patients were randomized and given capsules according to the study protocol. The cumulative adherence for each patient was computed as a percentage of the estimated number of capsules actually taken over the total number that should have been taken according to the protocol during the first five years of follow-up or until death (if death occurred during the first five years). Here, we classify a patient as 'taking' the assigned treatment if the cumulative adherence of this patient is over or equal to 80 %. For illustration purposes only, we assume that the effect of 'not taking Clofibrate', is the same as that of 'taking the placebo'. We summarize the data in Table 2.2. In the placebo group there were noncompliers (of whom some might be always-takers), but who did not take Clofibrate. Hence the exclusion restriction assumption $\pi_{1|A}^{(1)} = \pi_{1|A}^{(0)}$ for always-takers may not hold. In this case, however, we can show that the expectation $E(\hat{\delta}) = \delta = \Delta_{CA}\pi_{+CA}$.

Table 2.2 The data taken from the Coronary Drug Project Research Group studying the effect of cholesterol lowering drug Clofibrate on reducing mortality from coronary heart disease.

Clofibrate arm ($g = 1$)

		Treatment actually	received	
		taking Clofibrate	not-taking Clofibrate	Total
Status	Alive	602 (56.53 %)	269 (25.26 %)	871 (81.78 %)
	Dead	106 (9.95 %)	88 (8.26 %)	194 (18.22 %)
	Total	708 (66.48 %)	357 (33.52 %)	1065 (100 %)

Placebo arm ($g = 0$)

		Treatment actually	received	
		taking placebo	taking no placebo	Total
Status	Alive	1539 (57.11 %)	633 (23.49 %)	2172 (80.59 %)
	Dead	274 (10.17 %)	249 (9.24 %)	523 (19.41 %)
	Total	1813 (67.27 %)	882 (32.73 %)	2695 (100 %)

Thus, we have $\delta = 0$ if and only if $\Delta_{CA} = 0$. This suggests that we be able to apply test statistics (2.3) and (2.4) to test $H_0 : \Delta_{CA} = 0$ (rather than $H_0 : \Delta = 0$).

Given the data in Table 2.2, we obtain the p-values of 0.403 and 0.402 using test statistics (2.3) and (2.4), respectively. Thus, there is no significant evidence that using Clofibrate can affect the survival rate among those patients who would accept the Clofibrate at the 5 % level. If the condition that $\pi_{1|C}^{(1)} - \pi_{1|C}^{(0)} = \pi_{1|A}^{(1)} - \pi_{1|A}^{(0)}$ were true, then Δ_{CA} would be identical to $\Delta(2.1)$. Under this additional assumption, test statistics (2.3) and (2.4) can still be used to test $H_0 : \Delta = 0$. Note that the exclusion restriction assumption for never-takers (who were classified as not taking Clofibrate based on the cumulative adherence) in this example may also be violated in this RCT. This is because never-takers who would possibly receive the partial treatment if they were assigned to the experimental group, while they would not receive the treatment at all if they were assigned to the placebo group. Thus, we should be cautious in our inference when dichotomizing patients into 'compliance' or 'noncompliance' categories based on the extent of compliance to a treatment (Jo, Asparouhov and Muthén, 2008).

Example 2.3   Consider the data (Table 2.3) taken from a randomized trial studying the effect of a multiple intervention program on mortality from CHD (Multiple Risk Factor Intervention Trial Research Group, 1982) for reducing the mortality of CHD. Eligible men aged 35–57 years at increased risk of death from CHD were randomly assigned to either the intervention or control group. Participants assigned to the intervention group were provided with dietary advice to reduce blood cholesterol, smoking cessation counseling, and hypertension medication, while participants assigned to the control group were referred to their usual physicians for treatment. Because only the program for cigarette smoking cessation was actually effective, we restrict our attention to the effect of quitting cigarette smoking (Mark and Robins, 1993; Matsui, 2005). For the purpose of illustration, we consider only patients with the number of smoked cigarettes less than 30 cigarettes per day at baseline. Based on these data, we obtain the estimate $\hat{\delta} = -0.0022$. When employing test procedures (2.3) and (2.4), we obtain a p-value of 0.705 in both cases. There is no evidence that quitting smoking can significantly reduce the mortality of CHD among compliers at the 5 % level.

Table 2.3   The data taken from a multiple risk factor intervention trial studying the intervention of quitting smoking in reducing mortality from coronary heart disease during 7 years of follow-up.

(a) Patients with the number of smoked cigarettes < 30 per day at baseline

Intervention group ($g = 1$)

		Quit Smoking		
		Yes	No	Total
Status	Dead	6 (0.48 %)	19 (1.51 %)	25 (1.98 %)
	Alive	448 (35.56 %)	787 (62.46 %)	1235 (98.01 %)
	Total	454 (36.03 %)	806 (63.97 %)	1260 (100 %)

Control group ($g = 0$)

Status	Dead	23 (1.95 %)	3 (0.25 %)	26 (2.20 %)
	Alive	998 (84.58 %)	156 (13.22 %)	1154 (97.80 %)
	Total	1021 (86.53 %)	159 (13.47 %)	1180 (100 %)

(b) Patients with the number of smoked cigarettes ≥ 30 per day at baseline

Intervention group ($g = 1$)

		Quit Smoking		
		Yes	No	Total
Status	Dead	5 (0.19 %)	39 (1.52 %)	44 (1.71 %)
	Alive	532 (20.68 %)	1997(77.61 %)	2529 (98.29 %)
	Total	537 (20.87 %)	2036(79.13 %)	2573 (100 %)

Control group ($g = 0$)

Status	Dead	47 (1.77 %)	1 (0.04 %)	48 (1.81 %)
	Alive	2388 (90.11 %)	214 (8.08 %)	2602 (98.19 %)
	Total	2435 (91.89 %)	215 (8.11 %)	2650 (100 %)

2.2   Testing noninferiority

When a new generic drug with fewer side effects or less expense to administer than the standard drug is developed, the new drug can be a useful and alternative drug to the standard drug if one can show that the former is noninferior to the latter. For certain drugs, such as anti-ulcer agents and topical anti-fungal agents, which do not produce an appreciable absorption into the systemic circulation, the pharmacokinetics parameters are no longer adequate for the assessment of noninferiority or bioequivalence. Thus, we may assess whether the generic drug is noninferior to the standard drug based on clinical endpoints, such as cure rate in the ulcer treatment trials or eradication rate in the anti-infective trials (Chen, Tsong and Kang, 2000; Tu, 1998; Liu and Chow, 1993). In other words, we may wish to find out whether the probability of a positive response for the new drug is not less than that for the standard drug by a pre-determined acceptable level of clinical significance. We may call this kind of trial the therapeutic noninferiority RCT with respect to clinical responses. This is the focus of noninferiority in this book.

2.2.1   Using the difference in proportions

To measure the relative treatment effect between an experimental treatment and a standard treatment in a RCT, the PD of a positive response between two treatments is probably the most commonly-used indices (Fleiss, 1981). In a RCT with noncompliance, the PD focused here is $\Delta = \pi_{1|C}^{(1)} - \pi_{1|C}^{(0)}$(2.1). The range of Δ is $-1 < \Delta < 1$. The parameter Δ is symmetric with respect to 0 when the outcomes of 'positive' and 'negative' responses are interchanged. In establishing noninferiority, we want to test $H_0 : \Delta \leq -\varepsilon_l$ versus $H_a : \Delta > -\varepsilon_l$, where $\varepsilon_l(> 0)$ is the maximum acceptable margin such that the experimental treatment can be regarded as noninferior to the standard treatment when $\pi_{1/C}^{(1)} > \pi_{1/C}^{(0)} - \varepsilon_l$ holds, and is usually pre-determined subjectively by clinicians based on their medical knowledge and expertise. In practice, it is generally desirable to shrink the acceptable margin ε_l as the underlying response rate increases from 0.50 to 1. As noted elsewhere (Rousson and Seifert, 2008; Garrett, 2003), the FDA (1997) recommended in a draft for establishing the effectiveness of a new *Helicobacter pylori* regimen using $\varepsilon_l = 0.20$,

0.15 or 0.10 depending on whether the highest of the two observed response rates was smaller 0.80, between 0.80 and 0.90, or larger than 0.90, respectively. Note that if $\Delta > -\varepsilon_l$ holds, then $\delta = \Delta \pi_{+C} > -\varepsilon_l$ will be true, but not vice versa (Exercise 2.7). Thus, when one wishes to test $H_0 : \Delta \le -\varepsilon_l$ for assessing noninferiority, it is no longer appropriate to employ the test statistic $\hat{\delta}$ for the ITT analysis to test $H_0 : \delta \le -\varepsilon_l$. We need to consider a test procedure directly based on the statistic $\hat{\Delta}$ (2.5), which is a consistent estimator of Δ under the above assumptions. Using the delta method (Agresti, 1990; Casella and Berger, 1990), we obtain an estimated asymptotic variance for $\hat{\Delta}$ (2.5) as (Exercise 2.8):

$$\hat{V}ar(\hat{\Delta}) = \{[\hat{\pi}_{1+}^{(1)}(1 - \hat{\pi}_{1+}^{(1)})/n_1 + \hat{\pi}_{1+}^{(0)}(1 - \hat{\pi}_{1+}^{(0)})/n_0]$$
$$+ \hat{\Delta}^2[\hat{\pi}_{+CA}^{(1)}(1 - \hat{\pi}_{+CA}^{(1)})/n_1 + \hat{\pi}_{+A}^{(0)}(1 - \hat{\pi}_{+A}^{(0)})/n_0]$$
$$- 2\hat{\Delta}[(\hat{\pi}_{1CA}^{(1)} - \hat{\pi}_{1+}^{(1)}\hat{\pi}_{+CA}^{(1)})/n_1 + (\hat{\pi}_{1A}^{(0)} - \hat{\pi}_{1+}^{(0)}\hat{\pi}_{+A}^{(0)})/$$
$$n_0]\}/(\hat{\pi}_{+CA}^{(1)} - \hat{\pi}_{+A}^{(0)})^2. \tag{2.6}$$

On the basis of (2.5) and (2.6) together with $\tanh^{-1}(\hat{\Delta})$ transformation, we consider the test statistic

$$Z = [\tanh^{-1}(\hat{\Delta}) + \tanh^{-1}(\varepsilon_l)]/\sqrt{\hat{V}ar(\tanh^{-1}(\hat{\Delta}))}, \tag{2.7}$$

where $\hat{V}ar(\tanh^{-1}(\hat{\Delta})) = \hat{V}ar(\hat{\Delta})/(1 - \hat{\Delta}^2)^2$. We will reject $H_0 : \Delta \le -\varepsilon_l$ at the α-level if the test statistic (2.7), $Z > Z_\alpha$. Because the range of Δ is between -1 and 1, as noted previously, the choice of the maximum clinically acceptable margin ε_l can heavily depend on the underlying value of $\pi_{1|C}^{(0)}$. For example, when $\pi_{1|C}^{(0)}$ equals 0.1, it would be senseless to choose ε_l to be larger than 0.1. Furthermore, a fixed value of ε_l can possess different clinical meanings and implications depending on the underlying value of $\pi_{1|C}^{(0)}$. This may lead us to consider use of alternative indices to the PD, such as PR or OR, to measure the relative treatment efficacy in establishing noninferiority.

2.2.2   Using the ratio of proportions

The PR provides us with the useful information on the number of manifolds for the response probability of interest between an experimental treatment and a standard treatment. When the PR is defined as the ratio of probabilities of an adverse event between an experimental treatment and a standard treatment (or placebo), the PR is called the risk ratio (RR), which is one of the most important indices in etiology (Fleiss, 1981; Lui, 2004 and 2006c). When the underlying value of RR is less than 1, 1-RR is also called the relative difference (Sheps, 1958 and 1959; Fleiss, 1981) or the relative risk reduction (Laupacis, Sackett and Roberts, 1988). Note that the PR is well known to lack symmetry when the 'positive' and 'negative' outcomes are interchanged. For clarity, we define the PR in a RCT with noncompliance considered here as

$$\gamma = \pi_{1|C}^{(1)}/\pi_{1|C}^{(0)} = \pi_{1C}^{(1)}/\pi_{1C}^{(0)}, \tag{2.8}$$

which is the ratio of probabilities of a positive response among compliers between the experimental and standard treatments. Note that the range for the PR is $0 < \gamma < \infty$. When $\gamma < 1$, the experimental treatment tends to decrease the probability of a positive response among compliers as compared with the standard treatment. When $\gamma = 1$, the effects on the probability of a positive response are equal between two treatments. When $\gamma > 1$, the experimental treatment tends to increase the probability of a positive response among compliers as compared with the standard treatment. By the functional invariance property of the MLE (Casella and Berger, 1990), we obtain the MLE of γ as given by

$$\hat{\gamma} = \hat{\pi}_{1|C}^{(1)}/\hat{\pi}_{1|C}^{(0)} = \hat{\pi}_{1C}^{(1)}/\hat{\pi}_{1C}^{(0)}$$
$$= (\hat{\pi}_{1CA}^{(1)} - \hat{\pi}_{1A}^{(0)})/(\hat{\pi}_{1CN}^{(0)} - \hat{\pi}_{1N}^{(1)}) \tag{2.9}$$

Note that $\hat{\gamma}$ (2.9) is actually the same estimator as that obtained by Cuzick, Edwards and Segnan (1997). Furthermore, using the delta method, we can easily show that an estimated asymptotic variance $\hat{Var}(\log(\hat{\gamma}))$ for the statistic $\log(\hat{\gamma})$ with the logarithmic transformation is given by (Exercise 2.9):

$$\hat{Var}(\log(\hat{\gamma})) = [\hat{\pi}_{1CA}^{(1)}(1 - \hat{\pi}_{1CA}^{(1)})/n_1 + \hat{\pi}_{1A}^{(0)}(1 - \hat{\pi}_{1A}^{(0)})/n_0]/$$
$$(\hat{\pi}_{1CA}^{(1)} - \hat{\pi}_{1A}^{(0)})^2 + [\hat{\pi}_{1N}^{(1)}(1 - \hat{\pi}_{1N}^{(1)})/n_1$$
$$+ \hat{\pi}_{1CN}^{(0)}(1 - \hat{\pi}_{1CN}^{(0)})/n_0]/(\hat{\pi}_{1CN}^{(0)} - \hat{\pi}_{1N}^{(1)})^2$$
$$- 2[\hat{\pi}_{1CA}^{(1)}\hat{\pi}_{1N}^{(1)}/n_1 + \hat{\pi}_{1CN}^{(0)}\hat{\pi}_{1A}^{(0)}/n_0]/$$
$$[(\hat{\pi}_{1CA}^{(1)} - \hat{\pi}_{1A}^{(0)})(\hat{\pi}_{1CN}^{(0)} - \hat{\pi}_{1N}^{(1)})]. \tag{2.10}$$

We consider testing $H_0 : \gamma \leq 1 - \gamma_l$ versus $H_a : \gamma > 1 - \gamma_l$, where γ_l is the maximum clinically acceptable margin such that the experimental treatment can be regarded as noninferior to the standard treatment when $\gamma > 1 - \gamma_l$ holds. When rejecting $H_0 : \gamma \leq 1 - \gamma_l$ at the α-level, we claim that the experimental treatment is noninferior to the standard treatment. As the number of patients n_g is large in both groups, we consider the following test statistic,

$$Z = (\log(\hat{\gamma}) - \log(1 - \gamma_l)) / \sqrt{\widehat{Var}(\log(\hat{\gamma}))}. \tag{2.11}$$

We reject $H_0 : \gamma \leq 1 - \gamma_l$ at the α-level when the test statistic (2.11), $Z > Z_\alpha$. Note that the noninferior margin $(1 - \gamma_l)$ for the PR corresponds to the noninferior margin $\varepsilon_l = \gamma_l \pi_{1|C}^{(0)}$ on the PD scale. The larger the underlying probability of a positive response $\pi_{1|C}^{(0)}$, the larger is the noninferior margin $\varepsilon_l (= \gamma_l \pi_{1|C}^{(0)})$ on the PD scale. This contradicts the general desirable guideline in a draft that the noninferior margin ε_l should shrink when the underlying response rates in a RCT become large (FDA, 1997). To illustrate this point, for example, set $\gamma_l = 0.50$. The acceptable margin ε_l increases from 0.25 to 0.45 when $\pi_{1|C}^{(0)}$ changes from 0.50 to 0.90. To alleviate this concern of using the PR, Garrett (2003) contended that the OR should be the most rational index to measure the relative treatment effect in establishing noninferiority or equivalence.

2.2.3   Using the odds ratio of proportions

The OR is invariant under various study designs (Fleiss, 1981; Lui, 2004), symmetric with respect to 0 on the log-scale when the outcomes of 'positive' and 'negative' responses are interchanged, and gives a good approximation to the RR for a rare disease. Thus, the OR is probably the most frequently used index to measure the strength of association between a risk factor and an outcome in epidemiology. Furthermore, since the OR can be expressed in terms of model parameters under the log-linear or logistic regression model (Bishop, Fienberg, and Holland, 1975; Agresti, 1990; Hosmer and Lemeshow, 1989), we can study the OR while controlling the effects of other confounders easily. In RCTs, the OR has been recommended to measure the relative treatment effect in establishing noninferiority (or equivalence) in a RCT or meta-analysis

(Tu, 1998 and 2003; Wang, Chow and Li, 2002; Garrett, 2003). Note that because the probability of a patient response of interest is generally not small in a RCT, however, the OR and PR cannot be regarded as a similar index as commonly done for a rare disease in epidemiology. For a RCT with noncompliance, we define the OR here as

$$\varphi = (\pi_{1|C}^{(1)}/\pi_{2|C}^{(1)})/(\pi_{1|C}^{(0)}/\pi_{2|C}^{(0)}) = (\pi_{1C}^{(1)}\pi_{2C}^{(0)})/(\pi_{2C}^{(1)}\pi_{1C}^{(0)}), \qquad (2.12)$$

which is the OR of probabilities of a positive response among compliers between two treatments. Note that the range for the OR is $\varphi > 0$. When the OR $\varphi < 1$, the experimental treatment tends to decrease the probability of a positive response among compliers as compared with the standard treatment. When the OR $\varphi = 1$, the experimental treatment has the same effect as the standard treatment on the probability of a positive response among compliers. When the OR $\varphi > 1$, the experimental treatment tends to increase the probability of a positive response among compliers as compared with the standard treatment. Based on the functional invariance property of the MLE (Casella and Berger, 1990) again, we obtain the MLE for φ (2.12) as

$$\begin{aligned}
\hat{\varphi} &= (\hat{\pi}_{1C}^{(1)}\hat{\pi}_{2C}^{(0)})/(\hat{\pi}_{2C}^{(1)}\hat{\pi}_{1C}^{(0)}) \\
&= [(\hat{\pi}_{1CA}^{(1)} - \hat{\pi}_{1A}^{(0)})(\hat{\pi}_{2CN}^{(0)} - \hat{\pi}_{2N}^{(1)})]/ \\
&\quad [(\hat{\pi}_{2CA}^{(1)} - \hat{\pi}_{2A}^{(0)})(\hat{\pi}_{1CN}^{(0)} - \hat{\pi}_{1N}^{(1)})]. \qquad (2.13)
\end{aligned}$$

Using the delta method (Agresti, 1990; Lui, 2004), we obtain an estimated asymptotic variance for $\log(\hat{\varphi})$ with the logarithmic transformation as (Exercise 2.10):

$$\begin{aligned}
\hat{Var}(\log(\hat{\varphi})) =& [\hat{\pi}_{1CA}^{(1)}(1-\hat{\pi}_{1CA}^{(1)})/n_1 + \hat{\pi}_{1A}^{(0)}(1-\hat{\pi}_{1A}^{(0)})/n_0]/(\hat{\pi}_{1CA}^{(1)} - \hat{\pi}_{1A}^{(0)})^2 \\
&+ [\hat{\pi}_{2CN}^{(0)}(1-\hat{\pi}_{2CN}^{(0)})/n_0 + \hat{\pi}_{2N}^{(1)}(1-\hat{\pi}_{2N}^{(1)})/n_1]/(\hat{\pi}_{2CN}^{(0)} - \hat{\pi}_{2N}^{(1)})^2 \\
&+ [\hat{\pi}_{2CA}^{(1)}(1-\hat{\pi}_{2CA}^{(1)})/n_1 + \hat{\pi}_{2A}^{(0)}(1-\hat{\pi}_{2A}^{(0)})/n_0]/(\hat{\pi}_{2CA}^{(1)} - \hat{\pi}_{2A}^{(0)})^2 \\
&+ [\hat{\pi}_{1CN}^{(0)}(1-\hat{\pi}_{1CN}^{(0)})/n_0 + \hat{\pi}_{1N}^{(1)}(1-\hat{\pi}_{1N}^{(1)})/n_1]/(\hat{\pi}_{1CN}^{(0)} - \hat{\pi}_{1N}^{(1)})^2 \\
&+ 2[\hat{\pi}_{1CA}^{(1)}\hat{\pi}_{2N}^{(1)}/n_1 + \hat{\pi}_{1A}^{(0)}\hat{\pi}_{2CN}^{(0)}/n_0]/[(\hat{\pi}_{1CA}^{(1)} - \hat{\pi}_{1A}^{(0)})(\hat{\pi}_{2CN}^{(0)} - \hat{\pi}_{2N}^{(1)})] \\
&+ 2[\hat{\pi}_{1CA}^{(1)}\hat{\pi}_{2CA}^{(1)}/n_1 + \hat{\pi}_{1A}^{(0)}\hat{\pi}_{2A}^{(0)}/n_0]/[(\hat{\pi}_{1CA}^{(1)} - \hat{\pi}_{1A}^{(0)})(\hat{\pi}_{2CA}^{(1)} - \hat{\pi}_{2A}^{(0)})] \\
&- 2[\hat{\pi}_{1CA}^{(1)}\hat{\pi}_{1N}^{(1)}/n_1 + \hat{\pi}_{1CN}^{(0)}\hat{\pi}_{1A}^{(0)}/n_0]/[(\hat{\pi}_{1CA}^{(1)} - \hat{\pi}_{1A}^{(0)})(\hat{\pi}_{1CN}^{(0)} - \hat{\pi}_{1N}^{(1)})] \\
&- 2[\hat{\pi}_{2CA}^{(1)}\hat{\pi}_{2N}^{(1)}/n_1 + \hat{\pi}_{2A}^{(0)}\hat{\pi}_{2CN}^{(0)}/n_0]/[(\hat{\pi}_{2CA}^{(1)} - \hat{\pi}_{2A}^{(0)})(\hat{\pi}_{2CN}^{(0)} - \hat{\pi}_{2N}^{(1)})]
\end{aligned}$$

$$+ 2[\hat{\pi}_{1N}^{(1)}\hat{\pi}_{2N}^{(1)}/n_1 + \hat{\pi}_{1CN}^{(0)}\hat{\pi}_{2CN}^{(0)}/n_0]/[(\hat{\pi}_{2CN}^{(0)} - \hat{\pi}_{2N}^{(1)})(\hat{\pi}_{1CN}^{(0)} - \hat{\pi}_{1N}^{(1)})]$$
$$+ 2[\hat{\pi}_{2CA}^{(1)}\hat{\pi}_{1N}^{(1)}/n_1 + \hat{\pi}_{2A}^{(0)}\hat{\pi}_{1CN}^{(0)}/n_0]/[(\hat{\pi}_{2CA}^{(1)} - \hat{\pi}_{2A}^{(0)})(\hat{\pi}_{1CN}^{(0)} - \hat{\pi}_{1N}^{(1)})].$$

$$(2.14)$$

We consider testing $H_0 : \varphi \leq 1 - \varphi_l$ versus $H_0 : \varphi > 1 - \varphi_l$, where φ_l is the maximum clinically acceptable margin such that the experimental treatment can be regarded as noninferior to the standard treatment when $\varphi > 1 - \varphi_l$ holds. Note that when setting $\varphi_l = 0.50$, for example, we can easily see that the corresponding noninferior margin ε_l for the PD would decrease from 0.17 to 0.08 when $\pi_{1|C}^{(0)}$ increases from 0.50 to 0.90. This generally agrees with the general guideline of a draft provided by the FDA (1997) that the noninferior margin on the PD scale should decrease as the underlying probability of responses increases. On the basis of (2.13) and (2.14), we consider the following test statistic:

$$Z = (\log(\hat{\varphi}) - \log(1 - \varphi_l))/\sqrt{\hat{Var}(\log(\hat{\varphi}))}. \qquad (2.15)$$

We will reject $H_0 : \varphi \leq 1 - \varphi_l$ at the α-level if the test statistic (2.15), $Z > Z_\alpha$, and claim that the experimental treatment is noninferior to the standard treatment.

Example 2.4   Consider the data (Table 2.3a) regarding the status of cigarette smoking and the incidence of death from CHD during 7 years of follow-up for patients with the number of cigarettes smoked fewer than 30 cigarettes per day at baseline taken from a multiple risk factor intervention trial. Suppose that we are interested in finding out whether the survival rate of patients who quitted smoking is noninferior to the survival rate of patients who did not quit smoking. Using these data, we obtain a point estimate for the OR of $\hat{\varphi} = 2.01$. This suggests that the survival rate of patients who quitted smoking should be higher than that for those who did not quit. When employing test statistic (2.15) with $\varphi_l = 0.50$ to test noninferiority, however, we obtain a p-value of 0.199. Thus, there is no significant evidence that 'quitting smoking' is noninferior to 'not-quitting smoking' with respect to the survival rate of CHD at the 5 % level. This example illustrates the case in which a high noncompliance rate, as considered in Table 2.3, can cause the loss of an opportunity to detect the noninferiority of an experimental treatment to a standard treatment, even when the former may have a better treatment efficacy than the latter as suggested by the resulting OR point estimate $\hat{\varphi}$. Thus, to avoid reaching this seemingly controversial situation, it is of critical importance to design a randomized encouragement design (RED) with a minimal probability of noncompliance.

2.3   Testing equivalence

When a generic drug is developed, we may often consider assessing whether the therapeutic efficacy of the generic drug is equivalent to that of the standard drug (Dunnett and Gent, 1977; Westlake, 1974 and 1979). A decrease in the response rate may suggest that the generic drug does not have the desired efficacy, while an increase may raise the concern that the generic drug is more toxic than the standard one. In this case, we may wish to test equivalence (Dunnett and Gent, 1977; Westlake, 1979; Schuirmann, 1987; Hauck and Anderson, 1984, 1986; Liu and Chow, 1992; Bristol, 1993) rather than test noninferiority between the treatment effects of two drugs. We may call this kind of trial the therapeutic equivalence RCT with respect to clinical endpoints. In addition to the drug development, the application of the idea for testing equivalence (or noninferiority) in other medically relevant areas can be found elsewhere (Dunnett and Gent, 1977; Obuchowski, 1997; Lui and Zhou, 2004).

2.3.1   Using the difference in proportions

When using the PD ($\Delta = \pi_{1|C}^{(1)} - \pi_{1|C}^{(0)}$) to measure the relative treatment effect in establishing equivalence, we want to test $H_0 : \Delta \leq -\varepsilon_l$ or $\Delta \geq \varepsilon_u$ versus $H_a : -\varepsilon_l < \Delta < \varepsilon_u$, where ε_l and ε_u (> 0) are the maximum clinically acceptable lower and upper margins that the experimental treatment (or drug) can be regarded as equivalent to the standard treatment (or drug) when the inequality $-\varepsilon_l < \Delta < \varepsilon_u$ holds. Using the Intersection-Union test (Casella and Berger, 1990), we will reject the null hypothesis $H_0 : \Delta \leq -\varepsilon_l$ or $\Delta \geq \varepsilon_u$ at the α-level and claim that the two treatments are equivalent if the test statistic $\tanh^{-1}(\hat{\Delta})$ simultaneously satisfies the following two inequalities:

$$(\tanh^{-1}(\hat{\Delta}) + \tanh^{-1}(\varepsilon_l))/\sqrt{\hat{Var}(\tanh^{-1}(\hat{\Delta}))} > Z_\alpha$$

$$\text{and} \quad (\tanh^{-1}(\hat{\Delta}) - \tanh^{-1}(\varepsilon_u))/\sqrt{\hat{Var}(\tanh^{-1}(\hat{\Delta}))} < -Z_\alpha, \quad (2.16)$$

where $\hat{Var}(\tanh^{-1}(\hat{\Delta})) = \hat{Var}(\hat{\Delta})/(1 - \hat{\Delta}^2)^2$, $\hat{\Delta}$ and $\hat{Var}(\hat{\Delta})$ are given in (2.5) and (2.6), respectively. Note that under the above assumptions, we have $0 \le |\delta| = |\Delta|\pi_{+C} \le |\Delta| < 1$. Thus, if the inequality $-\varepsilon_l < \Delta < \varepsilon_u$ is true, then the inequality $-\varepsilon_l < \delta < \varepsilon_u$ will hold, but not vice versa. In other words, if two treatment effects are equivalent, then the corresponding programmatic effectiveness between these two treatments, given a fixed acceptable range $(-\varepsilon_l, \varepsilon_u)$, will be equivalent, while the converse is not true.

2.3.2   Using the ratio of proportions

When using the PR $(\gamma = \pi_{1|C}^{(1)}/\pi_{1|C}^{(0)})$ to measure the relative treatment effect among compliers in establishing equivalence, we want to test $H_0 : \gamma \le 1 - \gamma_l$ or $\gamma \ge 1 + \gamma_u$ versus $H_a : 1 - \gamma_l < \gamma < 1 + \gamma_u$, where γ_l and γ_u (> 0) are the maximum clinically acceptable lower and upper margins that the experimental treatment can be regarded as equivalent to the standard treatment when the inequality $1 - \gamma_l < \gamma < 1 + \gamma_u$ holds. We will reject $H_0 : \gamma \le 1 - \gamma_l$ or $\gamma \ge 1 + \gamma_u$ at the α-level and claim that the two treatments are equivalent if the test statistic $\log(\hat{\gamma})$ simultaneously satisfies the following two inequalities:

$$(\log(\hat{\gamma}) - \log(1 - \gamma_l))/\sqrt{\hat{Var}(\log(\hat{\gamma}))} > Z_\alpha \text{ and}$$

$$(\log(\hat{\gamma}) - \log(1 + \gamma_u))/\sqrt{\hat{Var}(\log(\hat{\gamma}))} < -Z_\alpha, \quad (2.17)$$

where $\hat{\gamma}$ and $\hat{Var}(\log(\hat{\gamma}))$ are given in (2.9) and (2.10), respectively. Using the PR as a measure of the relative treatment effect in establishing equivalence may contradict, as noted previously, the general guidelines in a draft provided by the FDA (1997). Thus, we may consider using the OR to measure the relative treatment effect in establishing equivalence.

2.3.3   Using the odds ratio of proportions

When using the OR ($\varphi = (\pi_{1|C}^{(1)}\pi_{2|C}^{(0)})/(\pi_{2|C}^{(1)}\pi_{1|C}^{(0)})$) to measure the relative treatment effect in establishing equivalence, we want to test $H_0 : \varphi \leq 1 - \varphi_l$ or $\varphi \geq 1 + \varphi_u$ versus $H_a : 1 - \varphi_l < \varphi < 1 + \varphi_u$, where φ_l and φ_u are the maximum clinically acceptable lower and upper margins that the experimental treatment can be regarded as equivalent to the standard treatment when the inequality $1 - \varphi_l < \varphi < 1 + \varphi_u$ is true. Using the Intersection-Union test, we will reject $H_0 : \varphi \leq 1 - \varphi_l$ or $\varphi \geq 1 + \varphi_u$ at the α-level if the test statistic $\log(\hat{\varphi})$ simultaneously satisfies the following two inequalities:

$$(\log(\hat{\varphi}) - \log(1 - \varphi_l))/\sqrt{\hat{V}ar(\log(\hat{\varphi}))} > Z_\alpha \text{ and}$$

$$(\log(\hat{\varphi}) - \log(1 + \varphi_u))/\sqrt{\hat{V}ar(\log(\hat{\varphi}))} < -Z_\alpha, \qquad (2.18)$$

where $\hat{\varphi}$ and $\hat{V}ar(\log(\hat{\varphi}))$ are given in (2.13) and (2.14), respectively. The choice of equivalence margins should usually be pre-determined by clinicians rather than statisticians. Rousson and Seifert (2008) provided a good overview of different choices of equivalence margins for the OR. For examples, Garrett (2003) noted that using $1 - \varphi_l = 0.50$ (and hence $1 + \varphi_u = 2$ so that $\log(1 - \varphi_l) = -\log(1 + \varphi_u)$ for a symmetric acceptance margin on the logarithm scale) appearing to embody the original philosophies of the FDA (1977). Senn (2000) suggested the choice of $1 - \varphi_l = 0.55$ (and hence $1 + \varphi_u = 1.82$) corresponding to a maximum possible difference of proportions between two treatments to be 0.15. Other possible alternative choices of equivalence margins can be found elsewhere (Tu, 1998).

2.4   Interval estimation

When the number of patients n_g for both the experimental ($g = 1$) and standard treatments ($g = 0$) is large, it is well known that one can still obtain statistical significance even when the underlying PD ($\neq 0$) between two treatments is small of no clinical significance (or equivalently, when the underlying PR or OR ($\neq 1$) is close to 1). Thus, it is important and useful to provide an interval estimator for the index of interest so that we can appreciate the magnitude of the relative treatment effect and the precision of our inference. To evaluate the performance of an interval estimator, we commonly use the coverage probability to measure its accuracy and the average length to measure its precision. An ideal asymptotic interval estimator is the one which can consistently have the coverage probability larger than or approximately equal to the desired confidence level and have the shortest average length among all interval estimators, subject to the coverage probability being larger than or approximately equal to the desired confidence level.

2.4.1   Estimation of the proportion difference

The PD ($\Delta = \pi_{1|C}^{(1)} - \pi_{1|C}^{(0)}$), that represents the excess benefits (or risks) of an experimental treatment compared to a standard treatment, is most easily understood by clinicians or investigators. In evidence-based medicine, the number needed to treat (NNT), which is a most recently proposed important index, is actually the reciprocal of the PD (Laupacis Sackett and Roberts, 1988; Lui, 2004). Thus, the interval estimators derived here can be easily modified to obtain the corresponding interval estimators for NNT (Lui, 2004).

Because of its simplicity, the interval estimator using Wald's statistic is often considered. On the basis of (2.5) and (2.6), we obtain an asymptotic $100(1 - \alpha)\%$ confidence interval for Δ ($= \pi_{1|C}^{(1)} - \pi_{1|C}^{(0)}$) as

$$[\max\{\hat{\Delta} - Z_{\alpha/2}(\hat{Var}(\hat{\Delta}))^{1/2}, -1\}, \min\{\hat{\Delta} + Z_{\alpha/2}(\hat{Var}(\hat{\Delta}))^{1/2}, 1\}], \quad (2.19)$$

where $\max\{a, b\}$ and $\min\{a, b\}$ denote the maximum and the minimum of the numerical values a and b, respectively. Since the sampling distribution of $\hat{\Delta}$ (2.5), which is a ratio of two random variables, can be skewed, the interval estimator (2.19) may not perform well, especially when n_g is not large. As done previously (Edwardes, 1995; Lui, 2002), we may consider using the $\tanh^{-1}(x)$ transformation. This leads us to obtain an asymptotic $100(1 - \alpha)\%$ confidence interval for Δ ($= \pi_{1|C}^{(1)} - \pi_{1|C}^{(0)}$) as

$$[\tanh(\tanh^{-1}(\hat{\Delta}) - Z_{\alpha/2}(\hat{Var}(\tanh^{-1}(\hat{\Delta})))^{1/2}),$$
$$\tanh(\tanh^{-1}(\hat{\Delta}) + Z_{\alpha/2}(\hat{Var}(\tanh^{-1}(\hat{\Delta})))^{1/2})], \quad (2.20)$$

where $\hat{V}ar(\tanh^{-1}(\hat{\Delta})) = \hat{V}ar(\hat{\Delta})/(1 - \hat{\Delta}^2)^2$. Note that the two inequalities (2.16) hold if and only if the $100(1 - 2\alpha)\%$ confidence interval using interval estimator (2.20) is completely contained in the acceptable range $(-\varepsilon_l, \varepsilon_u)$ (Exercise 2.11). Thus, the test procedure (2.16) for detecting equivalence at the α-level is identical to the statement that we claim the two treatments under comparison are equivalent if the resulting $100(1 - 2\alpha)\%$ confidence interval (2.20) is completely contained in the acceptable range.

To also account for the concern that the sampling distribution of the MLE $\hat{\Delta}$ can be skewed when n_g is small, we may use the idea of Fieller's Theorem (Casella and Berger, 1990). Define $Z^* = (\hat{\pi}_{1+}^{(1)} - \hat{\pi}_{1+}^{(0)}) - \Delta(\hat{\pi}_{+CA}^{(1)} - \hat{\pi}_{+A}^{(0)})$. Note that the expectation $E(Z^*)$ is equal to 0. The variance of Z^* is

$$Var(Z^*) = \pi_{1+}^{(1)}(1 - \pi_{1+}^{(1)})/n_1 + \pi_{1+}^{(0)}(1 - \pi_{1+}^{(0)})/n_0$$
$$+ \Delta^2[\pi_{+CA}^{(1)}(1 - \pi_{+CA}^{(1)})/n_1 + \pi_{+A}^{(0)}(1 - \pi_{+A}^{(0)})/n_0]$$
$$- 2\Delta[(\pi_{1CA}^{(1)} - \pi_{1+}^{(1)}\pi_{+CA}^{(1)})/n_1 + (\pi_{1A}^{(0)} - \pi_{1+}^{(0)}\pi_{+A}^{(0)})/n_0].$$
$$(2.21)$$

Thus, when both n_g are large, the probability $P((Z^*)^2/Var(Z^*) \leq Z_{\alpha/2}^2) \approx 1 - \alpha$. This leads us to consider the following quadratic equation:

$$A^*\Delta^2 - 2B^*\Delta + C^* \leq 0, \qquad (2.22)$$

where

$$A^* = (\hat{\pi}_{+CA}^{(1)} - \hat{\pi}_{+A}^{(0)})^2 - Z_{\alpha/2}^2[\hat{\pi}_{+CA}^{(1)}(1 - \hat{\pi}_{+CA}^{(1)})/n_1$$
$$+ \hat{\pi}_{+A}^{(0)}(1 - \hat{\pi}_{+A}^{(0)})/n_0],$$
$$B^* = (\hat{\pi}_{1+}^{(1)} - \hat{\pi}_{1+}^{(0)})(\hat{\pi}_{+CA}^{(1)} - \hat{\pi}_{+A}^{(0)}) - Z_{\alpha/2}^2[(\hat{\pi}_{1CA}^{(1)} - \hat{\pi}_{+CA}^{(1)}\hat{\pi}_{1+}^{(1)})/n_1$$
$$+ (\hat{\pi}_{1A}^{(0)} - \hat{\pi}_{+A}^{(0)}\hat{\pi}_{1+}^{(0)})/n_0], \quad \text{and}$$
$$C^* = (\hat{\pi}_{1+}^{(1)} - \hat{\pi}_{1+}^{(0)})^2 - Z_{\alpha/2}^2[\hat{\pi}_{1+}^{(1)}(1 - \hat{\pi}_{1+}^{(1)})/n_1 + \hat{\pi}_{1+}^{(0)}(1 - \hat{\pi}_{1+}^{(0)})/n_0].$$

If $A^* > 0$ and $(B^*)^2 - A^*C^* > 0$, then an asymptotic $100(1 - \alpha)\%$ confidence interval for Δ would be given by

$$[\max\{(B^* - \sqrt{(B^*)^2 - A^*C^*})/A^*, -1\},$$
$$\min\{(B^* + \sqrt{(B^*)^2 - A^*C^*})/A^*, 1\}]. \qquad (2.23)$$

Note that under the simple noncompliance RCT (i.e. $\pi_{+A} = 0$), Lui (2006b) considered and evaluated the performance of six asymptotic interval estimators, including interval estimators (2.19), (2.20), and (2.23), in a variety of situations. Lui (2006b) found that interval estimator (2.20) can not only perform well, but also be generally preferable to the other estimators. We refer readers to the publication (Lui, 2006b) for details.

Example 2.5   Consider the simple noncompliance RCT studying vitamin A supplementation to reduce mortality among preschool children in rural Indonesia (Sommer, Tarwotjo and Djunaedi *et al.*, 1986) in Table 2.1. As noted previously, we assume the proportion π_{+A} of always-takers to be 0. For the purpose of illustration, we ignore clusters here. Since children assigned to the control group were precluded from receiving a placebo for ethical reasons. We assume that the placebo effect is minimal in the following discussion. Suppose we are interested in estimation of the PD Δ in the survival rates between patients receiving vitamin A supplements and patients receiving no vitamin A supplements. Given the above data, the MLE $\hat{\Delta}$ (2.5) is 0.0032, which is larger than the MLE of the programmatic effectiveness $\hat{\delta}(= \hat{\pi}_{1+}^{(1)} - \hat{\pi}_{1+}^{(0)}) = 0.0026$. When applying interval estimators (2.19), (2.20), and (2.23), we obtain 95 % confidence intervals all to be [0.0010, 0.0055]. Since the total number of children in this randomized trial is quite large, we can see that the resulting 95 % confidence interval using interval estimators (2.19), (2.20), and (2.23) are essentially identical. Because all the above lower limits fall above 0, there is significant evidence at the 5 % level to support the hypothesis that taking vitamin A supplementation can increase the survival rate for preschool children. This is consistent with findings based on test procedures (2.3) and (2.4). Since the upper limits of these resulting confidence intervals are close to 0, however, the magnitude of the increase in the survival rate due to taking vitamin A supplementation is small.

2.4.2 Estimation of the proportion ratio

The PR $(\gamma = \pi_{1|C}^{(1)}/\pi_{1|C}^{(0)})$ represents the ratio of probabilities of a positive response among compliers between the experimental treatment and the standard treatment (or placebo). On the basis of $\hat{\gamma}$(2.9) and $\hat{Var}(\log(\hat{\gamma}))$(2.10), we obtain an asymptotic $100(1 - \alpha)\%$ confidence interval using Wald's statistic for the PR as

$$[\max\{\hat{\gamma} - Z_{\alpha/2}(\hat{Var}(\hat{\gamma}))^{1/2}, 0\}, \hat{\gamma} + Z_{\alpha/2}(\hat{Var}(\hat{\gamma}))^{1/2}], \qquad (2.24)$$

where $\hat{Var}(\hat{\gamma}) = \hat{\gamma}^2 \hat{Var}(\log(\hat{\gamma}))$. Since the sampling distribution of $\hat{\gamma}$ (2.9) (which is a ratio of two proportion estimates) can be skewed, we often consider use of a logarithmic transformation (Fleiss, 1981; Lui, 2004). This leads us to obtain an asymptotic $100(1 - \alpha)\%$ confidence interval using the logarithmic transformation for the PR as

$$[\hat{\gamma}\exp(-Z_{\alpha/2}(\hat{Var}(\log(\hat{\gamma})))^{1/2}), \hat{\gamma}\exp(Z_{\alpha/2}(\hat{Var}(\log(\hat{\gamma})))^{1/2})]. \quad (2.25)$$

Note that when there is perfect compliance (i.e. $\pi_{+C} = 1$), the interval estimator (2.25) reduces to that proposed elsewhere (Katz, Baptista and Azen et al., 1978; Fleiss, 1981; Lui, 2004). Note also that using the interval estimator (2.25) can sometimes cause a loss of precision. For example, consider the situation in which the denominator $\pi_{1C}^{(0)}(= \pi_{1CN}^{(0)} - \pi_{1N}^{(1)})$ of γ is small. The MLE $\hat{\gamma}$, if it exists, can be large by chance, and so is the estimated asymptotic variance $\hat{Var}(\log(\hat{\gamma}))$. This will produce a wide confidence interval using (2.25) especially when the exponential transformation is involved. To alleviate the possible loss of accuracy when using (2.24) and the possible loss of precision when using (2.25), Lui (2007a) considered an ad hoc procedure of combining (2.24) and (2.25). Define the indicator random variable $I(\hat{\gamma}, \hat{Var}(\hat{\gamma}))$ to be 1 if the length $\hat{\gamma}(\exp(Z_{\alpha/2}(\hat{Var}(\log(\hat{\gamma})))^{1/2}) - \exp(-Z_{\alpha/2}(\hat{Var}(\log(\hat{\gamma})))^{1/2}))$ of using (2.25) is larger than or equal to K times the length $(\hat{\gamma} + Z_{\alpha/2}\sqrt{\hat{Var}(\hat{\gamma})} - \max\{\hat{\gamma} - Z_{\alpha/2}\sqrt{\hat{Var}(\hat{\gamma})}, 0\})$ of using (2.24), and 0, otherwise. We then obtain an asymptotic $100(1 - \alpha)\%$ confidence interval for γ as

$$[\gamma_l, \gamma_u], \qquad (2.26)$$

where

$$\gamma_l = I(\hat{\gamma}, \hat{Var}(\hat{\gamma})) \max\{\hat{\gamma} - Z_{\alpha/2}(\hat{Var}(\hat{\gamma}))^{1/2}, 0\}$$
$$+ (1 - I(\hat{\gamma}, \hat{Var}(\hat{\gamma})))\hat{\gamma} \exp(-Z_{\alpha/2}(\hat{Var}(\log(\hat{\gamma})))^{1/2}), \quad \text{and}$$
$$\gamma_u = I(\hat{\gamma}, \hat{Var}(\hat{\gamma}))(\hat{\gamma} + Z_{\alpha/2}(\hat{Var}(\hat{\gamma}))^{1/2})$$
$$+ (1 - I(\hat{\gamma}, \hat{Var}(\hat{\gamma})))\hat{\gamma} \exp(Z_{\alpha/2}(\hat{Var}(\log(\hat{\gamma})))^{1/2})$$

Note that interval estimators (2.24) and (2.25) are limiting cases of (2.26) as K goes to 0 and ∞, respectively. When we choose a value for K too small, the interval estimator (2.26) tends to perform like the interval estimator (2.24) and hence can be liberal. On the other hand, when we choose a value for K too large, the interval estimator (2.26) tends to perform like the interval estimator (2.25) and hence can lose precision. When the number of patients n_g in both assigned treatments is large, because the performances of interval estimators (2.24) and (2.25) tend to be similar, the choice of a value for K has little effect on the performance of (2.26). In this case, the performances of interval estimators (2.24), (2.25), and (2.26) should be similar to one another. On the basis of some empirical evaluations of the coverage probability and average length using Monte Carlo simulations in other situations (Lui, 2007a), the constant $K = 2.5$ is recommended. For the simple noncompliance RCT, Lui (2007a) considered and evaluated the performance of five asymptotic interval estimators, including interval estimators (2.24)–(2.26). As what one would expect, Lui (2007a) noted that the use of interval estimator (2.24) could be liberal, while the interval estimator (2.25) could lose precision. Lui further noted that the interval estimator (2.26) could perform well and hence the interval estimator (2.26) was recommended for general use.

Example 2.6   To illustrate the use of $\hat{\gamma}$ (2.9) and interval estimators (2.24), (2.25), and (2.26), we again consider the simple noncompliance RCT studying vitamin A supplementation to reduce mortality among preschool children in Table 2.1. For illustration purposes, we ignore clusters and assume $\pi_{+A} = 0$. Suppose that we are interested in estimation of the ratio γ (= RR) (2.8) of mortality rates (rather than survival rates) between patients receiving vitamin A supplementation and patients without receiving any vitamin A supplementation. Given these data, we obtain the MLE $\hat{\gamma}(2.9)$ of 0.278. When applying interval estimators (2.24), (2.25), and (2.26), we obtain 95 % confidence intervals for γ of [0.071, 0.484], [0.132, 0.584], and [0.132, 0.584], respectively. We can see that the interval estimate (2.24) based on Wald's statistic tends to shift to the left as compared with the interval estimator (2.25) using the logarithmic transformation. Because all the above resulting upper limits are less than 1, we may conclude that there is significant evidence that taking vitamin A supplementation can reduce mortality among preschool children at the 5 % level.

Example 2.7   Consider the data in Table 2.3b studying the effect of quitting smoking in a multiple risk factor intervention randomized trial on the mortality of CHD among patients with the number of smoked cigarettes larger than 30 cigarettes per day at baseline (Multiple Risk Factor Intervention Trial Research Group, 1982). Using these data, we obtain $\hat{\gamma}(2.9)$ of 0.607, which suggests that patients who quitted smoking have a risk of CHD death lower than those who did not quit smoking. When applying interval estimators (2.24), (2.25) and (2.26), we obtain 95 % confidence intervals for γ as [0.000, 2.381], [0.033, 11.264], [0.000, 2.381], respectively. Because all these interval estimates contain $\gamma = 1$, there is no significant evidence at the 5 % level to support that quitting smoking can reduce the risk of CHD death. This example also illustrates the situation in which using the interval estimator (2.25) may sometimes cause a substantial loss of precision as compared with using interval estimator (2.24).

2.4.3   Estimation of the odds ratio

Recall that the OR $(\varphi = (\pi_{1|C}^{(1)}\pi_{2|C}^{(0)})/(\pi_{2|C}^{(1)}\pi_{1|C}^{(0)}))$ considered here is defined as the ratio of the odds of a positive response probability among compliers between the experimental and standard treatments. On the basis of $\hat{\varphi}$ (2.13) and $\hat{Var}(\log(\hat{\varphi}))$(2.14), we may obtain an asymptotic $100(1 - \alpha)$ % confidence interval using Wald's statistic for the OR as

$$[\max\{\hat{\varphi} - Z_{\alpha/2}(\hat{Var}(\hat{\varphi}))^{1/2}, 0\}, \hat{\varphi} + Z_{\alpha/2}(\hat{Var}(\hat{\varphi}))^{1/2}], \qquad (2.27)$$

where $\hat{Var}(\hat{\varphi}) = \hat{\varphi}^2 \hat{Var}(\log(\hat{\varphi}))$. Because the sampling distribution of $\hat{\varphi}$ can be skewed, as noted previously, we may consider use of the logarithmic transformation to improve the normal approximation. This leads us to obtain the following asymptotic $100(1 - \alpha)\%$ confidence interval for the OR with the logarithmic transformation as

$$[\hat{\varphi} \exp\left(-Z_{\alpha/2}(\hat{Var}(\log(\hat{\varphi})))^{1/2}\right), \quad \hat{\varphi} \exp\left(Z_{\alpha/2}(\hat{Var}(\log(\hat{\varphi})))^{1/2}\right)]. \tag{2.28}$$

Note that under perfect compliance the interval estimator (2.28) reduces to the most commonly used asymptotic interval estimator for the OR using the logarithmic transformation discussed elsewhere (Fleiss, 1981; Lui, 2004).

Although the logarithmic transformation may improve the coverage probability of a confidence interval for a ratio of two proportions, it can also cause a loss of precision. For example, consider the situation in which the denominator $(\hat{\pi}_{2CA}^{(1)} - \hat{\pi}_{2A}^{(0)})(\hat{\pi}_{1CN}^{(0)} - \hat{\pi}_{1N}^{(1)})$ of $\hat{\varphi}$ (2.13) is close to 0 and hence the estimated asymptotic variance $\hat{Var}(\log(\hat{\varphi}))$ can be large. This will produce a wide confidence interval using the interval estimator (2.28). To alleviate the possible loss of accuracy for using (2.27) and the possible loss of precision for using (2.28), we consider use of an ad hoc procedure of combining (2.27) and (2.28). Following the same arguments as that for deriving the interval estimator (2.26), we may obtain an asymptotic $100(1 - \alpha)\%$ confidence interval for φ as

$$[\varphi_l, \varphi_u], \tag{2.29}$$

where

$$\varphi_l = I(\hat{\varphi}, \hat{Var}(\hat{\varphi})) \max\{\hat{\varphi} - Z_{\alpha/2}(\hat{Var}(\hat{\varphi}))^{1/2}, 0\}$$
$$+ (1 - I(\hat{\varphi}, \hat{Var}(\hat{\varphi})))\hat{\varphi} \exp(-Z_{\alpha/2}(\hat{Var}(\log(\hat{\varphi})))^{1/2}), \quad \text{and}$$
$$\varphi_u = I(\hat{\varphi}, \hat{Var}(\hat{\varphi}))(\hat{\varphi} + Z_{\alpha/2}(\hat{Var}(\hat{\varphi}))^{1/2})$$
$$+ (1 - I(\hat{\varphi}, \hat{Var}(\hat{\varphi})))\hat{\varphi} \exp(Z_{\alpha/2}(\hat{Var}(\log(\hat{\varphi})))^{1/2}),$$

where $I(\hat{\varphi}, \hat{Var}(\hat{\varphi}))$ is an indicator random variable: $I(\hat{\varphi}, \hat{Var}(\hat{\varphi}))$ is 1 if the length $\hat{\varphi}(\exp(Z_{\alpha/2}(\hat{Var}(\log(\hat{\varphi})))^{1/2}) - \exp(-Z_{\alpha/2}(\hat{Var}(\log(\hat{\varphi})))^{1/2}))$ of (2.28) is larger than or equal to K times the length $(\hat{\varphi} + Z_{\alpha/2}(\hat{Var}(\hat{\varphi}))^{1/2} - \max\{\hat{\varphi} - Z_{\alpha/2}(\hat{Var}(\hat{\varphi}))^{1/2}, 0\})$ of (2.27), and is 0, otherwise. When using the interval estimator (2.29), we need to choose a value for K. As suggested in use of (2.26), we set the constant K to equal to 2.5 when employing (2.29).

Example 2.8   Consider the data (Table 2.3a) regarding the status of cigarette smoking and the incidence of death due to CHD during 7 years of follow-up for patients with the number of smoked cigarettes fewer than 30 cigarettes per day at baseline taken from a multiple risk factor intervention trial. Suppose that we are interested in estimation of the OR of the mortality rate between patients who quitted smoking and patients who did not quit smoking. When applying the MLE $\hat{\varphi}$ (2.13), we obtain $\hat{\varphi} = 0.498$. When employing interval estimators (2.27), (2.28), and (2.29), we obtain 95 % confidence intervals for φ as [0.000, 2.102], [0.020, 12.462], and [0.000, 2.102], respectively. Because all these interval estimates contain $\varphi = 1$, there is no significant evidence at the 5 % level to support that quitting smoking can reduce the risk of CHD death. Note that the length of (2.28) is approximately 6 times that of (2.27) and (2.29). This example illustrates the situation in which using interval estimator (2.28) can sometimes cause a loss of precision as compared with using (2.27), although the former may generally be preferable to the latter with respect to accuracy.

2.5   Sample size determination

In designing a RCT, it is essentially important to obtain an adequate number of patients so that we have an opportunity to detect the primary goal of interest in our trials. For a given test procedure at a nominal α-level, in fact, we can develop a corresponding sample size calculation procedure for a desired power $(1 - \beta)$ of detecting our study goal with a given specified parameter value of clinical interest. To assure that the estimate of the minimum required sample size is appropriate to achieve the desired power, we may need to be consistent between the test procedure used for calculation of the required sample size and the test procedure used for our data analysis. An estimate of the minimum required sample size calculated for a RCT with perfect compliance will certainly not be accurate for a RCT with many patients not complying with their assigned treatment. Thus, it is critical that one can incorporate noncompliance into sample size determination when it is expected to encounter some noncompliers in designing a RCT for testing superiority, noninferiority, and equivalence. Note that in testing superiority based on the ITT analysis, the conventional sample size formula (Sato, 2000), which does not account for the possible difference in the proportions of responses between compliers and noncompliers for a RCT with noncompliance, can be inappropriate for use.

Define $k = n_0/n_1$ the ratio of sample allocations between the standard and experimental treatments. The commonly used equal sample allocation simply corresponds to $k = 1$. Given a fixed ratio k, we focus our attention on calculating the minimum required number of patients n_1 from the experimental treatment. The corresponding estimates of the minimum required number of patients from the standard treatment and the total minimum required number of patients for the entire trial are then given by $n_0 = kn_1$ and $n_T = (k + 1)n_1$, respectively.

2.5.1   Sample size calculation for testing superiority

Consider using statistic (2.4) to test the null hypothesis $H_0 : \Delta = 0$ versus $H_a : \Delta = \Delta_0 \neq 0$, where Δ_0 is a specified magnitude of clinical significance which we wish to detect. Given Δ_0, π_{+C} and $\pi_{1+}^{(0)}$, note that we can uniquely determine $\pi_{1+}^{(1)}$ by $\Delta_0 \pi_{+C} + \pi_{1+}^{(0)}$. Thus, the variance $Var(\hat{\delta}|H_0)$ of test statistic $\hat{\delta}$(2.2) for the ITT analysis under $H_0 : \Delta = 0$ can be re-expressed as

$$S_0(\pi_{1+}^{(0)}, \Delta_0, \pi_{+C}, k)/n_1, \tag{2.30}$$

where $S_0(\pi_{1+}^{(0)}, \Delta_0, \pi_{+C}, k) = \bar{\pi}_{1+}^{(p)}(1 - \bar{\pi}_{1+}^{(p)})(1 + 1/k)$ and $\bar{\pi}_{1+}^{(p)} = (\pi_{1+}^{(1)} + k\pi_{1+}^{(0)})/(1 + k)$. Since the test statistic (2.4) can be generally more powerful than the test statistic (2.3) (Lui, 2006a), we calculate the minimum required number of patients based on the test statistic (2.4) to possibly save the number of patients needed. On the basis of the test statistic (2.4) at a nominal α-level, we obtain an estimate of the minimum required number of patients n_1 from the experimental treatment for a desired power $(1 - \beta)$ of detecting a given specified value $\Delta_0 (\neq 0)$ as (Exercise 2.16):

$$n_1 = Ceil\{(Z_{\alpha/2}\sqrt{S_0(\pi_{1+}^{(0)}, \Delta_0, \pi_{+C}, k)} + Z_\beta \sqrt{S_1(\pi_{1+}^{(0)}, \Delta_0, \pi_{+C}, k)}/$$
$$[1 - (\Delta_0 \pi_{+C})^2])^2/(\tanh^{-1}(\Delta_0 \pi_{+C}))^2\}, \qquad (2.31)$$

where $Ceil\{x\}$ is the smallest integer $\geq x$ and

$$S_1(\pi_{1+}^{(0)}, \Delta_0, \pi_{+C}, k) = [\pi_{1+}^{(1)}(1 - \pi_{1+}^{(1)}) + \pi_{1+}^{(0)}(1 - \pi_{1+}^{(0)})/k].$$

To study the effect due to noncompliance on $n_1(2.31)$, we summarize in Table 2.4 the estimate of the minimum required sample size n_1 derived from statistic (2.4) for testing superiority at the 5 %-level for a desired power 80 % of detecting the underlying PD $\Delta_0 = 0.05, 0.10$ in situations in which the proportion of compliers $\pi_{+C} = 1.0, 0.90, 0.80, 0.70$; the underlying probability of a positive response in the standard treatment $\pi_{1+}^{(0)} = 0.30, 0.50, 0.70$; and the ratio of sample allocation $k = 1, 2, 3, 4, 8$. When the benefits and risks of taking the experimental treatment are uncertain, we may wish to assign more patients to the standard treatment in a RCT for ethical reasons. As seen from Table 2.4, we note that the extent of reduction in the estimate of the minimum required number of patients n_1 from the experimental treatment via an increase in the number of patients assigned to the standard treatment seems to decrease quickly when the ratio of sample allocation k reaches 4. For example, when $\pi_{+C} = 0.90$, $\Delta_0 = 0.05$, and $\pi_{1+}^{(0)} = 0.50$, a single one unit increase in k from $(k =) 1$ to $(k =) 2$ results in a reduction of n_1 by $482 (= 1933 - 1451)$. In other words, for reducing a single one patient assigned to the experimental treatment, we need to assign $2(\approx (1451 \times 2 - 1933)/482)$ more patients on average to the standard treatment in this case. However, a unit increase in k from $(k =) 3$ to $(k =) 4$ results in a reduction of n_1 by only 81 patients $(= 1290 - 1209)$ in the same situation as above. This means that saving one patient assigned to the experimental treatment requires assigning approximately $12(\approx (1209 \times 4 - 1290 \times 3)/(1290 - 1209))$ more patients on average to the standard treatment. Therefore, we may seldom employ a quite unbalanced sample allocation (i.e. $k \geq 5$) in practice. Table 2.4 also shows that the estimate of the minimum required number n_1 (2.31) of patients (or equivalently,

Table 2.4   The estimate of the minimum required sample size n_1 (2.31) from the experimental treatment derived from statistic (2.4) for testing superiority at the 0.05-level for a desired power 80% of detecting the underlying PD $\Delta_0 = 0.05, 0.10$ in situations, in which the subpopulation proportion of compliers $\pi_{+C} = 1.0, 0.90, 0.80, 0.70$; the underlying probability of a positive response in the standard treatment $\pi_{1+}^{(0)} = 0.30$, 0.50, 0.70; and the ratio of sample allocation $k = 1, 2, 3, 4, 8$.

π_{+C}	Δ_0	$\pi_{1+}^{(0)}$	$k =$	1	2	3	4	8
1.00	0.05	0.30		1377	1027	910	852	764
		0.50		1565	1174	1044	979	881
		0.70		1251	945	843	792	715
	0.10	0.30		356	265	234	219	195
		0.50		388	291	259	243	219
		0.70		293	224	200	189	171
0.90	0.05	0.30		1693	1263	1120	1048	941
		0.50		1933	1451	1290	1209	1088
		0.70		1553	1173	1045	982	886
	0.10	0.30		437	325	287	269	240
		0.50		480	360	320	301	270
		0.70		367	279	250	235	213
0.80	0.05	0.30		2134	1593	1413	1323	1187
		0.50		2448	1837	1633	1531	1378
		0.70		1977	1491	1329	1248	1126
	0.10	0.30		549	409	362	338	303
		0.50		608	457	406	381	343
		0.70		471	358	320	301	272
0.70	0.05	0.30		2776	2074	1839	1722	1546
		0.50		3199	2400	2133	2000	1800
		0.70		2597	1957	1744	1637	1477
	0.10	0.30		713	531	470	439	394
		0.50		796	598	531	498	448
		0.70		623	472	422	397	359

the estimate of the total number $n_T = (k+1)n_1$ of patients) can increase substantially as the proportion of compliers π_{+C} decreases. For example, when $\Delta_0 = 0.05$, $\pi_{1+}^{(0)} = 0.50$, and $k = 1$, the number n_1 increases from 1565 to 2448 as π_{+C} drops from 1.0 (i.e. perfect compliance) to 0.80; the percentage of this increase in n_1 is approximately 56 % ($\approx (2448 - 1565)/1565$). Thus, it is crucial that we can minimize the probability of noncompliance if we wish to save the number of patients needed for a RCT. For the convenience of readers, the SAS program for producing Table 2.4 is included in the Appendix. Readers may modify this program to accommodate the situation of their interest easily.

Example 2.9   Suppose we know that the underlying positive response rate for the standard treatment $\pi_{1+}^{(0)} = 0.50$ and the proportion of compliers in the sampling population $\pi_{+C} = 0.80$ from a pilot study. Recall that $\pi_{+C} = \pi_{+CA}^{(1)} + \pi_{+CN}^{(0)} - 1$ and thereby, the proportion of compliers π_{+C} can be determined by the sum of the sample proportion of compliance to the two assigned treatments under comparison minus 1 in practice. Say, we wish to find out an estimate of the minimum required sample size for a desired power 80 % of detecting a given difference $\Delta_0 = 0.10$ on the basis of the test statistic (2.4) at the 0.05-level. From Table 2.4, the estimates of the minimum required number of patients n_1 from the experimental treatment for the ratio of sample allocation $k = 1, 2, 3, 4$ are 608, 457, 406, and 381, respectively. These produce estimates of the total minimum required number of patients ($= (k+1)n_1$) to be 1216, 1371, 1624, and 1905 patients for the entire RCT.

2.5.2   Sample size calculation for testing noninferiority

When measuring the relative treatment effect, we may consider use of the PD, PR, or OR in establishing noninferiority. Because the PD is most easily understood, we begin with sample size calculation for testing noninferiority based on the PD. Recall that we want to demonstrate that the difference Δ in the probabilities of a positive response between two treatments is $> -\varepsilon_l$, where the acceptable margin ε_l is provided by clinicians and is usually selected on the basis of their subjective medical knowledge.

2.5.2.1   Using the difference in proportions

Consider use of the test procedure based on statistic (2.7). Note that given the set of parameters $\{\pi_{+C}, \pi_{+A}, \pi_{1|C}^{(0)}, \pi_{1|A}, \pi_{1|N}, \Delta\}$, we can completely determine all the cell probabilities $\pi_{rS}^{(g)}$ ($r = 1, 2, S = CA$, N for $g = 1$ and $S = CN$, A for $g = 0$) (Exercise 2.18) and hence $Var(\tanh^{-1}(\hat{\Delta}))$ which is a function of these cell probabilities. For example, we can uniquely determine $\pi_{1CA}^{(1)}$ by $(\pi_{1|C}^{(0)} + \Delta)\pi_{+C} + \pi_{1|A}\pi_{+A}$. As another example, we can uniquely determine $\pi_{1+}^{(1)} = (\pi_{1|C}^{(0)} + \Delta)\pi_{+C} + \pi_{1|A}\pi_{+A} + \pi_{1|N}(1 - \pi_{+C} - \pi_{+A})$. Thus, we can re-express the asymptotic variance $Var(\tanh^{-1}(\hat{\Delta}))$ for the test statistic $\tanh^{-1}(\hat{\Delta})$ as

$$V_{PD}(\pi_{+C}, \pi_{+A}, \pi_{1|C}^{(0)}, \pi_{1|A}, \pi_{1|N}, \Delta, k)/[n_1(1 - \Delta^2)^2], \qquad (2.32)$$

where

$$\begin{aligned}
V_{PD}(\pi_{+C}, \pi_{+A}, \pi_{1|C}^{(0)}, \pi_{1|A}, \pi_{1|N}, \Delta, k) = & \{[\pi_{1+}^{(1)}(1 - \pi_{1+}^{(1)}) \\
& + \pi_{1+}^{(0)}(1 - \pi_{1+}^{(0)})/k] + \Delta^2[\pi_{+CA}^{(1)}(1 - \pi_{+CA}^{(1)}) \\
& + \pi_{+A}(1 - \pi_{+A})/k] - 2\Delta[(\pi_{1CA}^{(1)} - \pi_{1+}^{(1)}\pi_{+CA}^{(1)}) \\
& + (\pi_{1A} - \pi_{1+}^{(0)}\pi_{+A})/k]\}/(\pi_{+C})^2.
\end{aligned}$$

Based on the test statistic (2.7) and the asymptotic variance (2.32), we obtain an estimate of the minimum required number of patients n_1 from the experimental treatment for a desired power $(1 - \beta)$ of detecting noninferiority with a given specified value Δ_0 $(> -\varepsilon_l)$ at a nominal α-level as given by (Exercise 2.19):

$$\begin{aligned}
n_1 = Ceil\{&((Z_\alpha + Z_\beta)^2 V_{PD}(\pi_{+C}, \pi_{+A}, \pi_{1|C}^{(0)}, \pi_{1|A}, \pi_{1|N}, \Delta_0, k)/ \\
& [(1 - \Delta_0^2)^2])/(\tanh^{-1}(\varepsilon_l) + \tanh^{-1}(\Delta_0))^2\}. \qquad (2.33)
\end{aligned}$$

Note that when each patient complied with his/her assigned treatment (i.e. perfect compliance), sample size graphs for testing noninferiority without use of the $\tanh^{-1}(\hat{\Delta})$ transformation based on the PD appeared elsewhere (Blackwelder and Chang, 1984).

2.5.2.2   Using the ratio of proportions

When using the PR to measure the relative treatment effect in establishing noninferiority, we want to demonstrate that the ratio γ of probabilities of a positive response between two treatments under comparison is larger than $1 - \gamma_l$, where γ_l is the pre-determined noninferior margin. Given the set of parameters $\{\pi_{+C}, \pi_{+A}, \pi_{1|C}^{(0)}, \pi_{1|A}, \pi_{1|N}, \gamma\}$, we can completely determine all the cell probabilities $\pi_{rS}^{(g)}$ ($r = 1, 2$, $S = CA$, N for $g = 1$, or $S = CN$, A for $g = 0$) and thereby $Var(\log(\hat{\gamma}))$ which is a function of these parameters as well. For example, we can uniquely determine $\pi_{1CA}^{(1)}$ by $\gamma \pi_{1|C}^{(0)} \pi_{+C} + \pi_{1|A} \pi_{+A}$. For a given ratio of sample allocation $k = n_0/n_1$, we can easily show that the asymptotic variance $Var(\log(\hat{\gamma}))$ for $\log(\hat{\gamma})$ can be re-expressed as

$$Var(\log(\hat{\gamma})) = V_{LPR}(\pi_{+C}, \pi_{+A}, \pi_{1|C}^{(0)}, \pi_{1|A}, \pi_{1|N}, \gamma, k)/n_1, \qquad (2.34)$$

where

$$\begin{aligned}
V_{LPR}(\pi_{+C}, \pi_{+A}, \pi_{1|C}^{(0)}, \pi_{1|A}, \pi_{1|N}, \gamma, k) &= [\pi_{1CA}^{(1)}(1 - \pi_{1CA}^{(1)}) \\
&+ \pi_{1A}(1 - \pi_{1A})/k]/(\pi_{1C}^{(1)})^2 + [\pi_{1N}(1 - \pi_{1N}) \\
&+ \pi_{1CN}^{(0)}(1 - \pi_{1CN}^{(0)})/k]/(\pi_{1C}^{(0)})^2 \\
&- 2[\pi_{1CA}^{(1)}\pi_{1N} + \pi_{1CN}^{(0)}\pi_{1A}/k]/[(\pi_{1C}^{(1)})(\pi_{1C}^{(0)})].
\end{aligned}$$

On the basis of the test statistic (2.11) and the asymptotic variance (2.34), we obtain an estimate of the minimum required number n_1 of patients from the experimental treatment for a desired power $(1 - \beta)$ of detecting noninferiority with a given specified value $\gamma_0(> 1 - \gamma_l)$ at a nominal α-level as (Exercise 2.20):

$$n_1 = Ceil\{(Z_\alpha + Z_\beta)^2 V_{LPR}(\pi_{+C}, \pi_{+A}, \pi_{1|C}^{(0)}, \pi_{1|A}, \pi_{1|N}, \gamma_0, k)/$$
$$(\log(\gamma_0) - \log(1 - \gamma_l))^2\}. \qquad (2.35)$$

2.5.2.3   Using the odds ratio of proportions

Note that using the OR to measure the relative treatment effect may naturally follow, as noted previously, the philosophies of the FDA (1997) in determination of the noninferior margin and hence the OR has been recently recommended for use in testing noninferiority or equivalence

(Garrett, 2003). Given the set of parameters $\{\pi_{+C}, \pi_{+A}, \pi_{1|C}^{(0)}, \pi_{1|A},$ $\pi_{1|N}, \varphi\}$, we can uniquely determine all the cell probabilities $\pi_{rS}^{(g)}$ ($r = 1, 2, S = CA, N$ for $g = 1$, and $S = CN, A$ for $g = 0$). For example, we can determine the cell probability $\pi_{1CA}^{(1)}$ by $(\varphi\pi_{1|C}^{(0)}\pi_{+C})/[\varphi\pi_{1|C}^{(0)} + (1 - \pi_{1|C}^{(0)})] + \pi_{1|A}\pi_{+A}$. Thus, for a given ratio of sample size allocation $k = n_0/n_1$, we can re-express the asymptotic variance $Var(\log(\hat{\varphi}))$ for $\hat{\varphi}$ as

$$Var(\log(\hat{\varphi})) = V_{LOR}(\pi_{+C}, \pi_{+A}, \pi_{1|C}^{(0)}, \pi_{1|A}, \pi_{1|N}, \varphi, k)/n_1, \quad (2.36)$$

where

$$
\begin{aligned}
V_{LOR}(\pi_{+C}, \pi_{+A}, \pi_{1|C}^{(0)}, \pi_{1|A}, \pi_{1|N}, \varphi, k) &= [\pi_{1CA}^{(1)}(1 - \pi_{1CA}^{(1)}) \\
&+ \pi_{1A}(1 - \pi_{1A})/k]/(\pi_{1C}^{(1)})^2 + [\pi_{2CN}^{(0)}(1 - \pi_{2CN}^{(0)})/k \\
&+ \pi_{2N}(1 - \pi_{2N})]/(\pi_{2C}^{(0)})^2 + [\pi_{2CA}^{(1)}(1 - \pi_{2CA}^{(1)}) \\
&+ \pi_{2A}(1 - \pi_{2A})/k]/(\pi_{2C}^{(1)})^2 + [\pi_{1CN}^{(0)}(1 - \pi_{1CN}^{(0)})/k \\
&+ \pi_{1N}(1 - \pi_{1N})]/(\pi_{1C}^{(0)})^2 + 2[\pi_{1CA}^{(1)}\pi_{2N} + \pi_{1A}\pi_{2CN}^{(0)}/k]/ \\
&[(\pi_{1C}^{(1)})(\pi_{2C}^{(0)})] + 2[\pi_{1CA}^{(1)}\pi_{2CA}^{(1)} + \pi_{1A}\pi_{2A}/k]/[(\pi_{1C}^{(1)})(\pi_{2C}^{(1)})] \\
&- 2[\pi_{1CA}^{(1)}\pi_{1N} + \pi_{1CN}^{(0)}\pi_{1A}/k]/[(\pi_{1C}^{(1)})(\pi_{1C}^{(0)})] - 2[\pi_{2CA}^{(1)}\pi_{2N} \\
&+ \pi_{2A}\pi_{2CN}^{(0)}/k]/[(\pi_{2C}^{(1)})(\pi_{2C}^{(0)})] + 2[\pi_{1N}\pi_{2N} + \pi_{1CN}^{(0)}\pi_{2CN}^{(0)}/k]/ \\
&[(\pi_{2C}^{(0)})(\pi_{1C}^{(0)})] + 2[\pi_{2CA}^{(1)}\pi_{1N} + \pi_{2A}\pi_{1CN}^{(0)}/k]/[(\pi_{2C}^{(1)})(\pi_{1C}^{(0)})].
\end{aligned}
$$

Based on the test statistic (2.15) and (2.36), we obtain an estimate of the minimum required number n_1 of patients for a desired power $(1 - \beta)$ of detecting noninferiority with a given specified value $\varphi_0(> 1 - \varphi_l)$ at a nominal α-level as

$$
\begin{aligned}
n_1 = Ceil\{&((Z_\alpha + Z_\beta)^2 V_{LOR}(\pi_{+C}, \pi_{+A}, \pi_{1|C}^{(0)}, \pi_{1|A}, \pi_{1|N}, \varphi_0, k))/ \\
&(\log(\varphi_0) - \log(1 - \varphi_l))^2\}. \quad (2.37)
\end{aligned}
$$

2.5.3   Sample size calculation for testing equivalence

As for testing noninferiority, it is important to obtain an adequate number of patients from each treatment so that we have the desired power of detecting equivalence between two treatments. When testing equivalence, however, we will need to make an additional approximation of the power function to obtain sample size calculation formulae in closed form when the underlying specified value of interest is not equal to the null value. Thus, if this approximation of the power function is not accurate, the closed-form sample size formulae as derived in the following may underestimate the minimum required number of patients.

2.5.3.1   Using the difference in proportions

When using the PD to measure the treatment effect in establishing equivalence, we want to demonstrate that the PD satisfies the inequality $-\varepsilon_l < \Delta < \varepsilon_u$, where ε_l and ε_u (>0) are the pre-determined lower and upper acceptable margins provided by clinicians. The power function for testing $H_0 : \Delta \leq -\varepsilon_l$ or $\Delta \geq \varepsilon_u$ at the α-level based on the test procedure (2.16) and the normal approximation is then given by (Exercise 2.21):

$$\phi_{PD}(\Delta_0) = \Phi(\frac{\tanh^{-1}(\varepsilon_u) - \tanh^{-1}(\Delta_0)}{\sqrt{Var(\tanh^{-1}(\hat{\Delta}))}} - Z_\alpha)$$
$$- \Phi(\frac{-\tanh^{-1}(\varepsilon_l) - \tanh^{-1}(\Delta_0)}{\sqrt{Var(\tanh^{-1}(\hat{\Delta}))}} + Z_\alpha), \quad (2.38)$$

where $-\varepsilon_l < \Delta_0 < \varepsilon_u$, and $\Phi(X)$ is the cumulative standard normal distribution. If the number of patients assigned to both treatments is large and $\Delta_0 < 0$, we can approximate the power function $\phi_{PD}(\Delta_0)$(2.38) by

$$1 - \Phi(\frac{-\tanh^{-1}(\varepsilon_l) - \tanh^{-1}(\Delta_0)}{\sqrt{Var(\tanh^{-1}(\hat{\Delta}))}} + Z_\alpha). \quad (2.39)$$

On the basis of the power function (2.39), we obtain an estimate of the minimum required number n_1 of patients from the experimental treatment such that we have the desired power $(1 - \beta)$ of detecting equivalence with a specified $-\varepsilon_l < \Delta_0 < 0$ at a nominal α-level as (Exercise 2.22):

$$n_1 = Ceil\{((Z_\alpha + Z_\beta)^2 V_{PD}(\pi_{+C}, \pi_{+A}, \pi_{1|C}^{(0)}, \pi_{1|A}, \pi_{1|N}, \Delta_0, k)/$$
$$[(1 - \Delta_0^2)^2])/(\tanh^{-1}(\varepsilon_l) + \tanh^{-1}(\Delta_0))^2\}. \quad (2.40)$$

If the number of patients assigned to both treatments is large and $0 < \Delta_0 < \varepsilon_u$, we can then approximate the power function $\phi_{PD}(\Delta_0)$ (2.38) by

$$\Phi(\frac{\tanh^{-1}(\varepsilon_u) - \tanh^{-1}(\Delta_0)}{\sqrt{Var(\tanh^{-1}(\hat{\Delta}))}} - Z_\alpha). \qquad (2.41)$$

On the basis of the power function (2.41), we obtain an estimate of the minimum required number n_1 of patients from the experimental treatment for a desired power $(1 - \beta)$ of detecting equivalence with a specified $\Delta_0 > 0$ at a nominal α-level as (Exercise 2.23):

$$n_1 = Ceil\{((Z_\alpha + Z_\beta)^2 V_{PD}(\pi_{+C}, \pi_{+A}, \pi_{1|C}^{(0)}, \pi_{1|A}, \pi_{1|N}, \Delta_0, k)/$$
$$[(1 - \Delta_0^2)^2])/(\tanh^{-1}(\varepsilon_u) - \tanh^{-1}(\Delta_0))^2\}. \qquad (2.42)$$

When $\Delta_0 = 0$, the power function $\phi_{PD}(\Delta_0)$ (2.38) simply becomes equal to

$$\phi_{PD}(\Delta_0) = \Phi(\frac{\tanh^{-1}(\varepsilon_u)}{\sqrt{Var(\tanh^{-1}(\hat{\Delta}))}} - Z_\alpha)$$
$$- \Phi(\frac{-\tanh^{-1}(\varepsilon_l)}{\sqrt{Var(\tanh^{-1}(\hat{\Delta}))}} + Z_\alpha). \qquad (2.43)$$

When $\varepsilon_l = \varepsilon_u$, we obtain an estimate of the minimum required number n_1 of patients from the experimental treatment such that we have the desired power $(1 - \beta)$ of detecting equivalence for a specified value $\Delta_0 = 0$ at a nominal α-level based on the power function (2.43) as (Exercise 2.24):

$$n_1 = Ceil\{((Z_\alpha + Z_{\beta/2})^2 V_{PD}(\pi_{+C}, \pi_{+A}, \pi_{1|C}^{(0)}, \pi_{1|A}, \pi_{1|N}, \Delta_0, k))/$$
$$(\tanh^{-1}(\varepsilon_u))^2\}. \qquad (2.44)$$

Note that when deriving n_1(2.40) and n_1(2.42), we need to assume that the approximation of the power function $\phi_{PD}(\Delta_0)$ (2.38) by those given in (2.39) and (2.41) is accurate. When the pre-determined equivalence margins ε_l and ε_u are not small, or the underlying $\Delta_0 (\neq 0)$ of interest is chosen to be in the neighborhood of 0, the resulting estimate of the minimum required number of patients n_1 may not be large enough to assure this approximation to be good. In this case, because the power function (2.39) (or the power function (2.41)) is larger than $\phi_{PD}(\Delta_0)$

(2.38), using n_1 (2.40) (or n_1 (2.42)) tends to underestimate the minimum required number of patients from the experimental treatment. To alleviate this concern, we may use n_1 (2.40) (or n_1 (2.42)) as the initial estimate and apply a trial-and-error procedure to find the minimum integer n_1 such that the power function $\phi_{PD}(\Delta_0)$ (2.38) is greater than or equal to the desired power $1 - \beta$. Note that when $\Delta_0 = 0$, the power function (2.43) and (2.38) are actually identical, and thereby, we do not have the above concern.

2.5.3.2   Using the ratio of proportions

When using the PR ($\gamma = \pi_{1|C}^{(1)}/\pi_{1|C}^{(0)}$) to measure the treatment effect in establishing equivalence, we want to demonstrate that the underlying ratio PR satisfies the inequality: $1 - \gamma_l < \gamma < 1 + \gamma_u$. On the basis of the test procedure (2.17), we may approximate the power function by

$$\phi_{PR}(\gamma_0) = \Phi(\frac{\log(1 + \gamma_u) - \log(\gamma_0)}{\sqrt{Var(\log(\hat{\gamma}))}} - Z_\alpha)$$
$$- \Phi(\frac{\log(1 - \gamma_l) - \log(\gamma_0)}{\sqrt{Var(\log(\hat{\gamma}))}} + Z_\alpha), \qquad (2.45)$$

where $1 - \gamma_l < \gamma_0 < 1 + \gamma_u$. Following the same arguments as that for deriving (2.40), (2.42), and (2.44), we obtain an estimate of the minimum required number n_1 of patients from the experimental treatment for a desired power $(1 - \beta)$ of detecting equivalence with a given specified value $1 - \gamma_l < \gamma_0 < 1 + \gamma_u$ at a nominal α-level as

$$n_1 = Ceil\{(Z_\alpha + Z_\beta)^2 V_{LPR}(\pi_{+C}, \pi_{+A}, \pi_{1|C}^{(0)}, \pi_{1|A}, \pi_{1|N}, \gamma_0, k)/$$
$$(\log(\gamma_0) - \log(1 - \gamma_l))^2\} \quad \text{for} \quad 1 - \gamma_l < \gamma_0 < 1, \qquad (2.46)$$
$$n_1 = Ceil\{(Z_\alpha + Z_\beta)^2 V_{LPR}(\pi_{+C}, \pi_{+A}, \pi_{1|C}^{(0)}, \pi_{1|A}, \pi_{1|N}, \gamma_0, k)/$$
$$(\log(\gamma_0) - \log(1 + \gamma_u))^2\} \quad \text{for} \quad 1 < \gamma_0 < 1 + \gamma_u, \qquad (2.47)$$

and

$$n_1 = Ceil\{(Z_\alpha + Z_{\beta/2})^2 V_{LPR}(\pi_{+C}, \pi_{+A}, \pi_{1|C}^{(0)}, \pi_{1|A}, \pi_{1|N}, \gamma_0, k)/$$
$$(\log(1 + \gamma_u))^2\} \quad \text{for} \quad \gamma_0 = 1 \quad \text{and} \quad \log(1 + \gamma_u) = -\log(1 - \gamma_l). \qquad (2.48)$$

Note that when the pre-determined equivalence margins γ_l and γ_u are not small (say, $\gamma_l = 0.5$) or the underlying $\gamma_0 (\neq 1)$ of interest is chosen to be in the neighborhood of 1, as previously noted for the PD, using n_1 (2.46) (or n_1 (2.47)) tends to underestimate the minimum required number of patients from the experimental treatment. To alleviate this concern, we may use n_1 (2.46) (or n_1 (2.47)) as the initial estimate and apply a trial-and-error procedure to find the minimum integer n_1 such that the power function $\phi_{PR}(\gamma_0)$ (2.45) is larger than or equal to the desired power $1 - \beta$.

2.5.3.3   Using the odds ratio of proportions

When using the OR ($\varphi = (\pi_{1|C}^{(1)}\pi_{2|C}^{(0)})/(\pi_{2|C}^{(1)}\pi_{1|C}^{(0)})$) to measure the treatment effect in establishing equivalence, we want to demonstrate that the OR satisfies the inequality: $1 - \varphi_l < \varphi < 1 + \varphi_u$. On the basis of the test procedure (2.18), we may approximate the power function by

$$\phi_{OR}(\varphi_0) = \Phi(\frac{\log(1 + \varphi_u) - \log(\varphi_0)}{\sqrt{Var(\log(\hat{\varphi}))}} - Z_\alpha)$$
$$- \Phi(\frac{\log(1 - \varphi_l) - \log(\varphi_0)}{\sqrt{Var(\log(\hat{\varphi}))}} + Z_\alpha), \qquad (2.49)$$

where $1 - \varphi_l < \varphi_0 < 1 + \varphi_u$. Following the same arguments as for deriving (2.40), (2.42), and (2.44), we obtain an estimate of the minimum required number n_1 of patients from the experimental treatment for a desired power $(1 - \beta)$ of detecting equivalence with a given specified value $1 - \varphi_l < \varphi_0 < 1 + \varphi_u$ at a nominal α-level as

$$n_1 = Ceil\{(Z_\alpha + Z_\beta)^2 V_{LOR}(\pi_{+C}, \pi_{+A}, \pi_{1|C}^{(0)}, \pi_{1|A}, \pi_{1|N}, \varphi_0, k)/$$
$$(\log(\varphi_0) - \log(1 - \varphi_l))^2\} \quad \text{for} \quad 1 - \varphi_l < \varphi_0 < 1, \qquad (2.50)$$
$$n_1 = Ceil\{(Z_\alpha + Z_\beta)^2 V_{LOR}(\pi_{+C}, \pi_{+A}, \pi_{1|C}^{(0)}, \pi_{1|A}, \pi_{1|N}, \varphi_0, k)/$$
$$(\log(\varphi_0) - \log(1 + \varphi_u))^2\} \quad \text{for} \quad 1 < \varphi_0 < 1 + \varphi_u, \qquad (2.51)$$

and

$$n_1 = Ceil\{(Z_\alpha + Z_{\beta/2})^2 V_{LOR}(\pi_{+C}, \pi_{+A}, \pi_{1|C}^{(0)}, \pi_{1|A}, \pi_{1|N}, \varphi_0, k)/$$
$$(\log(1 + \varphi_u))^2\} \quad \text{for} \quad \varphi_0 = 1 \quad \text{and} \quad \log(1 + \varphi_u) = -\log(1 - \varphi_l).$$
$$(2.52)$$

Note that when $\pi_{+C} = 1.0$ (or equivalently, $\pi_{+A} = \pi_{+N} = 0$) for a RCT under perfect compliance, sample size formulae (2.46)–(2.48) and (2.50)–(2.52) for testing equivalence reduce to those published elsewhere (Tu, 1998; Wang, Chow and Li, 2002).

When the pre-determined margins φ_l and φ_u are not small (e.g. $\varphi_l = 0.50$ and $\varphi_u = 1$) or when the underlying $\varphi_0 (\neq 1)$ of interest is chosen to be in the neighborhood of 1, the approximation of the power function $\phi_{OR}(\varphi_0)$ (2.49) needed to derive n_1 (2.50) and n_1 (2.51) can be inaccurate. In this case, using n_1 (2.50) (or n_1 (2.51)) tends to underestimate the minimum required number of patients from the experimental treatment. As noted previously, we can use n_1 (2.50) (or n_1 (2.51)) as the initial estimate and employ a trial-and-error procedure to find the minimum integer n_1 such that the power function $\phi_{OR}(\varphi_0)$ (2.49) is larger than or equal to the desired power $1 - \beta$.

To investigate the effect due to noncompliance on the estimate of the minimum required number of patients n_1, we arbitrarily consider the pre-determined equivalence margins: $\varphi_l = 0.20$ and $\varphi_u = 0.25$ so that $\log(1 + \varphi_u) = -\log(1 - \varphi_l)$, and summarize in Table 2.5 the estimate of the minimum required number of patients from the experimental treatment for a desired power 80 % of detecting equivalence $\varphi_0 = 0.90$, 1.0, 1.10 at the 0.05-level in situations in which $(\pi_{1|C}^{(0)}, \pi_{1|A}, \pi_{1|N}) = \mathbf{A}, \mathbf{B}$, where $\mathbf{A} = (0.20, 0.35, 0.25)$, $\mathbf{B} = (0.50, 0.20, 0.30)$; $(\pi_{+C}, \pi_{+A}, \pi_{+N}) = \mathbf{I}, \mathbf{II}$, where $\mathbf{I} = (0.95, 0.03, 0.02)$, $\mathbf{II} = (0.80, 0.15, 0.05)$; and $k(= n_0/n_1) = 1, 2, 3, 4$. As found previously, we can see from Table 2.5 that the extent of the reduction in the minimum required number of patients n_1 from the experimental treatment through an increase of the number of patients assigned to the standard treatment decreases quickly as the ratio of sample allocation k reaches 4. We can also see that the estimate of the minimum required number n_1 of patients can increase substantially as the proportion of compliers π_{+C} decreases. Given that the pre-determined equivalence margins $\varphi_l = 0.20$ and $\varphi_u = 0.25$ considered here are small, we note that the sample size formulas (2.50)–(2.52) can actually perform well. However, we find that if we consider $\varphi_l = 0.50$ and $\varphi_u = 1.0$, then using the sample size formulae (2.50) and (2.51) can be inaccurate. Thus, in this case, we may wish to use the resulting (2.50) or (2.51) as the preliminary estimate, and apply a trial-and-error procedure to find the minimum required number of patients for the trial. For

Table 2.5   The estimate of the minimum required number n_1 of patients from the experimental treatment for a desired power 80 % of detecting equivalence $0.80 < \varphi_0 < 1.25$, where $\varphi_0 = 0.90, 1.0, 1.10$, at the 0.05-level in situations in which the vector of conditional probabilities of a positive response in various subpopulations $(\pi_{1|C}^{(0)}, \pi_{1|A}, \pi_{1|N}) = $ **A, B**, where **A** $= (0.20, 0.35, 0.25)$, **B** $= (0.50, 0.20, 0.30)$; the distribution of subpopulations $(\pi_{+C}, \pi_{+A}, \pi_{+N})' = $ **I, II**, where **I** $= (0.95, 0.03, 0.02)$, **II** $= (0.80, 0.15, 0.05)$; and the ratio of sample allocation $k(= n_0/n_1) =$ 1, 2, 3, 4.

π_{+C}	π_{+A}	π_{+N}	φ_0	$k=$	1	2	3	4
					A $= (0.20, 0.35, 0.25)$			
0.95	0.03	0.02	0.90		6543	4956	4427	4163
			1.00		2431	1824	1621	1520
			1.10		5183	3854	3411	3189
0.80	0.15	0.05	0.90		10039	7588	6771	6362
			1.00		3661	2746	2441	2289
			1.10		7691	5728	5074	4747
					B $= (0.50, 0.20, 0.30)$			
0.95	0.03	0.02	0.90		3947	2962	2633	2469
			1.00		1524	1143	1016	953
			1.10		3362	2522	2243	2103
0.80	0.15	0.05	0.90		5473	4106	3651	3423
			1.00		2124	1593	1416	1328
			1.10		4714	3537	3145	2948

convenience, the SAS program for producing Table 2.5 is included in the Appendix.

Example 2.10   Consider designing a RCT for testing equivalence with respect to the treatment efficacy measured by the OR in the presence of noncompliance. Suppose that the acceptable equivalence margins $\varphi_l = 0.20$ and $\varphi_u = 0.25$ are provided by clinicians. Say, we have the vector of conditional probabilities of patient response among various subpopulations $(\pi_{1|C}^{(0)}, \pi_{1|A}, \pi_{1|N}) = (0.50, 0.20, 0.30)$, and the distribution of subpopulations $(\pi_{+C}, \pi_{+A}, \pi_{+N}) = (0.95, 0.03, 0.02)$ based on our previous trials. From Table 2.5, we obtain the estimates of the minimum required number n_1 (2.51) of patients from the experimental treatment for a desired power 80 % of detecting equivalence when the underlying OR $\varphi_0 = 1.0$ at the 0.05-level for $k(= n_0/n_1) = 1, 2, 3, 4$ as 1524, 1143, 1016 and 953, respectively.

2.6   Risk model-based approach

On the basis of the fundamental idea in Rubin's causal model (Rubin, 1974, 1977; Holland, 1986; Robins, 1994), Sato (2000, 2001) and Matsuyama (2002) employed a semi-parametric model-based approach and defined the treatment effect in terms of model parameters. By contrast, we define the relative treatment effect by the parameters of the patient response distributions among compliers without modeling the treatment effect on the probability of individual patient response. To help readers easily appreciate the basic ideas behind use of the causal model-based approach, we begin with concentrating our discussions on constant risk models assumed and considered elsewhere (Sato, 2000, 2001; Matsuyama, 2002; Matsui, 2005; Lui, 2007b, 2007g, 20008a, 2008b; Lui and Chang, 2007) for simplicity. We then note the limitation of using these constant risk models, but show that the estimators and their estimated asymptotic variance derived under the constant risk models can still hold under more general risk models (Lui, 2007c). We note that Δ (2.1) defined here actually corresponds to the complier average causal effect (CACE) defined in Rubin's causal model under the monotonicity assumption. We show that the model parameters representing the PD and PR and their corresponding estimators based on the model-based approach are identical to those presented in the previous sections under the monotonicity assumption. Note that the constant risk models proposed by Sato (2000, 2001) and Matsuyama (2002) are actually special cases of the general class of the structural mean models (SMMs) (Robins, 1994) when there is no effect modification by treatment assignment (Clarke and Windmeijer, 2010; Hernan and Robins, 2006). The researches on using the SMM model to analyze complicated data for a RCT with noncompliance have been quite intensive (Robins and Rotnitzky, 2004; Fischer-Lapp and Goetghebeur, 1998; Vansteelandt and Goetghebeur, 2003; Ten Have, Joffe and Cary, 2003; Goetghebeur and Vansteelandt, 2005; Clarke and Windmeijer, 2010). Recently, Bellamy, Lin and Ten Have (2007) have provided an overview of the SMM and principal stratification approaches, as well as a list of publications in both of these two areas. We refer readers to the above publications for details.

Suppose that we randomly assign n_1 and n_0 patients to the experimental treatment $(g = 1)$ and the standard treatment (or placebo) $(g = 0)$, respectively. Let $Y_i^{(g)}$ denote the random variable of outcome for the *ith* $(i = 1, 2, 3, \ldots, n_g)$ patient assigned to treatment g, where $Y_i^{(g)} = 1$ if the patient has a positive response, and $= 0$, otherwise. Let $Z_i^{(g)}$ denote the random variable of the potential treatment receipt for the corresponding patient, where $Z_i^{(g)} = 1$ if the *ith* patient assigned to treatment g receives the experimental treatment, and $= 0$, otherwise. Note that the total number of studied patients in the trial is $n_1 + n_0$.

2.6.1   Constant risk additive model

Following Sato (2000, 2001) and Matsuyama (2002), we assume that the probability of a positive response is given by $P(Y_i^{(g)} = 1 | p_i^{(g)}, z_i^{(g)}) = p_i^{(g)} + Dz_i^{(g)}$, where $p_i^{(g)}$ denotes the probability of a positive response when the *ith* patient assigned to treatment g receives the standard treatment (or placebo); and D represents the excess effect due to the experimental treatment $(z_i^{(g)} = 1)$ over the standard treatment (or placebo) $(z_i^{(g)} = 0)$. In other words, patient i assigned to treatment g would have the probability $p_i^{(g)} + D$ of a positive response if he/she took the experimental treatment, or would have the probability $p_i^{(g)}$ of a positive response if he/she took the standard treatment (or placebo). Note that the expectation $E(p_i^{(1)})$ represents the underlying basic probability of a positive response for a randomly selected patient i from the assigned experimental treatment $(g = 1)$ when patients assigned to the experimental treatment are all assumed to receive the standard treatment. Similarly, the expectation $E(p_{i'}^{(0)})$ represents the underlying basic probability of a positive response for a randomly selected patient i' from the assigned standard treatment ($g = 0$) when patients assigned to the standard treatment are all assumed to receive their assigned (standard) treatment. Because patients are randomly assigned to either the experimental or standard treatment, we may claim that $E(p_i^{(1)}) = E(p_{i'}^{(0)})$, which is, in fact, also equal to the underlying basic probability of a positive response for a randomly selected patient from the sampling population when patients are assumed to all receive the standard treatment.

Note that since a given patient can receive one and only one of the two treatments, only one of the two potential positive responses corresponding to either the probability $p_i^{(g)} + D$ or the probability $p_i^{(g)}$ for each patient can be observed. Furthermore, note that the probability $p_i^{(g)}$ of a positive response and the random variable $Z_i^{(g)}$ of the potentially received treatment can be dependent, and hence using the difference in the two sample proportions of response as done in the AT analysis is likely to produce a biased estimator of D. To illustrate this point, consider the situation in which patients with higher $p_i^{(g)}$ tend to choose, for example, the experimental treatment. In this case, the difference in the sample proportions of response between patients who actually received the experimental treatment and patients who actually received the standard treatment in the AT analysis tends to be positive even when D is 0.

Let $n_{rc}^{(g)}$ denote the number of patients with $(Y_i^{(g)} = r, Z_i^{(g)} = c)$ (where $r = 1, 0$; and $c = 1, 0$) among n_g patients assigned to treatment g. Then the random vector $(n_{11}^{(g)}, n_{10}^{(g)}, n_{01}^{(g)}, n_{00}^{(g)})$ follows a multinomial distribution with parameters n_g and $(\pi_{11}^{(g)}, \pi_{10}^{(g)}, \pi_{01}^{(g)}, \pi_{00}^{(g)})$, where $\pi_{rc}^{(g)}$ denotes the cell probability that a randomly selected patient i assigned to treatment g has random vector $(Y_i^{(g)} = r, Z_i^{(g)} = c)$. Note that a commonly-used unbiased and consistent estimator for the cell probability $\pi_{rc}^{(g)}$ is simply the sample proportion $\hat{\pi}_{rc}^{(g)} = n_{rc}^{(g)}/n_g$. This leads us to estimate the marginal probabilities $P(Y_i^{(g)} = r) = \pi_{r+}^{(g)}$ and $P(Z_i^{(g)} = c) = \pi_{+c}^{(g)}$ by $\hat{\pi}_{r+}^{(g)} = \sum_c \hat{\pi}_{rc}^{(g)}$ and $\hat{\pi}_{+c}^{(g)} = \sum_r \hat{\pi}_{rc}^{(g)}$, respectively.

Given D, we define $U_i^{(g)} = Y_i^{(g)} - DZ_i^{(g)}$ for $i = 1, 2, \ldots, n_g$ and $g = 1, 0$. We can regard $U_i^{(g)}$ as the random variable of a positive response $Y_i^{(g)}$ adjusted with the experimental treatment effect D so that $U_i^{(g)}$ is centered around $E(p_i^{(g)})$. We consider the difference $\bar{U}_+^{(1)} - \bar{U}_+^{(0)}$, where $\bar{U}_+^{(g)} = \bar{Y}_+^{(g)} - D\bar{Z}_+^{(g)}$, $\bar{Y}_+^{(g)} = \sum_{i=1}^{n_g} Y_i^{(g)}/n_g$ and $\bar{Z}_+^{(g)} = \sum_{i=1}^{n_g} Z_i^{(g)}/n_g$, for $g = 1$, 0. Note that $E(\bar{U}_+^{(g)}) = E(U_i^{(g)}) = E(E(Y_i^{(g)}|p_i^{(g)}, z_i^{(g)}) - Dz_i^{(g)}) =$

$E(p_i^{(g)} + Dz_i^{(g)} - Dz_i^{(g')}) = E(p_i^{(g)})$. Recall that $E(p_i^{(1)}) = E(p_{i'}^{(0)})$ and hence we have $E(\bar{U}_+^{(1)} - \bar{U}_+^{(0)}) = 0$. This leads us to obtain the following equality:

$$D = (E(\bar{Y}_+^{(1)}) - E(\bar{Y}_+^{(0)}))/(E(\bar{Z}_+^{(1)}) - E(\bar{Z}_+^{(0)}))$$
$$= (\pi_{1+}^{(1)} - \pi_{1+}^{(0)})/(\pi_{+1}^{(1)} - \pi_{+1}^{(0)}). \qquad (2.53)$$

Note that $\pi_{1+}^{(g)}$ represents the probability of a positive response for patients assigned to treatment g ($g = 1, 0$). Note also that $\pi_{+1}^{(1)}$ represents the probability of compliance for patients assigned to the experimental treatment ($g = 1$), while $\pi_{+1}^{(0)}(= 1 - \pi_{+0}^{(0)})$ represents the probability of noncompliance for patients assigned to the standard treatment ($g = 0$).

When substituting $\hat{\pi}_{1+}^{(g)}$ for $\pi_{1+}^{(g)}$ and $\hat{\pi}_{+1}^{(g)}$ for $\pi_{+1}^{(g)}$ (for $g = 1, 0$) in D (2.53), we obtain the following estimator as

$$\hat{D} = (\hat{\pi}_{1+}^{(1)} - \hat{\pi}_{1+}^{(0)})/(\hat{\pi}_{+1}^{(1)} - \hat{\pi}_{+1}^{(0)}). \qquad (2.54)$$

Under the monotonicity assumption, we can easily see that the probabilities $\pi_{+1}^{(1)}$ and $\pi_{+1}^{(0)}$ are, by definition, identical to $\pi_{+CA}^{(1)}$ and $\pi_{+A}^{(0)}$, respectively. Therefore, the parameter D (2.53) and the estimator $\hat{D}$ (2.54) are actually the same as Δ (2.1) and $\hat{\Delta}$ (2.5), respectively. Note also that the estimator $\hat{D}$ (2.54) is, in fact, a special case of the estimator for the PD when there is only a single measurement per patient (Sato, 2001; Matsuyama, 2002). Using the delta method, we obtain an asymptotic variance of $\hat{D}$ (2.54) as given by

$$Var(\hat{D}) = \sum_g \{\pi_{1+}^{(g)}(1 - \pi_{1+}^{(g)}) + D^2\pi_{+1}^{(g)}(1 - \pi_{+1}^{(g)})$$
$$- 2D(\pi_{11}^{(g)} - \pi_{1+}^{(g)}\pi_{+1}^{(g)})\}/[n_g(\pi_{+1}^{(1)} - \pi_{+1}^{(0)})^2] \qquad (2.55)$$

When substituting $\hat{\pi}_{rc}^{(g)}$ for $\pi_{rc}^{(g)}$, $\hat{\pi}_{r+}^{(g)}$ for $\pi_{r+}^{(g)}$, $\hat{\pi}_{+c}^{(g)}$ for $\pi_{+c}^{(g)}$, and $\hat{D}$ for D in $Var(\hat{D})$ (2.55), we obtain the estimated asymptotic variance $\hat{Var}(\hat{D})$. Again, we can easily see that $\hat{Var}(\hat{D})$ is identical to $\hat{Var}(\hat{\Delta})$ (2.6) under the monotonicity assumption.

2.6.2   Constant risk multiplicative model

When the effect of an experimental treatment relative to that of a standard treatment (or placebo) is believed to be multiplicative, we may assume that the conditional probability of a positive response for patient i assigned to treatment g, given the treatment status $z_i^{(g)}(= 1$ for experimental; and $= 0$ for standard or placebo), is given by $P(Y_i^{(g)} = 1|z_i^{(g)}, p_i^{(g)}) = p_i^{(g)} \exp(\xi z_i^{(g)}) = p_i^{(g)} R^{z_i^{(g)}}$, where $p_i^{(g)}$ denotes the probability of a positive response when patient i assigned to treatment g is assumed to receive the standard treatment (or placebo); ξ represents the effect due to the experimental treatment and $R = \exp(\xi)$ represents the ratio of probabilities of a positive response when patient i receives the experimental treatment (i.e. $z_i^{(g)} = 1$) relative to that when he/she receives the standard treatment or placebo (i.e. $z_i^{(g)} = 0$). In other words, the probability of a positive response for patient i assigned to treatment g would equal $p_i^{(g)} R$ if he/she took the experimental treatment, and would equal $p_i^{(g)}$, otherwise.

Note that the underlying probabilities $p_i^{(g)}$ of a positive response for patients who are all assumed to receive the standard treatment (or placebo) like other pre-randomization covariates are expected to be balanced through randomization between the two treatments. That is, we have $E(p_i^{(1)}) = E(p_{i'}^{(0)})$ for patients i and i' randomly selected from the experimental and standard treatments, respectively. Note that for a randomly selected patient i from treatment g, we have

$$
\begin{aligned}
E(Y_i^{(g)} \exp(-\xi Z_i^{(g)})) &= E(E(Y_i^{(g)} \exp(-\xi Z_i^{(g)})|z_i^{(g)}, p_i^{(g)})) \\
&= E(\exp(-\xi z_i^{(g)})E(Y_i^{(g)}|z_i^{(g)}, p_i^{(g)})) \\
&= E(\exp(-\xi z_i^{(g)})p_i^{(g)} \exp(\xi z_i^{(g)})) = E(p_i^{(g)}).
\end{aligned}
$$

On the basis of the above results, we obtain

$$
E(Y_i^{(1)} \exp(-\xi Z_i^{(1)})) = E(Y_{i'}^{(0)} \exp(-\xi Z_{i'}^{(0)})). \tag{2.56}
$$

Note also that because $Y_i^{(g)} \exp(-\xi Z_i^{(g)}) = Y_i^{(g)}(Z_i^{(g)} \exp(-\xi) + (1 - Z_i^{(g)}))$, we can rewrite Equation (2.56) as

$$
E(X_1^{(1)} - X_{i'}^{(0)} + R(X_i^{(1)*} - X_{i'}^{(0)*})) = 0, \tag{2.57}
$$

where $X_i^{(g)} = Y_i^{(g)} Z_i^{(g)}$ and $X_i^{(g)*} = Y_i^{(g)}(1 - Z_i^{(g)})$. Therefore, we have

$$
R = [E(X_i^{(1)}) - E(X_{i'}^{(0)})]/[E(X_{i'}^{(0)*}) - E(X_i^{(1)*})]. \tag{2.58}
$$

Note that the possible values for random variables $X_i^{(g)}$ and $X_i^{(g)*}$ are either 0 or 1. Let $n_{rc}^{(g)}$ denote the number of patients among n_g patients with $(X_i^{(g)} = r, X_i^{(g)*} = c)$ assigned to treatment g. By the definition of $X_i^{(g)}$ and $X_i^{(g)*}$, the probability of obtaining a patient with $(X_i^{(g)} = 1, X_i^{(g)*} = 1)$ is 0. Note further that the random vector $\underline{n}_g' = (n_{10}^{(g)}, n_{01}^{(g)}, n_{00}^{(g)})$ may be assumed to follow the trinomial distribution with parameters n_g and $\underline{\theta}_g' = (\theta_{10}^{(g)}, \theta_{01}^{(g)}, \theta_{00}^{(g)})$, where $\theta_{rc}^{(g)}$ denotes the cell probability that a randomly selected patient assigned to treatment g has $(X_i^{(g)} = r, X_i^{(g)*} = c)$ for $(r, c) = (1, 0), (0, 1), (0, 0)$. Thus, the commonly employed unbiased consistent estimators for $P(X_i^{(g)} = 1) = \theta_{10}^{(g)}$ and $P(X_i^{(g)*} = 1) = \theta_{01}^{(g)}$ are $\hat{\theta}_{10}^{(g)} = n_{10}^{(g)}/n_g$ and $\hat{\theta}_{01}^{(g)} = n_{01}^{(g)}/n_g$, respectively. Note that we can rewrite (2.58) in terms of parameters $\theta_{rc}^{(g)}$'s as

$$R = (\theta_{10}^{(1)} - \theta_{10}^{(0)})/(\theta_{01}^{(0)} - \theta_{01}^{(1)}). \tag{2.59}$$

Thus, we can substitute $\hat{\theta}_{rc}^{(g)} = n_{rc}^{(g)}/n_g$ for $\theta_{rc}^{(g)}$ in R (2.59) and obtain the estimator

$$\hat{R} = (\hat{\theta}_{10}^{(1)} - \hat{\theta}_{10}^{(0)})/(\hat{\theta}_{01}^{(0)} - \hat{\theta}_{01}^{(1)}). \tag{2.60}$$

Note that $X_i^{(g)} = 1$ if and only if $Y_i^{(g)} = 1$ and $Z_i^{(g)} = 1$. Thus, the cell probability $P(X_i^{(1)} = 1) = \theta_{10}^{(1)}$ represents the probability of a randomly selected patient i assigned to the experimental treatment, who has a positive response and receives his/her assigned (experimental) treatment. Under the monotonicity assumption, this probability $\theta_{10}^{(1)}$ is simply identical to the cell probability $\pi_{1CA}^{(1)}$ as defined in the previous section. Following similar arguments, we can show under the monotonicity assumption that the probabilities $\theta_{01}^{(1)}, \theta_{10}^{(0)}$ and $\theta_{01}^{(0)}$ are, by definition, the same as $\pi_{1N}^{(1)}, \pi_{1A}^{(0)}$, and $\pi_{1CN}^{(0)}$, respectively. Thus, the parameter R (2.59) and the estimator $\hat{R}$ (2.60) are identical to γ (2.8) and $\hat{\gamma}$ (2.9) under the monotonicity assumption. Using the delta method (Casella and Berger, 1990), we can show that the asymptotic variance $Var(\log(\hat{R}))$ for $\log(\hat{R})$ is given by

$$\sum_g [\theta_{10}^{(g)}(1 - \theta_{10}^{(g)}) - 2R\theta_{10}^{(g)}\theta_{01}^{(g)} + R^2\theta_{01}^{(g)}(1 - \theta_{01}^{(g)})]/$$
$$[n_g(\theta_{01}^{(0)} - \theta_{01}^{(1)})^2 R^2]. \tag{2.61}$$

When substituting $\hat{\theta}_{rc}^{(g)}$ for $\theta_{rc}^{(g)}$ and $\hat{R}$ for R in (2.61), we obtain the estimated asymptotic variance $\hat{Var}(\log(\hat{R}))$, which is, in fact, the same as $\hat{Var}(\log(\hat{\gamma}))$ (2.10).

Note that using the model-based approach may help us appreciate the 'causal' effect due to the experimental treatment versus the standard treatment (or placebo) on the probability of individual patient response. Although each patient has two potential responses or outcomes, as noted before, we can only observe one of these two potential responses in reality. We often call this the counterfactual approach. By contrast, using the approach adopted in the previous sections does not require us to assume different structural risk models for various indices. All indices used to measure the relative treatment effect are directly expressed in terms of the parameters relevant to the patient response distributions among compliers and thereby, the derivation of test procedures and estimators as presented in the previous sections should be easier for readers to follow than the structural risk model-based or counterfactual approach.

Note also that one of the major concerns using the above constant risk models is that the relative treatment effect on the probability of patient response is assumed to be constant for all patients (Lui, 2007c; Sjölander, 2008). This is unlikely to be true in most practically encountered situations, although the indices and their estimators derived from these constant risk models coincide with those derived previously. To alleviate this concern, we may consider the following more general risk models, accounting for the variation of the relative treatment effect between subpopulations and individual patients (Lui, 2007c).

2.6.3   Generalized risk additive model

Recall that under the monotonicity assumption, our sampling population consists of compliers (C), always-takers (A), and never-takers (N). To account for the possible variation of the relative treatment effect between patients and subpopulations in the risk additive model, we may assume that

$$
\begin{aligned}
P(Y_i^{(g)} = 1 | p_i^{(g)}, z_i^{(g)}) &= p_i^{(g)} + D_{iC} Z_i^{(g)} \quad \text{if} \quad i \in C \\
&= p_i^{(g)} + D_{iA} Z_i^{(g)} \quad \text{if} \quad i \in A, \\
&= p_i^{(g)} + D_{iN} Z_i^{(g)} \quad \text{if} \quad i \in N, \quad (2.62)
\end{aligned}
$$

where D_{iS} represents the excess effect due to an experimental treatment over a standard treatment on the probability of a positive response for patient i from subpopulation S, $S = C, A, N$. We assume $E(D_{iS}|S) = D_S$. Note that the parameter D_C is called CACE. Note also that, by definition, if $i \in A$(always-takers), then $Z_i^{(g)} = 1$ regardless of his/her assigned treatment g ($g = 1, 0$). Similarly, if $i \in N$(never-takers), then $Z_i^{(g)} = 0$ despite that he/she is assigned to either of two treatments g. Also, if $i \in C$ (compliers), then we have $Z_i^{(1)} = 1$ and $Z_i^{(0)} = 0$. Because $E(Y_i^{(1)}) = E(E(Y_i^{(1)}|S))$, we can show that the expectation of $Y_i^{(1)}$ for a randomly selected patient i assigned to the experimental treatment ($g = 1$) is

$$E(Y_i^{(1)}) = P(C)[E(p_i^{(1)}|C) + D_C] + P(A)[E(p_i^{(1)}|A) + D_A]$$
$$+ P(N)E(p_i^{(1)}|N) = E(p_i^{(1)}) + P(C)D_C + P(A)D_A,$$

$$(2.63)$$

where $P(S)$ denotes the proportion of subpopulation S in the sampling population, where $S = C, A$, and N. Similarly, the expectation of $Y_{i'}^{(0)}$ for a randomly selected patient i' assigned to the standard treatment ($g = 0$) is given by

$$E(Y_{i'}^{(0)}) = P(C)E(p_{i'}^{(0)}|C) + P(A)[E(p_{i'}^{(0)}|A) + D_A]$$
$$+ P(N)E(p_{i'}^{(0)}|N) = E(p_{i'}^{(0)}) + P(A)D_A. \quad (2.64)$$

Furthermore, we can easily show that the corresponding expectations $E(Z_i^{(1)}) = P(C) + P(A) (= \pi_{+CA})$ and $E(Z_{i'}^{(0)}) = P(A) (= \pi_{+A})$ under the monotonicity assumption. On the basis of (2.63) and (2.64), as well as the above results, we obtain

$$D_C = [E(Y_i^{(1)}) - E(Y_{i'}^{(0)})]/[E(Z_i^{(1)}) - E(Z_{i'}^{(0)})]$$
$$= (\pi_{1+}^{(1)} - \pi_{1+}^{(0)})/(\pi_{+1}^{(1)} - \pi_{+1}^{(0)}). \quad (2.65)$$

In other words, the estimator $\hat{D}$ (2.54) derived under a constant risk additive model (or equivalently, $\hat{\Delta}$ (2.5) under the monotonicity assumption) is a consistent estimator of the CACE D_C under the generalized risk additive model (2.62).

2.6.4   Generalized risk multiplicative model

To account for a possible variation of an experimental effect between patients and subpopulations in the risk multiplicative model, we may assume that the generalized risk multiplicative model for the probability of a positive response on patient i assigned to treatment g is given by

$$P(Y_i^{(g)} = 1 | p_i^{(g)}, z_i^{(g)}) = p_i^{(g)} R_{iC}^{Z_i^{(g)}} \quad \text{if} \quad i \in C,$$
$$= p_i^{(g)} R_{iA}^{Z_i^{(g)}} \quad \text{if} \quad i \in A,$$
$$= p_i^{(g)} R_{iN}^{Z_i^{(g)}} \quad \text{if} \quad i \in N, \quad (2.66)$$

where R_{iS} represents the experimental effect relative to the standard treatment on the probability of a positive response for patient i from subpopulation S for $S = C, A, N$. We assume that $E(R_{iS}|S) = R_S$. Here, we need to make the additional assumption that $E(p_i^{(g)} R_{iS}|S) = E(p_i^{(g)}|S)E(R_{iS}|S)$ for $S = C, A$. If $R_{iS} = R_S$ for all i (i.e. there is no variation in the treatment effect between patients within a subpopulation S, $S = C, A$), or R_{iS} and $p_i^{(g)}$ are conditionally independent, given S, then this assumption will be satisfied. Based on the above assumptions, for a randomly selected patient i assigned to the experimental treatment ($g = 1$), we have the expectation

$$E(X_i^{(1)}) = P(Y_i^{(1)} = 1, Z_i^{(1)} = 1)$$
$$= P(C)E(p_i^{(1)}|C)R_C + P(A)E(p_i^{(1)}|A)R_A, \quad (2.67)$$

and

$$E(X_i^{(1)*}) = P(Y_i^{(1)} = 1, Z_i^{(1)} = 0) = P(N)E(p_i^{(1)}|N). \quad (2.68)$$

Similarly, for a randomly selected patient i' assigned to the standard treatment ($g = 0$), we have the following expectations,

$$E(X_{i'}^{(0)}) = P(Y_{i'}^{(0)} = 1, Z_{i'}^{(0)} = 1) = P(A)E(p_{i'}^{(0)}|A)R_A, \quad (2.69)$$

and

$$E(X_{i'}^{(0)*}) = P(Y_{i'}^{(0)} = 1, Z_{i'}^{(0)} = 0)$$
$$= P(C)E(p_{i'}^{(0)}|C) + P(N)E(p_{i'}^{(0)}|N). \quad (2.70)$$

Because of randomization, we may assume that $E(p_i^{(1)}|S) = E(p_{i'}^{(0)}|S)$ for $S = C$, A, and N. Therefore, when substituting (2.67)–(2.70), we obtain

$$R_C = [E(X_i^{(1)}) - E(X_{i'}^{(0)})]/[E(X_{i'}^{(0)*}) - E(X_i^{(1)*})]$$
$$= (\theta_{10}^{(1)} - \theta_{10}^{(0)})/(\theta_{01}^{(0)} - \theta_{01}^{(1)}). \tag{2.71}$$

Thus, the estimator $\hat{R}$ (2.60) derived from the constant risk multiplicative model is a consistent estimator of R_C defined in the generalized risk multiplicative model (2.66).

Exercises

2.1 Under SUTVA, the monotonicity assumption and the exclusion restriction assumption for always-takers and never-takers, show that the programmatic effectiveness δ is equal to $\Delta\pi_{+C}$, where Δ is defined in (2.1).

2.2 Using the delta method, show that the asymptotic variance of $\tanh^{-1}(\hat{\delta})$ is given by $Var(\tanh^{-1}(\hat{\delta})) = Var(\hat{\delta})/(1 - \delta^2)^2$.

2.3 Show that the MLE $\hat{\Delta}$ for Δ is given by $\hat{\Delta} = (\hat{\pi}_{1+}^{(1)} - \hat{\pi}_{1+}^{(0)})/(\hat{\pi}_{+CA}^{(1)} - \hat{\pi}_{+A}^{(0)})$ (hint: using the functional invariance property of the MLE (Casella and Berger, 1990) and the fact that the model assumed here is a saturated model containing 6 free parameters. For example, given the set of parameters $\{\pi_{+C}, \pi_{+A}, \pi_{1|C}^{(0)}, \pi_{1|A}, \pi_{1|N}, \Delta\}$, we can uniquely determine the underlying cell probabilities of observed data, and vice versa).

2.4 Show that the equality $\pi_{1|CA}^{(1)} - \pi_{1|CA}^{(0)} = \pi_{1|C}^{(1)} - \pi_{1|C}^{(0)}$ holds if and only if $\pi_{1|C}^{(1)} - \pi_{1|C}^{(0)} = \pi_{1|A}^{(1)} - \pi_{1|A}^{(0)}$.

2.5 Under the SCRD, show that an asymptotic variance of $\hat{\Delta}_{CA} = (\hat{\pi}_{1+}^{(1)} - \hat{\pi}_{1+}^{(0)})/\hat{\pi}_{+CA}^{(1)}$ is given by

$$Var(\hat{\Delta}_{CA}) = [\pi_{1+}^{(1)}(\pi_{1N}^{(1)} + \pi_{2CA}^{(1)}) + \pi_{1|}^{(0)}(\pi_{1|}^{(0)}\pi_{|N}^{(1)} - 2\pi_{1N}^{(1)})]/$$
$$[n_1(\pi_{+CA}^{(1)})^3] + \pi_{1+}^{(0)}(1 - \pi_{1+}^{(0)})/[n_0(\pi_{+CA}^{(1)})^2].$$

Thus, under the null hypothesis $H_0 : \Delta_{CA} = 0$, Lui (2006a) proposed the following estimated asymptotic variance

$$\hat{Var}(\hat{\Delta}_{CA}|H_0) = \hat{\pi}_{1+}^{(p)}[(\hat{\pi}_{1N}^{(1)} + \hat{\pi}_{2CA}^{(1)}) - (2\hat{\pi}_{1N}^{(1)} - \hat{\pi}_{1+}^{(p)}\hat{\pi}_{+N}^{(1)})]/$$
$$[n_1(\hat{\pi}_{+CA}^{(1)})^3] + \hat{\pi}_{1+}^{(p)}(1 - \hat{\pi}_{1+}^{(p)})/[n_0(\hat{\pi}_{+CA}^{(1)})^2]$$

for $\hat{\Delta}_{CA}$ and two simple test statistics, including $\hat{\Delta}_{CA}/\sqrt{\hat{Var}(\hat{\Delta}_{CA}|H_0)}$ and $\tanh^{-1}(\hat{\Delta}_{CA})/\sqrt{\hat{Var}(\hat{\Delta}_{CA}|H_0)}$, for testing $H_0 : \Delta_{CA} = 0$. Lui (2006a) found that these two test statistics can be more powerful than test statistic (2.3).

2.6 Based on the data in Table 2.1 regarding use of vitamin A supplementation to reduce the mortality among pre-school children and the results in Exercise 2.5, what are the p-values of using

$\hat{\Delta}_{CA}/\sqrt{\hat{Var}(\hat{\Delta}_{CA}|H_0)}$ and $\tanh^{-1}(\hat{\Delta}_{CA})/\sqrt{\hat{Var}(\hat{\Delta}_{CA}|H_0)}$ for testing $H_0 : \Delta_{CA} = 0$?

2.7 Show that under the monotonicity assumption and the exclusion restriction assumption for always-takers and never-takers, if $\Delta > -\varepsilon_l$ holds, then $\delta > -\varepsilon_l$ is true, where $\varepsilon_l > 0$, but not vice versa.

2.8 Using the delta method, show that an estimated asymptotic variance of $\hat{\Delta}$ (2.5) is given in (2.6).

2.9 Show that an estimated asymptotic variance $\hat{Var}(\log(\hat{\gamma}))$ for the statistic $\log(\hat{\gamma})$ is given by

$$
\begin{aligned}
\hat{Var}(\log(\hat{\gamma})) = {} & [\hat{\pi}_{1CA}^{(1)}(1 - \hat{\pi}_{1CA}^{(1)})/n_1 + \hat{\pi}_{1A}^{(0)}(1 - \hat{\pi}_{1A}^{(0)})/n_0]/ \\
& (\hat{\pi}_{1CA}^{(1)} - \hat{\pi}_{1A}^{(0)})^2 + [\hat{\pi}_{1N}^{(1)}(1 - \hat{\pi}_{1N}^{(1)})/n_1 \\
& + \hat{\pi}_{1CN}^{(0)}(1 - \hat{\pi}_{1CN}^{(0)})/n_0]/(\hat{\pi}_{1CN}^{(0)} - \hat{\pi}_{1N}^{(1)})^2 \\
& - 2[\hat{\pi}_{1CA}^{(1)}\hat{\pi}_{1N}^{(1)}/n_1 + \hat{\pi}_{1CN}^{(0)}\hat{\pi}_{1A}^{(0)}/n_0]/ \\
& [(\hat{\pi}_{1CA}^{(1)} - \hat{\pi}_{1A}^{(0)})(\hat{\pi}_{1CN}^{(0)} - \hat{\pi}_{1N}^{(1)})].
\end{aligned}
$$

2.10 Show that an estimated asymptotic variance $\hat{Var}(\log(\hat{\varphi}))$, where

$$
\hat{\varphi} = [(\hat{\pi}_{1CA}^{(1)} - \hat{\pi}_{1A}^{(0)})(\hat{\pi}_{2CN}^{(0)} - \hat{\pi}_{2N}^{(1)})]/[(\hat{\pi}_{2CA}^{(1)} - \hat{\pi}_{2A}^{(0)})(\hat{\pi}_{1CN}^{(0)} - \hat{\pi}_{1N}^{(1)})]
$$

is given in (2.14).

2.11 Show that the two inequalities (2.16) hold if and only if the $100(1 - 2\alpha)\%$ confidence interval using interval estimator (2.20) is completely contained in $(-\varepsilon_l, \varepsilon_u)$.

2.12 Consider the data in Table 2.6 taken from a RCT studying the treatments for carotid stenosis. Patients were randomized to carotid endarterectomy or medical care (Barnett and NASCET collaborators, 1991; Walter, Guyatt and Montori et al., 2006). The primary outcome was the occurrence of any fatal or nonfatal ipsilateral stroke.

(a) What is the ITT estimate $\hat{\delta}$ of the PD between the assigned medical care and surgery groups?

(b) What is the estimate $\hat{\Delta}$ of the PD between the assigned medical care and surgery groups?

(c) What are the 95% confidence intervals of Δ using (2.19), (2.20), and (2.23)?

(d) What is the MLE $\hat{\gamma}$ in (2.9)?

Table 2.6 The data on strokes taken from the North American Symptomatic Carotid Endarterectomy Trial (NASCET) study of carotid stenosis.

Assigned treatment: medical care ($g = 1$)

		Treatment received		
		Medical care	Surgery	Total
Stroke	Yes	61 (18.43 %)	1 (0.30 %)	62 (18.73 %)
	No	255 (77.04 %)	14 (4.22 %)	269 (81.27 %)
	Total	316 (95.47 %)	15 (4.53 %)	331 (100 %)

Assigned treatment: surgery ($g = 0$)

		Treatment received		
		Surgery	Medical care	Total
Stroke	Yes	26 (7.93 %)	1 (0.3 %)	27 (8.23 %)
	No	301 (91.77 %)	0 (0.0 %)	301 (91.77 %)
	Total	327 (99.70 %)	1 (0.3 %)	328 (100 %)

(e) What are the 95 % confidence intervals of the PR γ using (2.24), (2.25), and (2.26)?

2.13 Consider the mortality data regarding a simple noncompliance RCT studying the efficacy of breast screening by mammography in the Swedish two-county trial in Table 2.7 (Cuzick, Edwards and Segnan, 1997; Tabár, Fagerberg and Day et al., 1987). There were approximately 13500 women of age 40–74 years old randomized to either mammographic screening every 2–3 years or control. As shown in Table 2.7, there were 11 % of women assigned to breast screening group who declined to be screened.

(a) What is the MLE $\hat{\gamma}$ in (2.9)?

(b) What are the 95 % confidence intervals for γ using (2.24), (2.25), and (2.26)? (hint: $\hat{\gamma} = 0.682$; [0.455, 0.908], [0.489, 0.951], [0.489, 0.951]).

Table 2.7 The frequency and the corresponding percentage (in parenthesis) taken from a simple noncompliance RCT studying the efficacy of breast cancer screening by mammography in the Swedish two-county trial.

Experimental group: breast screening by mammography ($g = 1$)

		Breast Screening		
		Yes	No	Total
Outcome	Death	85 (0.11 %)	39 (0.05 %)	124 (0.16 %)
	Survival	69410 (88.89 %)	8551 (10.95 %)	77961 (99.84 %)
	Total	69495 (89.00 %)	8590 (11.00 %)	78085 (100 %)

Control group: no breast screening by mammography ($g = 0$)

		Breast Screening		
		No	Yes	Total
Outcome	Death	119 (0.21 %)	0	119 (0.21 %)
	Survival	56663 (99.79 %)	0	56663 (99.79 %)
	Total	56782 (100 %)	0	56782 (100 %)

2.14 Show that (a) the estimator $\hat{\gamma}$ (2.9) becomes $\hat{\pi}_{1CA}^{(1)}/(\hat{\pi}_{1+}^{(0)} - \hat{\pi}_{1N}^{(1)})$ under the simple noncompliance RCT assuming $\pi_{+A} = 0$ (Lui, 2007a). (b) When the placebo effect is minimal, show that $\hat{\pi}_{1CA}^{(1)}/(\hat{\pi}_{1+}^{(0)} - \hat{\pi}_{1N}^{(1)})$ will actually be a consistent estimator of $\gamma_{CA} = \pi_{1|CA}^{(1)}/\pi_{1|CA}^{(0)}$ if $\pi_{+A} > 0$ and always-takers assigned to the placebo treatment do not receive any treatment due to the built-in feature in the design. (c) Show that $\gamma_{CA} = \gamma$ if and only if $\pi_{1|C}^{(1)}/\pi_{1|C}^{(0)} = \pi_{1|A}^{(1)}/\pi_{1|A}^{(0)}$.

2.15 Under the simple noncompliance RCT (with $\pi_{+A} = 0$), we may use $\Delta^* = \pi_{1|C}^{(0)} - \pi_{1|N}^{(0)}$, the difference in the conditional probabilities of a positive response between compliers and never-takers in the control group to measure the selection effect.

(a) Show that under the exclusion restriction assumption for never-takers, we have $\pi_{1+}^{(0)} - \pi_{1N}/\pi_{+N} = \Delta^*\pi_{+C}$. Thus, the MLE for Δ^* is $\hat{\Delta}^* = (\hat{\pi}_{1+}^{(0)} - \hat{\pi}_{1N}^{(1)}/\hat{\pi}_{+N}^{(1)})/\hat{\pi}_{+C}$.

(b) Show that the asymptotic variance $\hat{Var}(\hat{\pi}_{1+}^{(0)} - \hat{\pi}_{1N}^{(1)}/\hat{\pi}_{+N}^{(1)})$ is given by

$$\hat{\pi}_{1+}^{(0)}(1 - \hat{\pi}_{1+}^{(0)})/n_0 + [\hat{\pi}_{1N}^{(1)}(1 - \hat{\pi}_{1N}^{(1)}) + (\hat{\pi}_{1|N}^{(1)})^2 \hat{\pi}_{+N}^{(1)}(1 - \hat{\pi}_{+N}^{(1)})$$
$$- 2\hat{\pi}_{1|N}^{(1)}\hat{\pi}_{1N}^{(1)}(1 - \hat{\pi}_{+N}^{(1)})]/[n_1(\hat{\pi}_{+N}^{(1)})^2],$$

where $\hat{\pi}_{1|N}^{(1)} = \hat{\pi}_{1N}^{(1)}/\hat{\pi}_{+N}^{(1)}$. Note that $\pi_{1+}^{(0)} - \pi_{1N}/\pi_{+N} = 0$ if and only if $\Delta^* = 0$. Thus, we can apply the statistic $\hat{\pi}_{1+}^{(0)} - \hat{\pi}_{1N}^{(1)}/\hat{\pi}_{+N}^{(1)}$ together with its estimated asymptotic variance $\hat{Var}(\hat{\pi}_{1+}^{(0)} - \hat{\pi}_{1N}^{(1)}/\hat{\pi}_{+N}^{(1)})$ to test $H_0 : \Delta^* = 0$.

(c) Discuss why we cannot use the difference $\pi_{1|C}^{(1)} - \pi_{1|N}^{(1)}$ to measure the selection effect.

2.16 Show that based on the test procedure (2.4) at a nominal α-level, the minimum required number of patients n_1 from the experimental treatment for a desired power $(1 - \beta)$ of detecting a given specified nonzero value Δ_0 is given by

$$n_1 = Ceil\{(Z_{\alpha/2}\sqrt{S_0(\pi_{1+}^{(0)}, \Delta_0, \pi_{+C}, k)}$$
$$+ Z_\beta\sqrt{S_1(\pi_{1+}^{(0)}, \Delta_0, \pi_{+C}, k)}/[1 - (\Delta_0\pi_{+C})^2])^2/$$
$$(\tanh^{-1}(\Delta_0\pi_{+C}))^2\},$$

where $Ceil\{x\}$ is the smallest integer $\geq x$ and

$$S_1(\pi_{1+}^{(0)}, \Delta_0, \pi_{+C}, k) = [\pi_{1+}^{(1)}(1 - \pi_{1+}^{(1)}) + \pi_{1+}^{(0)}(1 - \pi_{1+}^{(0)})/k].$$

2.17 To test $H_0 : \Delta = 0$ versus $H_a : \Delta \neq 0$, we can also apply a test statistic directly based on $\hat{\Delta}$ (2.5) with the $\tanh^{-1}(x)$ transformation, $Z = \tanh^{-1}(\hat{\Delta})/\sqrt{\hat{Var}(\hat{\Delta}|H_0)}$, where

$$\hat{Var}(\hat{\Delta}|H_0) = (n_1 + n_0)\hat{\pi}_{1+}^{(p)}(1 - \hat{\pi}_{1+}^{(p)})/[(\hat{\pi}_{+CA}^{(1)} - \hat{\pi}_{+A}^{(0)})^2(n_1n_0)],$$

and

$$\hat{\pi}_{1+}^{(p)} = (n_1\hat{\pi}_{1+}^{(1)} + n_0\hat{\pi}_{1+}^{(0)})/(n_1 + n_0),$$

and reject $H_0 : \Delta = 0$ at the α-level if $Z > Z_{\alpha/2}$ or $Z < -Z_{\alpha/2}$. On the basis of this test procedure, show that an estimate of the minimum required sample size n_1 from the experimental treatment for a desired power $1 - \beta$ of detecting a given nonzero difference Δ_0 at the α-level is equal to

$$n_1 = Ceil\{[Z_{\alpha/2}\sqrt{V_{PD|H_0}} + Z_\beta\sqrt{V_{PD}}/(1 - \Delta_0^2)]^2/[\tanh^{-1}(\Delta_0)]^2\},$$

where $Ceil\{x\}$ is the smallest integer $\geq x$,

$$V_{PD|H_0} = V_{PD}(\pi_{+C}, \pi_{+A}, \pi_{1|C}^{(0)}, \pi_{1|A}, \pi_{1|N}, \Delta_0, k|H_0)$$
$$= \bar{\pi}_{1+}^{(p)}(1 - \bar{\pi}_{1+}^{(p)})(1 + 1/k)/(\pi_{+C})^2,$$
$$\bar{\pi}_{1+}^{(p)} = (\pi_{1+}^{(1)} + k\pi_{1+}^{(0)})/(1 + k),$$

and

$$V_{PD} = V_{PD}(\pi_{+C}, \pi_{+A}, \pi_{1|C}^{(0)}, \pi_{1|A}, \pi_{1|N}, \Delta_0, k)$$
$$= \{[\pi_{1+}^{(1)}(1 - \pi_{1+}^{(1)}) + \pi_{1+}^{(0)}(1 - \pi_{1+}^{(0)})/k]$$
$$+ \Delta^2[\pi_{+CA}^{(1)}(1 - \pi_{+CA}^{(1)}) + \pi_{+A}(1 - \pi_{+A})/k] - 2\Delta$$
$$[(\pi_{1CA}^{(1)} - \pi_{1+}^{(1)}\pi_{+CA}^{(1)}) + (\pi_{1A} - \pi_{1+}^{(0)}\pi_{+A})/k]\}/(\pi_{+C})^2.$$

2.18 Show that given the set of parameters $\{\pi_{+C}, \pi_{+A}, \pi_{1|C}^{(0)}, \pi_{1|A}, \pi_{1|N}, \Delta\}$, we can uniquely determine all the cell probabilities $\pi_{rS}^{(g)}$ ($r = 1, 2, S = CA, N$ for $g = 1$ and $S = CN, A$ for $g = 0$) under the monotonicity assumption and the exclusion restriction assumption for always-takers and never-takers.

2.19 Based on the test statistic (2.7) and the asymptotic variance (2.32), show that an estimate of the minimum required number of patients n_1 from the experimental treatment for a desired power $(1 - \beta)$ of detecting noninferiority with a given specified value $\Delta_0(> -\varepsilon_l)$ at a nominal α-level is

$$n_1 = Ceil\{((Z_\alpha + Z_\beta)^2 V_{PD}(\pi_{+C}, \pi_{+A}, \pi_{1|C}^{(0)}, \pi_{1|A}, \pi_{1|N}, \Delta_0, k)/$$
$$[(1 - \Delta_0^2)^2])/(\tanh^{-1}(\varepsilon_l) + \tanh^{-1}(\Delta_0))^2\}.$$

2.20 On the basis of the test statistic (2.11) and the asymptotic variance (2.34), show that an estimate of the minimum required number n_1 of patients for a desired power $(1 - \beta)$ of detecting noninferiority with a given specified value $\gamma_0(> 1 - \gamma_l)$ at a nominal α-level is given by

$$n_1 = Ceil\{(Z_\alpha + Z_\beta)^2 V_{LPR}(\pi_{+C}, \pi_{+A}, \pi_{1|C}^{(0)}, \pi_{1|A}, \pi_{1|N}, \gamma_0, k)/$$
$$(\log(\gamma_0) - \log(1 - \gamma_l))^2\}.$$

2.21 Show that the power function $\phi_{PD}(\Delta_0)$ for testing $H_0 : \Delta \le -\varepsilon_l$ or $\Delta \ge \varepsilon_u$ at the α-level based on the test procedure (2.16) is given by

$$\phi_{PD}(\Delta_0) = \Phi(\frac{\tanh^{-1}(\varepsilon_u) - \tanh^{-1}(\Delta_0)}{\sqrt{Var(\tanh^{-1}(\hat{\Delta}))}} - Z_\alpha)$$
$$- \Phi(\frac{-\tanh^{-1}(\varepsilon_l) - \tanh^{-1}(\Delta_0)}{\sqrt{Var(\tanh^{-1}(\hat{\Delta}))}} + Z_\alpha),$$

where $\Phi(X)$ is the cumulative standard normal distribution.

2.22 On the basis of the power function (2.39) and (2.32), show that an estimate of the minimum required number of patients n_1 from the experimental treatment such that we have the desired power $(1 - \beta)$ of detecting equivalence for a specified $-\varepsilon_l < \Delta_0 < 0$ at a nominal α-level is given by

$$n_1 = Ceil\{((Z_\alpha + Z_\beta)^2 V_{PD}(\pi_{+C}, \pi_{+A}, \pi_{1|C}^{(0)}, \pi_{1|A}, \pi_{1|N}, \Delta_0, k)/$$
$$[(1 - \Delta_0^2)^2])/(\tanh^{-1}(\varepsilon_l) + \tanh^{-1}(\Delta_0))^2\}.$$

2.23 On the basis of the power function (2.41) and (2.32), show that an estimate of the minimum required number n_1 of patients from the experimental treatment such that we have the desired power $(1 - \beta)$ of detecting equivalence for a given specified $0 < \Delta_0 < \varepsilon_u$ at a nominal α-level is given by

$$n_1 = Ceil\{((Z_\alpha + Z_\beta)^2 V_{PD}(\pi_{+C}, \pi_{+A}, \pi_{1|C}^{(0)}, \pi_{1|A}, \pi_{1|N}, \Delta_0, k)/$$
$$[(1 - \Delta_0^2)^2])/(\tanh^{-1}(\varepsilon_u) - \tanh^{-1}(\Delta_0))^2\}.$$

2.24 When $\varepsilon_l = \varepsilon_u$, show that an estimate of the minimum required number n_1 of patients from the experimental treatment such that we have the desired power $(1 - \beta)$ of detecting equivalence for a given specified $\Delta_0 = 0$ at a nominal α-level based on the power function (2.43) is given by

$$n_1 = Ceil\{((Z_\alpha + Z_{\beta/2})^2 V_{PD}(\pi_{+C}, \pi_{+A}, \pi_{1|C}^{(0)}, \pi_{1|A}, \pi_{1|N}, \Delta_0, k))/$$
$$(\tanh^{-1}(\varepsilon_u))^2\}.$$

2.25 This exercise is regarding estimation of the PR when the dose level of the experimental treatment is trichotomous in a RCT with noncompliance (Lui and Chang, 2009a). Consider comparing two treatments, an experimental drug ($g = 1$) and a placebo ($g = 0$) in a RCT. Suppose that each patient assigned to the experimental group is planned to receive a total of two doses of the experimental drug. However, some patients assigned to the experimental group may receive fewer than two doses, while some patients assigned to the placebo group may even switch and receive one or two doses of the experimental drug. We assume that the effect of receiving no doses of the experimental drug on the patient response is the same as that of receiving the placebo. For each given patient, we define the vector $(d(1), d(0))$ as the status of his/her potential treatment receipt: $d(g) = t$ if the patient assigned to treatment g ($= 1$ for experimental, $= 0$ for placebo) receives t ($= 0, 1, 2$) doses of the experimental drug.

(a) Under the assumption of monotonicity (i.e. $d(1) \geq d(0)$) for all patients, show that we can divide the population into 6 subpopulations: full compliers (FC) (i.e. $d(1) = 2, d(0) = 0$), partial compliers of Type I (PCI) (i.e. $d(1) = 1, d(0) = 0$), partial compliers of Type II (PCII) (i.e. $d(1) = 2, d(0) = 1$), always-takers (AT) (i.e. $d(1) = 2, d(0) = 2$), never-takers (NT) (i.e. $d(1) = 0, d(0) = 0$), and always noncompliers (AN) (i.e. $d(1) = 1, d(0) = 1$). We let $p_{1S}^{(g)}$ (and $p_{2S}^{(g)}$) denote the cell probability of having (and not having) an outcome of interest for a randomly selected patient assigned to treatment g in category S: $S = $ FC, PCI, PCII, AT, NT, and AN. We define $p_{+S}^{(g)} = p_{1S}^{(g)} + p_{2S}^{(g)}$.

(b) Argue why it may be reasonable to assume that $p_{1AT}^{(1)} = p_{1AT}^{(0)}$, $p_{1NT}^{(1)} = p_{1NT}^{(0)}$ and $p_{1AN}^{(1)} = p_{1AN}^{(0)}$. This can be called the exclusion restriction assumption for always-takers, never-takers, and always noncompliers.

(c) State the reason why we may reasonably assume that $p_{+S}^{(1)} = p_{+S}^{(0)}$ (for $S =$ FC, PCI, PCII, AT, NT, and AN), which is identical to the distribution of subpopulation S in the sampling population. Thus, when there is no confusion in referring to the above particular probabilities, we will delete their superscripts for simplicity. Note that because patients who are AT, NT, or AN will always take, by definition, the same dose level of the experimental drug despite the treatment group to which they are assigned, the effect due to the experimental drug on these patients is of less interest. Thus, we focus attention on estimation of the experimental effect on the outcome of interest among patients who are FC, PCI, or PCII. To measure the effect of the experimental drug on these patients, we define the risk ratio, $RR_S = p_{1|S}^{(1)}/p_{1|S}^{(0)} = p_{1S}^{(1)}/p_{1S}^{(0)}$, where $p_{1|S}^{(g)} = p_{1S}^{(g)}/p_{+S}$ is the conditional probability of having the outcome of interest given patients assigned to treatment group g in category S ($S =$ FC, PCI and PCII). Suppose that we assume that the effect of the experimental drug depends on only the difference in dose levels which a patient received (i.e. $RR_{PCI} = RR_{PCII}$). We denote this common value by γ.

(d) Show that $RR_{FC} = \gamma^2$. Based on the assumption of monotonicity, we can summarize the observed data of patients assigned to the experimental and standard treatments by use of the following tables:

Experimental group ($g = 1$)

Outcomes of interest	Zero dose ($t = 0$)	One dose ($t = 1$)	Two doses ($t = 2$)
Yes	p_{1NT}	$p_{1PCI}^{(1)} + p_{1AN}$	$p_{1FC}^{(1)} + p_{1PCII}^{(1)} + p_{1AT}$
No	p_{2NT}	$p_{2PCI}^{(1)} + p_{2AN}$	$p_{2FC}^{(1)} + p_{2PCII}^{(1)} + p_{2AT}$
Total	p_{+NT}	$p_{+PCI} + p_{+AN}$	$p_{+FC} + p_{+PCII} + p_{+AT}$

Placebo group ($g = 0$)

Outcome of interest	Zero dose ($t = 0$)	One dose ($t = 1$)	Two doses ($t = 2$)
Yes	$p_{1NT} + p_{1FC}^{(0)} + p_{1PCI}^{(0)}$	$p_{1PCII}^{(0)} + p_{1AN}$	p_{1AT}
No	$p_{2NT} + p_{1FC}^{(0)} + p_{2PCI}^{(0)}$	$p_{2PCII}^{(0)} + p_{2AN}$	p_{2AT}
Total	$p_{+NT} + p_{+FC} + p_{+PCI}$	$p_{+PCII} + p_{+AN}$	p_{+AT}

We let $\pi_{100}^{(g)}$, $\pi_{010}^{(g)}$, and $\pi_{001}^{(g)}$ denote the cell probability of having the outcome of interest for a randomly selected patient assigned to treatment group g ($= 1, 0$) receiving the dose level of $t = 0, 1$, and 2, respectively. That is, $\pi_{100}^{(1)} = p_{1NT}$, $\pi_{010}^{(1)} = p_{1PCI}^{(1)} + p_{1AN}$, $\pi_{001}^{(1)} = p_{1FC}^{(1)} + p_{1PCII}^{(1)} + p_{1AT}$ for the experimental group, as well as $\pi_{100}^{(0)} = p_{1NT} + p_{1FC}^{(0)} + p_{1PCI}^{(0)}$, $\pi_{010}^{(0)} = p_{1PCII}^{(0)} + p_{1AN}$, and $\pi_{001}^{(0)} = p_{1AT}$ for the placebo group. We further define $\pi_{000}^{(g)} = 1 - (\pi_{100}^{(g)} + \pi_{010}^{(g)} + \pi_{001}^{(g)})$ as the probability of having no outcome of interest for a patient assigned to treatment group g. Suppose that we randomly assign $n_g (g = 1,0)$ patients to treatment group g. We let $n_{ijk}^{(g)}$ denote the number of patients among n_g patients corresponding to the cell probability $\pi_{ijk}^{(g)}$, where $(i, j, k) = (1, 0, 0), (0, 1, 0), (0, 0, 1), (0, 0, 0)$. Thus, the random vector $\underline{n}_g = (n_{100}^{(g)}, n_{010}^{(g)}, n_{001}^{(g)}, n_{000}^{(g)})$ follows a multinomial distribution with parameters n_g and $\underline{\pi}_g = (\pi_{100}^{(g)}, \pi_{010}^{(g)}, \pi_{001}^{(g)}, \pi_{000}^{(g)})$. An unbiased consistent estimator for $\pi_{ijk}^{(g)}$ is then $\hat{\pi}_{ijk}^{(g)} = n_{ijk}^{(g)}/n_g$.

(e) Show that $\gamma = -(B + \sqrt{B^2 - 4AC})/(2A)$, where $A = \pi_{100}^{(1)} - \pi_{100}^{(0)} = -(p_{1FC}^{(0)} + p_{1PCI}^{(0)})$, $B = \pi_{010}^{(1)} - \pi_{010}^{(0)} = p_{1PCI}^{(1)} - p_{1PCII}^{(0)} = \gamma p_{1PCI}^{(0)} - p_{1PCII}^{(0)}$, and $C = \pi_{001}^{(1)} - \pi_{001}^{(0)} = p_{1FC}^{(1)} + p_{1PCII}^{(1)} = \gamma^2 p_{1FC}^{(0)} + \gamma p_{1PCII}^{(0)}$. Thus, we may obtain a consistent estimator for γ as $\hat{\gamma} = -(\hat{B} + \sqrt{\hat{B}^2 - 4\hat{A}\hat{C}})/(2\hat{A})$ by simply substituting $\hat{\pi}_{ijk}^{(g)}$ for $\pi_{ijk}^{(g)}$, where $\hat{A} = \hat{\pi}_{100}^{(1)} - \hat{\pi}_{100}^{(0)}$, $\hat{B} = \hat{\pi}_{010}^{(1)} - \hat{\pi}_{010}^{(0)}$, and $\hat{C} = \hat{\pi}_{001}^{(1)} - \hat{\pi}_{001}^{(0)}$.

(f) Show that $B^2 - 4AC = (\gamma p_{1PCI}^{(0)} + 2\gamma p_{1FC}^{(0)} + p_{1PCII}^{(0)})^2$. Thus, as long as any of subpopulation proportions, $p_{1FC}^{(0)}$, $p_{1PCI}^{(0)}$, and $p_{1PCII}^{(0)}$, is > 0, the inequality $B^2 - 4AC > 0$ will hold.

(g) Show that when the treatment level is dichotomous (i.e. $\pi_{001}^{(1)} - \pi_{001}^{(0)} = 0$ and hence $\hat{\pi}_{001}^{(1)} - \hat{\pi}_{001}^{(0)} = 0$), $\hat{\gamma}$ reduces to (2.9) derived for a dichotomous treatment level.

(h) Show that, using the delta method, we obtain an estimated asymptotic variance for the MLE $\hat{\gamma}$ as given by

$$
\begin{aligned}
\hat{Var}(\hat{\gamma}) = &[\hat{C}(\hat{B}^2 - 4\hat{A}\hat{C})^{-1/2} - \hat{\gamma}]^2 [\hat{\pi}_{100}^{(1)}(1 - \hat{\pi}_{100}^{(1)})/n_1 \\
&+ \hat{\pi}_{100}^{(0)}(1 - \hat{\pi}_{100}^{(0)})/n_0]/\hat{A}^2 + [1 + \hat{B}(\hat{B}^2 - 4\hat{A}\hat{C})^{-1/2}]^2 \\
&\times [\hat{\pi}_{010}^{(1)}(1 - \hat{\pi}_{010}^{(1)})/n_1 + \hat{\pi}_{010}^{(0)}(1 - \hat{\pi}_{010}^{(0)})/n_0]/(4\hat{A}^2) \\
&+ (\hat{B}^2 - 4\hat{A}\hat{C})^{-1}[\hat{\pi}_{001}^{(1)}(1 - \hat{\pi}_{001}^{(1)})/n_1 + \hat{\pi}_{001}^{(0)}(1 - \hat{\pi}_{001}^{(0)})/n_0] \\
&+ [\hat{C}(\hat{B}^2 - 4\hat{A}\hat{C})^{-1/2} - \hat{\gamma}][1 + \hat{B}(\hat{B}^2 - 4\hat{A}\hat{C})^{-1/2}] \\
&\times [\hat{\pi}_{100}^{(1)}\hat{\pi}_{010}^{(1)}/n_1 + \hat{\pi}_{100}^{(0)}\hat{\pi}_{010}^{(0)}/n_0]/\hat{A}^2 \\
&- 2[\hat{C}(\hat{B}^2 - 4\hat{A}\hat{C})^{-1/2} - \hat{\gamma}](\hat{B}^2 - 4\hat{A}\hat{C})^{-1/2} \\
&\times [\hat{\pi}_{100}^{(1)}\hat{\pi}_{001}^{(1)}/n_1 + \hat{\pi}_{100}^{(0)}\hat{\pi}_{001}^{(0)}/n_0]/\hat{A} \\
&+ [1 + \hat{B}(\hat{B}^2 - 4\hat{A}\hat{C})^{-1/2}](\hat{B}^2 - 4\hat{A}\hat{C})^{-1/2} \\
&\times [\hat{\pi}_{010}^{(1)}\hat{\pi}_{001}^{(1)}/n_1 + \hat{\pi}_{010}^{(0)}\hat{\pi}_{001}^{(0)}/n_0]/\hat{A}.
\end{aligned}
$$

Thus, we can use the above results to derive an asymptotic $100(1 - \alpha)\%$ confidence interval for γ (Lui and Chang, 2009a). Note that when the dose level is ordinal, Goetghebeur, Molenberghs and Katz (1998) assumed monotone dose response and discussed estimation of the causal effect of compliance in a RCT on the basis of likelihood methods (Goetghebeur and Molenberghs, 1996).

2.26 Under the monotonicity and exclusion restriction assumptions for always-takers and never-takers with $0 < \pi_{+C} < 1$, using the ITT analysis tends to underestimate the relative treatment effect based on all three important indices, including the PD, PR, and OR. Confirming this by showing that: (a) If $\Delta > 0$, then $\Delta > \delta > 0$ and if $\Delta < 0$, then $\Delta < \delta < 0$, where Δ is defined in (2.1) and $\delta = \pi_{1+}^{(1)} - \pi_{1+}^{(0)}$. (b) If $\gamma > 1$, then $\gamma > \gamma_{ITT} > 1$, and if $\gamma < 1$, then $\gamma < \gamma_{ITT} < 1$, where γ is defined in (2.8) and $\gamma_{ITT} = \pi_{1+}^{(1)}/\pi_{1+}^{(0)}$.

(c) If $\varphi > 1$, then $\varphi > \varphi_{ITT} > 1$, and if $\varphi < 1$, then $\varphi < \varphi_{ITT} < 1$, where φ is defined in (2.12) and $\varphi_{ITT} = \pi_{1+}^{(1)}\pi_{2+}^{(0)}/(\pi_{2+}^{(1)}\pi_{1+}^{(0)})$. (d) Also, show that the following conditions are all equivalent (i.e. any one of the conditions implies the others): $\Delta = 0$, $\delta = 0$, $\gamma = 1$, $\gamma_{ITT} = 1$, $\varphi = 1$, and $\varphi_{ITT} = 1$.

2.27 Under SUTVA, the monotonicity assumption and exclusion restriction assumption for always-takers and never-takers, because $E(\hat{\delta}) = \Delta\pi_{+C} < \Delta$, the ITT estimate $\hat{\delta}$ tends to underestimate the treatment efficacy Δ. However, when the exclusion restriction assumption for always-takers or never-takers violates, the ITT estimate can overestimate treatment efficacy. For example, consider a population consisting of 50 % of compliers, 30 % of always-takers and 20 % of never-takers. Suppose that the conditional probabilities among compliers for the experimental and standard treatments are $P(survival|complier, g = 1) = 0.15$ and $P(survival|complier, g = 0) = 0.05$, respectively. Thus, the underlying PD for Δ here is 0.10. Suppose further that the exclusion restriction assumption for always-takers is violated. Say, we have $P(survival|always-takers, g = 1) = 0.50$, and $P(survival|always-takers, g = 0) = 0.10$, respectively. On the other hand, we assume that the exclusion restriction assumption for never-takers holds. Show that δ for the programmatic effectiveness in the ITT analysis is 0.17, which is larger than $\Delta = 0.10$. Readers should not confuse this note with the comments (Lui, 2009; Bang and Davis, 2007).

2.28 When using the OR to measure the relative treatment effect, we may consider use of the logistic model and assume that the conditional probability of a positive response for patient i assigned to treatment g, given the received-treatment $z_i^{(g)}(= 1$ for experimental; and $= 0$ for standard or placebo), is given by $P(Y_i^{(g)} = 1|z_i^{(g)}, p_i^{(g)}) = \exp(p_i^{(g)} + \psi_S z_i^{(g)})/(1 + \exp(p_i^{(g)} + \psi_S z_i^{(g)}))$ if patient $i \in S$ (where $S = C$, A, and N). Under the assumed logistic model, we can easily see that the OR of the probabilities of a positive response when patient i ($\in S$) receives the experimental treatment (i.e. $z_i^{(g)} = 1$) relative to that when he/she receives the standard treatment or placebo (i.e. $z_i^{(g)} = 0$) is $\exp(\psi_S)$. Show that the OR of the probabilities of a positive response among compliers $\varphi = (\pi_{1C}^{(1)}\pi_{2C}^{(0)})/(\pi_{2C}^{(1)}\pi_{1C}^{(0)})$ (2.12) is generally different from $\exp(\psi_C)$ due to the noncollapsibility of the OR. In other words, the parameter φ focused here no longer corresponds to a parameter in the structural logistic risk model. Some discussions on use of the logistic SMM model can be found elsewhere (Clarke and Windmeijer, 2010; Robins and Rotnitzky, 2004; Vansteelandt and Goetghebeur, 2003).

Appendix

The following SAS program is used to calculate the estimate of the minimum required number of patients n_1 (2.31) from the experimental treatment presented in Table 2.4 for testing superiority based on the test statistic (2.4).

```
data step1;
 za=probit(0.975); ** two-sided test at 0.05 level;
 zb=probit(0.80); ** desired power of 0.80;
 array nk(ii) nsam1-nsam5;
 put @25 "k=" @31 "1" @41 "2" @51 "3" @61 "4" @71 "8";
 do compr=1.0,0.90, 0.80, 0.70; ** proportion of subpopulation compliers;
 do delta=0.05,0.10; ** proportion difference of clinical interest among
compliers;
 do p1sdot=0.30, 0.50, 0.70; ** marginal proportion of a positive response
in the standard treatment or placebo;
 do k=1,2,3,4,8; ** sample allocation between the experimental and standard
treatments;
 p1edot=p1sdot+delta*compr; ** marginal proportion of a positive response
in the experimental treatment;
 p1pdot=(p1edot+k*p1sdot)/(1+k);
 s0=p1pdot*(1-p1pdot)*(1+1/k);
 s1=p1edot*(1-p1edot)+p1sdot*(1-p1sdot)/k;
 num=(za*sqrt(s0)+zb*sqrt(s1)/(1-(delta*compr)**2))**2;
 den=(0.5*log((1+delta*compr)/(1-delta*compr)))**2;
 if k = 1 then ii = 1;
 if k = 2 then ii = 2;
 if k = 3 then ii = 3;
 if k = 4 then ii = 4;
 if k = 8 then ii = 5;
 nk=ceil(num/den);
 if k = 8 then do;
 put compr 1-5 2 delta 8-13 2 p1sdot 16-20 2 nsam1 25-32 nsam2 35-42 nsam3
45-52 nsam4 55-62 nsam5 65-72 ;
 end;
 end; ** end of do k;
 end; ** end of do p1sdot;;
 end; ** end of do delta;
 end; ** end of do compr;
```

The following program is used to calculate the estimate of the minimum required number n_1 of patients from the experimental treatment for testing equivalence with respect to the OR presented in Table 2.5. This program uses the estimates n_1 (2.50)–(2.52) as the initial estimate and employs a trial-and-error procedure to find the minimum integer n_1 such that the power is larger than or equal to the desired power 80 %.

```
data step1;
 array fn(w1) fnx1-fnx4;
 za=probit(0.95);
 zb=probit(0.80);
 zb2=probit(0.90);
 ldellow=log(0.80); ** lower margin for OR on the logarithmic scale;
 ldelup=log(1.25); ** upper margin for OR on the logarithmic scale;
 do rprob=1,2; ** patterns of conditional prob of a positive response;
 ** for different subpopulations in standard treatment;
 if rprob =1 then do;
 rpc=0.20; rpa=0.35; rpn=0.25;
 end;
 if rprob = 2 then do;
 rpc=0.50; rpa=0.20; rpn=0.30;
 end;
 put rprob 20-50;
 do pattern=1,2; ** patterns of subpopulation distribution;
 if pattern= 1 then do;
 psc=0.95; psa=0.03; psn=0.02;
 end;
 if pattern = 2 then do;
 psc=0.80; psa=0.15; psn=0.05;
 end;
 do or=0.90,1.0,1.1;
 do sratio=1,2,3,4; ** ratio of sample allocation;
 rpce=or*rpc/(1+(or-1)*rpc);
 pi1cae=psc*rpce+psa*rpa;
 pi2cae=psc*(1-rpce)+psa*(1-rpa);
 pi1ne=psn*rpn;
 pi2ne=psn*(1-rpn);
 pi1cns=psc*rpc+psn*rpn;
 pi2cns=psc*(1-rpc)+psn*(1-rpn);
 pi1as=psa*rpa;
 pi2as=psa*(1-rpa);
 s1=(pi1cae*(1-pi1cae)+pi1as*(1-pi1as)/(sratio))/(pi1cae-pi1as)**2;
 s2=(pi2ne*(1-pi2ne)+pi2cns*(1-pi2cns)/(sratio))/(pi2cns-pi2ne)**2;
 s3=(pi2cae*(1-pi2cae)+pi2as*(1-pi2as)/(sratio))/(pi2cae-pi2as)**2;
 s4=(pi1ne*(1-pi1ne)+pi1cns*(1-pi1cns)/(sratio))/(pi1cns-pi1ne)**2;
 s12=(pi1cae*pi2ne+pi1as*pi2cns/(sratio))/((pi1cae-pi1as)*(pi2cns-pi2ne));
 s13=(pi1cae*pi2cae+pi1as*pi2as/(sratio))/((pi1cae-pi1as)*(pi2cae-pi2as));
 s14=(pi1cae*pi1ne+pi1cns*pi1as/(sratio))/((pi1cae-pi1as)*(pi1cns-pi1ne));
 s23=(pi2cae*pi2ne+pi2as*pi2cns/(sratio))/((pi2cae-pi2as)*(pi2cns-pi2ne));
 s24=(pi1ne*pi2ne+pi1cns*pi2cns/(sratio))/((pi2cns-pi2ne)*(pi1cns-pi1ne));
 s34=(pi2cae*pi1ne+pi2as*pi1cns/(sratio))/((pi2cae-pi2as)*(pi1cns-pi1ne));
 svar=s1+s2+s3+s4+2*s12+2*s13-2*s14-2*s23+2*s24+2*s34;
 if or lt 1 then n1s=ceil((za+zb)**2*svar/((ldellow-log(or))**2));
 if or gt 1 then n1s=ceil((za+zb)**2*svar/((ldelup-log(or))**2));
 if or eq 1 then n1s=ceil((za+zb2)**2*svar/(ldelup**2));
```

```
power=probnorm((ldelup-log(or))/sqrt(svar/n1s)-za)-
probnorm((ldellow-log(or))/sqrt(svar/n1s)+za);
do while (power lt 0.80);
n1s+1;
power=probnorm((ldelup-log(or))/sqrt(svar/n1s)-za)-
probnorm((ldellow-log(or))/sqrt(svar/n1s)+za);
end;
n1=n1s;
n0=n1*sratio;
if sratio eq 1 then w1=1;
if sratio eq 2 then w1=2;
if sratio eq 3 then w1=3;
if sratio eq 4 then w1=4;
fn=n1;
if sratio eq 4 then
put psc 1-5 2 psa 6-10 2 psn 11-15 2 or 16-20 2 fnx1 26-35 fnx2 36-45
fnx3 46-55 fnx4 56-65;
end; ** end of do sratio;
end; ** do or;
end; ** do pattern;
end; ** do rprob;
```

3

Randomized clinical trials with noncompliance in stratified sampling

When assessing the efficacy of an experimental treatment in a randomized clinical trial (RCT), we may encounter the situation in which one needs to account for the effects due to both confounders and noncompliance. For example, consider the multiple risk factor intervention trial (Multiple Risk Factor Intervention Trial Research Group, 1982) to reduce the mortality of coronary heard disease (CHD). Eligible men aged 35–57 years at increased risk of death from CHD were randomly assigned to either the intervention program, including smoking cessation counseling and other risk factor modification, or the control group in which patients were referred to their usual physicians for treatments. There were in the intervention group participants who continued smoking, while there were in the control group participants who quitted smoking. The extent of noncompliance also varies between strata formed by the number of cigarettes smoked per day at baseline. Thus, we may need to do stratified analysis to incorporate the effects due to noncompliance and the number of cigarettes smoked per day at baseline into estimation of the smoking effect to avoid making a possibly biased inference (Cuzick, Edwards and Segnan, 1997). Similarly,

Binary Data Analysis of Randomized Clinical Trials with Noncompliance, First Edition. Kung-Jong Lui.
© 2011 John Wiley & Sons, Ltd. Published 2011 by John Wiley & Sons, Ltd.

in practice we may have the difficulty in recruiting an appropriate number of patients from a single medical center into a RCT. To facilitate the collection of data, we often employ a multiple-center design, in which patients are enrolled from several centers into a trial under a common study protocol with independent randomization within each center. Because patients attending various centers may possess different characteristics and various noncompliance rates, we want to apply stratified analysis with strata formed by centers to control the center effects on patient responses (Fleiss, 1981). Using the intent-to-treat (ITT) analysis ignoring the information on noncompliance, we can use all statistical methods for stratified sampling discussed elsewhere (Fleiss, 1981; Lui, 2004). As noted in the previous chapters, however, the ITT analysis estimates the programmatic effectiveness rather than the treatment efficacy, and may lead us to obtain a biased inference when the latter is our interest.

Under the assumption that the underlying index used to measure the relative treatment effect is homogeneous across strata (i.e. there is no interaction between treatment and stratum effects), we discuss testing superiority between two treatments for a RCT with noncompliance in stratified analysis in Section 3.1. We further discuss testing noninferiority in Section 3.2 and testing equivalence in Section 3.3 based on the proportion difference (PD), the proportion ratio (PR) and the odds ratio (OR) in the presence of noncompliance under stratified sampling. We consider interval estimation of the underlying common PD, PR and OR in a stratified RCT with noncompliance in Section 3.4. Finally, we address testing the homogeneity of the PD, PR and OR across strata, while accounting for noncompliance in Section 3.5.

Consider comparing an experimental treatment ($g = 1$) with a standard treatment ($g = 0$) in a RCT with K strata formed by centers in a multi-center study or determined by the combined levels of several confounders. Suppose that for each stratum k ($k = 1, 2, \ldots, K$), we randomly assign n_{gk} ($g = 1$ for experimental, and $= 0$ for standard) patients to either of these two treatments, but some of these patients do not comply with their assigned treatment. To estimate the relative treatment effect, we make the stable unit treatment value assumption (SUTVA) – there is no interference between patients such that the outcome of a patient does not depend on either the outcome or the received-treatment of the other patients. For each patient, we define the vector $(d(1), d(0))$ as the status of his/her potential treatment receipt: $d(g) = 1$ if the patient assigned to treatment g ($g = 1, 0$) actually receives the experimental treatment, and $d(g) = 0$ otherwise. Thus, we may divide our population into four subpopulations. These include compliers ($d(1) = 1$ and $d(0) = 0$), never-takers ($d(1) = d(0) = 0$), always-takers ($d(1) = d(0) = 1$), and defiers ($d(1) = 0$ and $d(0) = 1$). We assume monotonicity ($d(1) \geq d(0)$) (i.e. no defiers). For stratum k ($k = 1, 2, \ldots, K$), let $\pi_{1S|k}^{(g)}$ denote the cell probability for a randomly selected patient assigned to treatment g ($= 1, 0$) who has a positive response and falls in category S: $S = C$ for compliers, $= A$ for always-takers, and $= N$ for never-takers. We further let $\pi_{2S|k}^{(g)}$ denote the corresponding cell probability of a negative response and treatment-received status S for a randomly selected patient assigned to treatment g in stratum k. To conveniently represent summation over a given subscript, we use '+' notation to designate summation of cell probabilities over that particular subscript. For example, we let $\pi_{+S|k}^{(1)}$ represent $\pi_{1S|k}^{(1)} + \pi_{2S|k}^{(1)}$.

Note that because we randomly assign patients to one of the two treatments within each stratum, we have $\pi_{+S|k}^{(1)} = \pi_{+S|k}^{(0)} = \pi_{+S|k}$ for $S = C$, A, N, where $\pi_{+S|k}$ denotes the proportion of subpopulation S in the sampling population for stratum k. We define $\pi_{1|Sk}^{(g)} = \pi_{1S|k}^{(g)}/\pi_{+S|k}$ ($g = 1, 0$, $S = C, A, N$; $k = 1, 2, \ldots, K$), the conditional probability of a positive response for patients assigned to treatment g ($g = 1, 0$) among subpopulation S in stratum k. Because patients are randomized to treatments and because always-takers (or never-takers) take the same experimental (or standard) treatment irrespective of their originally assigned treatment, the exclusion restriction assumption (Angrist, Imbens and Rubin, 1996) for always-takers and never-takers: $\pi_{1|Ak}^{(1)} = \pi_{1|Ak}^{(0)} (= \pi_{1|Ak})$ and $\pi_{1|Nk}^{(1)} = \pi_{1|Nk}^{(0)} (= \pi_{1|Nk})$, is likely to hold, especially for a double-blind study design. This together with $\pi_{+S|k}^{(1)} = \pi_{+S|k}^{(0)} = \pi_{+S|k}$ for $S = C$, A, N implies that $\pi_{rA|k}^{(1)} = \pi_{rA|k}^{(0)}$ and $\pi_{rN|k}^{(1)} = \pi_{rN|k}^{(0)}$ (for $r = 1, 2$, $k = 1, 2, 3, \ldots, K$). For simplicity, we may denote these common values by $\pi_{rA|k}$ and $\pi_{rN|k}$ whenever there is no confusion. For clarity, we may summarize in the following table the latent probability structure for the observed data of patients assigned to the experimental treatment ($g = 1$) in stratum k under the above assumptions:

In stratum k $(k = 1, 2, \ldots, K)$
Patients assigned to the experimental treatment $(g = 1)$

		Treatment actually received		
		Experimental treatment (CA)	Standard treatment (N)	Total
Outcome	Positive	$\pi^{(1)}_{1CA|k} = \pi^{(1)}_{1C|k} + \pi_{1A|k}$	$\pi_{1N|k}$	$\pi^{(1)}_{1+|k}$
	Negative	$\pi^{(1)}_{2CA|k} = \pi^{(1)}_{2C|k} + \pi_{2A|k}$	$\pi_{2N|k}$	$\pi^{(1)}_{2+|k}$
	Total	$\pi^{(1)}_{+CA|k} = \pi_{+C|k} + \pi_{+A|k}$	$\pi_{+N|k}$	1.0

For example, the parameter $\pi^{(1)}_{1CA|k} = \pi^{(1)}_{1C|k} + \pi_{1A|k}$ represents the cell probability that a randomly selected patient assigned to the experimental treatment $(g = 1)$ has a positive response and receives his/her assigned (experimental) treatment in stratum k. As another example, the parameter $\pi^{(1)}_{+CA|k} = \pi^{(1)}_{+C|k} + \pi_{+A|k}$ represents the compliance probability that a randomly selected patient assigned to the experimental treatment complies with his/her assigned (experimental) treatment in stratum k. Similarly, we may summarize in the following table the latent probability structure for the observed data of patients assigned to the standard treatment $(g = 0)$ in stratum k:

In stratum k $(k = 1, 2, \ldots, K)$
Patients assigned to the standard treatment $(g = 0)$

		Treatment actuallyreceived		
		Standard treatment (CN)	Experimental treatment (A)	Total
Outcome	Positive	$\pi^{(0)}_{1CN|k} = \pi^{(0)}_{1C|k} + \pi_{1N|k}$	$\pi_{1A|k}$	$\pi^{(0)}_{1+|k}$
	Negative	$\pi^{(0)}_{2CN|k} = \pi^{(0)}_{2C|k} + \pi_{2N|k}$	$\pi_{2A|k}$	$\pi^{(0)}_{2+|k}$
	Total	$\pi^{(0)}_{+CN|k} = \pi_{+C|k} + \pi_{+N|k}$	$\pi_{+A|k}$	1.0

Thus, the parameter $\pi^{(0)}_{1CN|k} = \pi^{(0)}_{1C|k} + \pi_{1N|k}$ represents the cell probability that a randomly selected patient assigned to the standard treatment

$(g = 0)$ has a positive response and receives his/her assigned (standard) treatment in stratum k. We let $n_{rS|k}^{(g)}$ denote the observed frequency of patients with the cell probability $\pi_{rS|k}^{(g)}$ among n_{gk} patients assigned to treatment g in stratum k ($r = 1, 2$; $S = CA, N$ for $g = 1$, and $S = CN$, A for $g = 0$). The random vector $(n_{1CA|k}^{(1)}, n_{1N|k}^{(1)}, n_{2CA|k}^{(1)}, n_{2N|k}^{(1)})$ then follows a multinomial distribution with parameters n_{1k} and $(\pi_{1CA|k}^{(1)}, \pi_{1N|k}^{(1)}, \pi_{2CA|k}^{(1)}, \pi_{2N|k}^{(1)})$, while the random vector $(n_{1CN|k}^{(0)}, n_{1A|k}^{(0)}, n_{2CN|k}^{(0)}, n_{2A|k}^{(0)})$ follows a multinomial distribution with parameters n_{0k} and $(\pi_{1CN|k}^{(0)}, \pi_{1A|k}^{(0)}, \pi_{2CN|k}^{(0)}, \pi_{2A|k}^{(0)})$, respectively. Therefore, the MLE for $\pi_{rS|k}^{(g)}$ is $\hat{\pi}_{rS|k}^{(g)} = n_{rS|k}^{(g)}/n_{gk}$. This leads the corresponding MLE for the marginal probabilities to be: $\hat{\pi}_{r+|k}^{(1)} = \hat{\pi}_{rCA|k}^{(1)} + \hat{\pi}_{rN|k}^{(1)}$, $\hat{\pi}_{r+|k}^{(0)} = \hat{\pi}_{rCN|k}^{(0)} + \hat{\pi}_{rA|k}^{(0)}$ ($r = 1, 2$), and $\hat{\pi}_{+S|k}^{(g)} = \hat{\pi}_{1S|k}^{(g)} + \hat{\pi}_{2S|k}^{(g)}$ ($S = CA, N$ for $g = 1$, and $S = CN, A$ for $g = 0$). Note that because $\pi_{+C|k} = \pi_{+CA|k} - \pi_{+A|k}$, the MLE for $\pi_{+C|k}$ is then given by $\hat{\pi}_{+C|k} = \hat{\pi}_{+CA|k}^{(1)} - \hat{\pi}_{+A|k}^{(0)} = \hat{\pi}_{+CA|k}^{(1)} + \hat{\pi}_{+CN|k}^{(0)} - 1$. Furthermore, because $\pi_{1C|k}^{(1)} = \pi_{1CA|k}^{(1)} - \pi_{1A|k}$ and $\pi_{1C|k}^{(0)} = \pi_{1CN|k}^{(0)} - \pi_{1N|k}$, we obtain the MLE for these parameters as $\hat{\pi}_{1C|k}^{(1)} = \hat{\pi}_{1CA|k}^{(1)} - \hat{\pi}_{1A|k}^{(0)}$ and $\hat{\pi}_{1C|k}^{(0)} = \hat{\pi}_{1CN|k}^{(0)} - \hat{\pi}_{1N|k}^{(1)}$, respectively. On the basis of the above results, the MLE for the conditional probability of a positive response among compliers assigned to treatment g in stratum k is $\hat{\pi}_{1|Ck}^{(g)} = \hat{\pi}_{1C|k}^{(g)}/\hat{\pi}_{+C|k}$, for $g = 1, 0$. We define the PD in the probabilities of a positive response among compliers between the two treatments in stratum k as

$$\Delta_k = \pi_{1|Ck}^{(1)} - \pi_{1|Ck}^{(0)}$$
$$= (\pi_{1+|k}^{(1)} - \pi_{1+|k}^{(0)})/\pi_{+C|k}. \tag{3.1}$$

Thus, the MLE for Δ_k is simply given by

$$\hat{\Delta}_k = \hat{\pi}_{1|Ck}^{(1)} - \hat{\pi}_{1|Ck}^{(0)}$$
$$= (\hat{\pi}_{1+|k}^{(1)} - \hat{\pi}_{1+|k}^{(0)})/(\hat{\pi}_{+CA|k}^{(1)} - \hat{\pi}_{+A|k}^{(0)}). \tag{3.2}$$

Note that under the monotonicity assumption and the exclusion restriction assumption for always-takers and never-takers, the PD, $\delta_k = \pi_{1+|k}^{(1)} - \pi_{1+|k}^{(0)}$, for the ITT analysis in stratum k can be easily shown to equal $\Delta_k \pi_{+C|k}$, which is an increasing function of the proportion of compliers $\pi_{+C|k}$. Because $0 < \pi_{+C|k} < 1$, we have $0 \le |\delta_k| \le |\Delta_k|$.

Thus, using the ITT analysis tends to attenuate the relative treatment effect. When $\pi_{+C|k} = 1$ (i.e. perfect compliance in stratum k), the PD δ_k for the ITT analysis is equal to the PD Δ_k for treatment efficacy in stratum k. On the other hand, if $\pi_{+C|k} \approx 0$, as noted in Chapter 2, the PD $\delta_k (= \Delta_k \pi_{+C|k})$ will be small regardless of a given fixed magnitude Δ_k of treatment efficacy.

Note that if the index used to measure the treatment effect is heterogeneous between strata, a summary test or estimator may mask the important treatment effect (Fleiss, 1981; Lui, 2004). For example, if a treatment has a positive effect on patient responses in some strata and a negative effect in other strata, a summary statistic may show no effect due to possibly canceling out between treatment effect estimates across strata. Therefore, we may not wish to provide a summary estimator of the underlying index in this case. This is because it is essentially important to allow investigators to see what situations under which the studied treatment has a beneficial effect and what situations under which the studied treatment has a harmful effect. In the following Sections 3.1–3.4, we assume that the underlying index used to measure the relative treatment effect is homogeneous across strata.

3.1   Testing superiority

When using the PD as the effect measure, the homogeneity assumption is equivalent to assume that $\Delta_1 = \Delta_2 = \cdots = \Delta_K$. We denote this common value by Δ_0. When comparing an experimental treatment with a standard treatment (or a placebo) in a multiple-centre trial, we are mostly interested in finding out whether the experimental treatment is better than the standard treatment (or the placebo) with respect to treatment efficacy over various centers. On the other hand, as noted in Chapter 2, we may wish to have an opportunity to detect that if the former should be unexpectedly worse than the latter for ethical and safety reasons (Fleiss, 1981). Thus, we consider testing $H_0 : \Delta_0 = 0$ versus $H_a : \Delta_0 \neq 0$. Note that $\Delta_k = 0$ if and only if $\delta_k = E(\hat{\pi}_{1+|k}^{(1)} - \hat{\pi}_{1+|k}^{(0)}) = 0$. Thus, for testing $H_0 : \Delta_0 (= \Delta_1 = \Delta_2 = \cdots = \Delta_K) = 0$, we can apply the ITT approach to test $H_0 : \delta_1 = \delta_2 = \cdots = \delta_K = 0$. This leads us to consider the statistic $\sum_k \hat{W}_k^{(RB)}(\hat{\pi}_{1+|k}^{(1)} - \hat{\pi}_{1+|k}^{(0)})$ with the estimated optimal weight $\hat{W}_k^{(RB)} = 1/\hat{Var}_{RB}(\hat{\pi}_{1+|k}^{(1)} - \hat{\pi}_{1+|k}^{(0)})$, where $\hat{Var}_{RB}(\hat{\pi}_{1+|k}^{(1)} - \hat{\pi}_{1+|k}^{(0)})$ is the randomization-based variance (Cochran, 1977) and is given by (Exercise 3.1) $\{(n_{1k} + n_{0k})^2/[n_{1k}n_{0k}(n_{1k} + n_{0k} - 1)]\}\hat{\pi}_{1+|k}^{(p)}(1 - \hat{\pi}_{1+|k}^{(p)})$, and $\hat{\pi}_{1+|k}^{(p)} = (n_{1k}\hat{\pi}_{1+|k}^{(1)} + n_{0k}\hat{\pi}_{1+|k}^{(0)})/(n_{1k} + n_{0k})$, the pooled estimate of the probability of a positive responses over the two treatments in stratum k. Note that when all n_{gk} are large, the variance of $\sum_k \hat{W}_k^{(RB)}(\hat{\pi}_{1+|k}^{(1)} - \hat{\pi}_{1+|k}^{(0)})$ can be approximated by $\sum_k \hat{W}_k^{(RB)}$ (Exercise 3.2). Therefore, we may use the following test statistic based on the ITT approach with the randomization-based variance to test $H_0 : \Delta_0(= \Delta_1 = \Delta_2 = \cdots = \Delta_K) = 0$,

$$Z = \sum_k \hat{W}_k^{(RB)}(\hat{\pi}_{1+|k}^{(1)} - \hat{\pi}_{1+|k}^{(0)})/\sqrt{\sum_k \hat{W}_k^{(RB)}}. \tag{3.3}$$

We will reject $H_0 : \Delta_0 = 0$ at the α-level if the test statistic (3.3), $Z > Z_{\alpha/2}$ or $Z < -Z_{\alpha/2}$. Furthermore, note that if the experimental treatment is superior to the standard treatment (i.e. $\Delta_0 > 0$), the PD $\delta_k(= \Delta_0\pi_{+C|k})$ for the ITT analysis will all tend to be positive and so is the test statistic (3.3). Thus, we will claim that the experimental treatment is superior to the standard treatment if the test statistic (3.3), $Z > Z_{\alpha/2}$. As noted elsewhere (Lui, 2007d), when the proportion $\pi_{+C|k}$ of compliers decreases, the expectation $E(\hat{\delta}_k) = \delta_k = \Delta_0\pi_{+C|k}$ becomes small, and hence the test statistic (3.3) can lack power. To alleviate this concern, we may consider use of the test statistic directly based on $\hat{\Delta}_k$ (3.2). Using the delta method (Casella and Berger, 1990; Agresti, 1990), we can show that an estimated asymptotic variance of $\hat{\Delta}_k$ under $H_0 : \Delta_0(= \Delta_1 = \Delta_2 = \cdots = \Delta_K) = 0$ is given by (Exercise 3.3),

$$\hat{Var}(\hat{\Delta}_k|H_0) = (n_{1k} + n_{0k})\hat{\pi}_{1+|k}^{(p)}(1 - \hat{\pi}_{1+|k}^{(p)})/[(\hat{\pi}_{+CA|k}^{(1)} - \hat{\pi}_{+A|k}^{(0)})^2 n_{1k}n_{0k}]. \tag{3.4}$$

Based on $\hat{\Delta}_k$ (3.2) and $\hat{Var}(\hat{\Delta}_k|H_0)$ (3.4), we obtain the following summary test statistic (Lui, 2007d),

$$Z = \sum_k \hat{W}_k(H_0)\hat{\Delta}_k/\sqrt{\sum_k \hat{W}_k(H_0)} \tag{3.5}$$

where $\hat{W}_k(H_0) = 1/\hat{Var}(\hat{\Delta}_k|H_0)$. When n_{gk} are all large, we will reject $H_0 : \Delta_0 (= \Delta_1 = \Delta_2 = \cdots = \Delta_K) = 0$ at the α-level if the test statistic

(3.5), $Z > Z_{\alpha/2}$ or $Z < -Z_{\alpha/2}$. Furthermore, we may claim that the experimental treatment is superior to the standard treatment if the test statistic (3.5), $Z > Z_{\alpha/2}$.

Attempting to improve the power of the test statistic (3.5), we may also consider the $\tanh^{-1}(x)$ $(= \frac{1}{2}\log((1+x)/(1-x)))$ transformation in use of $\hat{\Delta}_k$ (3.2) (Edwardes, 1995; Lui, 2002). Because the asymptotic variance $Var(\tanh^{-1}(\hat{\Delta}_k)|H_0) = Var(\hat{\Delta}_k|H_0)$ under $H_0 : \Delta_0(= \Delta_1 = \Delta_2 = \cdots = \Delta_K) = 0$, we obtain the following test statistic with the $\tanh^{-1}(x)$ transformation,

$$Z = [\sum_k \hat{W}_k(H_0) \tanh^{-1}(\hat{\Delta}_k)]/\sqrt{\sum_k \hat{W}_k(H_0)} \qquad (3.6)$$

We will reject $H_0 : \Delta_0(= \Delta_1 = \Delta_2 = \cdots = \Delta_K) = 0$ at the α-level if the test statistic (3.6), $Z > Z_{\alpha/2}$ or $Z < -Z_{\alpha/2}$. Furthermore, we may claim that the experimental treatment is superior to the standard treatment if the test statistic (3.6), $Z > Z_{\alpha/2}$.

When the number of patients n_{gk} is not moderate and the probability of a positive response $\pi_{1+|k}^{(p)}$ does not vary much between strata, one may consider weights similar as that used for the Mantel-Haenszel (MH) type estimator (Sato, 1995; Greenland and Robins, 1985) in the ITT analysis, and obtain the following test statistic,

$$Z = \sum_k \hat{W}_k^{(MH)}(\hat{\pi}_{1+|k}^{(1)} - \hat{\pi}_{1+|k}^{(0)})/\sqrt{\sum_k \hat{W}_k^{(MH)}\hat{\bar{\pi}}_{1+|k}^{(p)}(1 - \hat{\bar{\pi}}_{1+|k}^{(p)})},$$

$$(3.7)$$

where $\hat{W}_k^{(MH)} = (n_{1k}n_{0k})/(n_{1k} + n_{0k})$. We will reject $H_0 : \Delta_0(= \Delta_1 = \Delta_2 = \cdots = \Delta_K) = 0$ at the α-level if the statistic (3.7), $Z > Z_{\alpha/2}$ or $Z < -Z_{\alpha/2}$. Again, we may claim that the experimental treatment is superior to the standard treatment if the test statistic (3.7), $Z > Z_{\alpha/2}$.

On the basis of Monte Carlo simulation, Lui (2007d) evaluated and compared the performance of test statistics (3.3) and (3.5)–(3.7). Lui found that the estimated Type I error for test statistics (3.3), (3.5) and (3.7) agrees reasonably well with the nominal 0.05-level, while the estimated Type I error of the test statistic (3.6) with the $\tanh^{-1}(x)$ transformation can be slightly larger than the latter when the mean stratum size per treatment is small or moderate. Lui (2007d) further found that when the mean stratum size per treatment is moderate, the test statistic (3.5) is generally preferable to the others with respect to power subject to controlling Type I error reasonably well. However, the test statistic (3.6) with the $\tanh^{-1}(x)$ transformation can outperform the other with respect to power when the proportion of compliers is high ($\pi_{+C|k} \geq 0.95$) and the mean stratum size per treatment is large without sacrificing the accuracy of Type I error. When the underlying PD is large or when the mean stratum size per treatment is large, powers for all test statistics considered here are essentially equivalent and close to 1. Also, all powers of test statistics (3.3) and (3.5)–(3.7) decrease as the proportion of compliers $\pi_{+C|k}$ drops. Therefore, designing a RCT with a high extent of compliance will be of critical importance if one wishes to avoid a loss of power.

Example 3.1   To illustrate the use of test statistics in (3.3) and (3.5)–(3.7), consider the mortality data regarding CHD in Table 2.3 taken from the multiple risk factor intervention trial on men aged 35–57 years (Multiple Risk Factor Intervention Trial Research Group, 1982; Lui, 2007d). Participants were randomly assigned to either the intervention or the control group. Participants assigned to the intervention group were provided with dietary advice to reduce blood cholesterol, smoking cessation counseling, and hypertension medication, while participants assigned to the control group were referred to their usual physicians for medical care. Although the trial attempted to investigate the intervention effects due to the reduction of multiple factors, only the counseling for cigarettes smoking cessation was actually effective, while the other factors changed minimal due to the intervention program. Thus, we focus our attention on the effect of quitting cigarette smoking. We base on the number of cigarettes per day at baseline (1–29, and $\geq$ 30 per day) to determine the strata. When applying test statistics in (3.3) and (3.5)–(3.7) to test whether there is an effect due to quitting smoking on reducing the CHD death incidence, we obtain test values Z as -0.467, -0.467, -0.437, and -0.449, respectively (2007d). Obviously, none of these resulting test values suggests that there be significant evidence to claim that quitting smoking can reduce the risk of CHD death at the 5 % in middle-aged men. This is consistent with the finding published elsewhere (Matsui, 2005).

3.2   Testing noninferiority

When establishing an experimental treatment to be effective against a disease or an infection, we may often consider testing superiority by investigating whether the new treatment improves the probability of a positive response as compared with a placebo group. It can be sometimes unethical, however, to have a placebo controlled group for a RCT. Thus, we may want to compare the experimental treatment with the standard treatment. Because it is more difficult to beat an established (standard) treatment than a placebo, we can be pleased if one demonstrates that the experimental treatment is noninferior to the standard treatment. This is true especially when the experimental treatment has fewer side effects or less expense to administer than the standard treatment (Rousson and Seifert, 2008). In this section, we discuss testing noninferiority based on the PD, PR and OR to measure the relative treatment effect in a stratified RCT with noncompliance. We focus our discussion on large strata, in which the number n_{gk} of patients assigned to both treatments $g \, (= 1, 0)$ is large for all strata.

Note that each statistic, which leads to produce a one-sided lower bound for an index, can be actually used to develop a corresponding test procedure for testing noninferiority. Generally speaking, we may claim that an experimental treatment is noninferior to a standard treatment with respect to a given index at the α-level as long as the corresponding $100(1-\alpha)$ % one-sided lower limit for this index is larger than or equal to the acceptable noninferior margin. For brevity, we will present only the test procedure based on the WLS approach for each of the indices in testing noninferiority.

3.2.1   Using the difference in proportions

To measure the relative treatment effect between an experimental treatment and a standard treatment in a RCT, the PD is probably the most frequently used index because of its easiness of understanding and interpretation. When establishing noninferiority, we want to test $H_0 : \Delta_0 \leq -\varepsilon_l$ versus $H_a : \Delta_0 > -\varepsilon_l$, where Δ_0 denotes the underlying common value Δ_k under the homogeneity assumption, and $\varepsilon_l \, (> 0)$ is the maximum acceptable margin such that the experimental drug can be regarded as noninferior to the standard treatment when the inequality $\Delta_0 > -\varepsilon_l$ holds.

First, we consider the following most commonly used weighted-least-squares (WLS) point estimator for Δ_0 with the estimated optimal weight minimizing the variance of linear combination of $\hat{\Delta}_k$ (Fleiss, 1981),

$$\hat{\Delta}_{WLS} = [\sum_k \hat{W}_k^{(WLSPD)} \hat{\Delta}_k]/ \sum_k \hat{W}_k^{(WLSPD)}, \qquad (3.8)$$

where $\hat{W}_k^{(WLSPD)} = 1/\hat{Var}(\hat{\Delta}_k)$ and

$$\hat{Var}(\hat{\Delta}_k) = \{[\hat{\pi}_{1+|k}^{(1)}(1 - \hat{\pi}_{1+|k}^{(1)})/n_{1k} + \hat{\pi}_{1+|k}^{(0)}(1 - \hat{\pi}_{1+|k}^{(0)})/n_{0k}]$$
$$+ \hat{\Delta}_k^2[\hat{\pi}_{+CA|k}^{(1)}(1 - \hat{\pi}_{+CA|k}^{(1)})/n_{1k} + \hat{\pi}_{+A|k}^{(0)}(1 - \hat{\pi}_{+A|k}^{(0)})/n_{0k}]$$
$$- 2\hat{\Delta}_k[(\hat{\pi}_{1CA|k}^{(1)} - \hat{\pi}_{1+|k}^{(1)}\hat{\pi}_{+CA|k}^{(1)})/n_{1k}$$
$$+ (\hat{\pi}_{1A|k}^{(0)} - \hat{\pi}_{1+|k}^{(0)}\hat{\pi}_{+A|k}^{(0)})/n_{0k}]\}/(\hat{\pi}_{+CA|k}^{(1)} - \hat{\pi}_{+A|k}^{(0)})^2.$$

Note that an estimated asymptotic variance $\hat{Var}(\hat{\Delta}_{WLS})$ of $\hat{\Delta}_{WLS}$ (3.8) can be shown to approximately equal $1/\sum_k \hat{W}_k^{(WLSPD)}$ (Exercise 3.4). On the basis of these results, we obtain the following test statistic,

$$Z = (\hat{\Delta}_{WLS} + \varepsilon_l)\sqrt{\sum_k \hat{W}_k^{(WLSPD)}}. \qquad (3.9)$$

We will reject $H_0 : \Delta_0 \leq -\varepsilon_l$ at the α-level and claim that the experimental treatment is noninferior to the standard treatment if the test statistic (3.9), $Z > Z_\alpha$.

Because the $\tanh^{-1}(x)$ transformation has been successfully applied to improve the performance of the test statistic relevant to the PD under other situations (Edwardes, 1995; Lui, 2002), we may also consider use of this transformation on $\hat{\Delta}_k$ in testing noninferiority. Furthermore, note that the asymptotic variance $Var(\tanh^{-1}(\hat{\Delta}_k))$ is given by $Var(\hat{\Delta}_k)$ $/ (1 - \Delta_0^2)^2$ under the assumption $\Delta_1 = \Delta_2 = \cdots = \Delta_K = \Delta_0$. Thus, the estimated optimal weight minimizing the variance of linear combination of $\tanh^{-1}(\hat{\Delta}_k)$ can be the same as that for the WLS estimator of $\hat{\Delta}_k$. This leads us to consider the following test statistic with the $\tanh^{-1}(\hat{\Delta}_k)$ transformation,

$$\hat{\Delta}_{WLS}^{(TR)} = [\sum_k \hat{W}_k^{(WLSPD)} \tanh^{-1}(\hat{\Delta}_k)]/ \sum_k \hat{W}_k^{(WLSPD)}. \qquad (3.10)$$

Note that as n_{gk} is all large, an estimated asymptotic variance of $\hat{\Delta}_{WLS}^{(TR)}$ is given by $\hat{Var}(\hat{\Delta}_{WLS}^{(TR)}) = 1/[(1 - \hat{\Delta}_{WLS}^2)^2 \sum_k \hat{W}_k^{(WLSPD)}]$ (Exercise 3.5). Thus, we obtain the following statistic for testing noninferiority,

$$Z = [(\hat{\Delta}_{WLS}^{(TR)}) + \tanh^{-1}(\varepsilon_l)]\sqrt{(1 - \hat{\Delta}_{WLS}^2)^2 \sum_k \hat{W}_k^{(WLSPD)}}. \qquad (3.11)$$

We will reject $H_0 : \Delta_0 \le -\varepsilon_l$ at the α-level if the test statistic (3.11), $Z > Z_\alpha$.

When employing statistics (3.9) and (3.11) to test noninferiority, we need to make the assumption of homogeneity with respect to the PD (i.e. $\Delta_1 = \Delta_2 = \cdots = \Delta_K = \Delta_0$). This assumption can be, however, commonly violated in practice, especially when the underlying probability of a positive response for the standard treatment varies between strata (Fleiss, 1981). By contrast, the indices PR and OR can be relatively more stable than the PD across strata. Thus, when doing stratified analysis or meta-analysis, we may consider using the PR or OR more frequently than using the PD to measure the relative treatment effect.

3.2.2   Using the ratio of proportions

Recall the PR which is well known to lack symmetry when the 'positive' and 'negative' outcomes are interchanged. For clarity, we define the PR in stratum k ($k = 1, 2, \ldots, K$) as the ratio of conditional probabilities of a positive response among compliers between the experimental and standard treatments here,

$$\gamma_k = \pi_{1|Ck}^{(1)}/\pi_{1|Ck}^{(0)} = \pi_{1C|k}^{(1)}/\pi_{1C|k}^{(0)}. \qquad (3.12)$$

Based on the data in stratum k, we can estimate γ_k by simply substituting $\hat{\pi}_{1|Ck}^{(g)}$ for $\pi_{1|Ck}^{(g)}$ in (3.12) to obtain the following estimator,

$$\begin{aligned} \hat{\gamma}_k &= \hat{\pi}_{1|Ck}^{(1)}/\hat{\pi}_{1|Ck}^{(0)} = \hat{\pi}_{1C|k}^{(1)}/\hat{\pi}_{1C|k}^{(0)} \\ &= (\hat{\pi}_{1CA|k}^{(1)} - \hat{\pi}_{1A|k}^{(0)})/(\hat{\pi}_{1CN|k}^{(0)} - \hat{\pi}_{1N|k}^{(1)}). \end{aligned} \qquad (3.13)$$

Note that the homogeneity assumption for the PR is to mean that $\gamma_1 = \gamma_2 = \cdots = \gamma_K$. We denote these common values of γ_k by γ_0. When establishing noninferiority, we want to test $H_0 : \gamma_0 \le 1 - \gamma_l$

versus $H_a : \gamma_0 > 1 - \gamma_l$, where γ_l is the maximum clinically acceptable margin such that the experimental treatment can be regarded as non-inferior to the standard treatment when the inequality $\gamma_0 > 1 - \gamma_l$ holds. When rejecting $H_0 : \gamma_0 \le 1 - \gamma_l$ at the α-level, we claim that the experimental treatment is noninferior to the standard treatment. As the number of patients n_{gk} assigned to treatment g in stratum k is large for all strata, we may consider the WLS test statistic with the logarithmic transformation,

$$\hat{\gamma}_{WLS}^{(LOG)} = [\sum_k \hat{W}_k^{(WLSLPR)} \log(\hat{\gamma}_k)] / \sum_k \hat{W}_k^{(WLSLPR)}, \qquad (3.14)$$

where $\hat{W}_k^{(WLSLPR)} = 1/\hat{Var}(\log(\hat{\gamma}_k))$ and

$$\hat{Var}(\log(\hat{\gamma}_k)) = [\hat{\pi}_{1CA|k}^{(1)}(1 - \hat{\pi}_{1CA|k}^{(1)})/n_{1k} + \hat{\pi}_{1A|k}^{(0)}(1 - \hat{\pi}_{1A|k}^{(0)})/n_{0k}]/$$
$$(\hat{\pi}_{1CA|k}^{(1)} - \hat{\pi}_{1A|k}^{(0)})^2 + [\hat{\pi}_{1N|k}^{(1)}(1 - \hat{\pi}_{1N|k}^{(1)})/n_{1k}$$
$$+ \hat{\pi}_{1CN|k}^{(0)}(1 - \hat{\pi}_{1CN|k}^{(0)})/n_{0k}]/(\hat{\pi}_{1CN|k}^{(0)} - \hat{\pi}_{1N|k}^{(1)})^2$$
$$- 2[\hat{\pi}_{1CA|k}^{(1)}\hat{\pi}_{1N|k}^{(1)}/n_{1k} + \hat{\pi}_{1CN|k}^{(0)}\hat{\pi}_{1A|k}^{(0)}/n_{0k}]/$$
$$[(\hat{\pi}_{1CA|k}^{(1)} - \hat{\pi}_{1A|k}^{(0)})(\hat{\pi}_{1CN|k}^{(0)} - \hat{\pi}_{1N|k}^{(1)})].$$

We can easily show that an estimated asymptotic variance $\hat{Var}(\hat{\gamma}_{WLS}^{(LOG)})$ is $1/\sum_k \hat{W}_k^{(WLSLPR)}$. Thus, we obtain the following test statistic based on $\hat{\gamma}_{WLS}^{(LOG)}$ (3.14),

$$Z = (\hat{\gamma}_{WLS}^{(LOG)} - \log(1 - \gamma_l))\sqrt{\sum_k \hat{W}_k^{(WLSLPR)}}. \qquad (3.15)$$

We will reject $H_0 : \gamma_0 \le 1 - \gamma_l$ at the α-level and claim that the experimental treatment is noninferior to the standard treatment if the test statistic (3.15), $Z > Z_\alpha$. When one employs the PR to measure the relative treatment effect, however, the noninferior margin for the PR may produce a corresponding noninferior margin on the PD scale against the FDA (1997) general guideline – the acceptable margin on the PD scale in a draft for establishing the effectiveness of a new *H. pylori* regimen should generally decrease as the probability of the underlying response increases from 0.50 to 0.90 (see Section 2.2.2). This leads us to consider use of the OR to measure the relative treatment effect in establishing noninferiority (Garrett, 2003).

3.2.3   Using the odds ratio of proportions

Because use of the OR to measure the relative treatment effect can lead us to obtain a clinically acceptable margin following well along with the general guideline of a draft provided by the FDA (1997) for testing noninferiority, the OR has been recommended for use (Garrett, 2003; Tu, 1998 and 2003; Wang, Chow and Li, 2002). In terms of the probability of a positive response among compliers between the experimental and standard treatments in stratum k, we define the OR as

$$\varphi_k = (\pi_{1|Ck}^{(1)}/\pi_{2|Ck}^{(1)})/(\pi_{1|Ck}^{(0)}/\pi_{2|Ck}^{(0)}) = (\pi_{1C|k}^{(1)}\pi_{2C|k}^{(0)})/(\pi_{2C|k}^{(1)}\pi_{1C|k}^{(0)}). \quad (3.16)$$

Thus, we may simply substitute $\hat{\pi}_{rC|k}^{(g)}$ for $\pi_{rC|k}^{(g)}$ in φ_k (3.16) and obtain the following estimator given by

$$\hat{\varphi}_k = (\hat{\pi}_{1C|k}^{(1)}\hat{\pi}_{2C|k}^{(0)})/(\hat{\pi}_{2C|k}^{(1)}\hat{\pi}_{1C|k}^{(0)})$$
$$= [(\hat{\pi}_{1CA|k}^{(1)} - \hat{\pi}_{1A|k}^{(0)})(\hat{\pi}_{2CN|k}^{(0)} - \hat{\pi}_{2N|k}^{(1)})]/$$
$$[(\hat{\pi}_{2CA|k}^{(1)} - \hat{\pi}_{2A|k}^{(0)})(\hat{\pi}_{1CN|k}^{(0)} - \hat{\pi}_{1N|k}^{(1)})]. \quad (3.17)$$

We assume the homogeneity of OR (i.e. $\varphi_1 = \varphi_2 = \cdots = \varphi_K$) and denote these common values of φ_k by φ_0. When testing noninferiority, we want to test $H_0 : \varphi_0 \le 1 - \varphi_l$ versus $H_0 : \varphi_0 > 1 - \varphi_l$, where φ_l is the maximum clinically acceptable margin such that the experimental treatment can be regarded as noninferior to the standard treatment when the inequality $\varphi_0 > 1 - \varphi_l$ holds. Because the sampling distribution of $\hat{\varphi}_k$ can be skewed, we consider the following test statistic using the WLS approach with the logarithmic transformation,

$$\hat{\varphi}_{WLS}^{(LOG)} = [\sum_k \hat{W}_k^{(WLSLOR)} \log(\hat{\varphi}_k)]/\sum_k \hat{W}_k^{(WLSLOR)}, \quad (3.18)$$

where $\hat{W}_k^{(WLSLOR)} = 1/\hat{Var}(\log(\hat{\varphi}_k))$ and

$$\hat{Var}(\log(\hat{\varphi}_k)) = [\hat{\pi}_{1CA|k}^{(1)}(1 - \hat{\pi}_{1CA|k}^{(1)})/n_{1k} + \hat{\pi}_{1A|k}^{(0)}(1 - \hat{\pi}_{1A|k}^{(0)})/n_{0k}]/$$
$$(\hat{\pi}_{1CA|k}^{(1)} - \hat{\pi}_{1A|k}^{(0)})^2 + [\hat{\pi}_{2CN|k}^{(0)}(1 - \hat{\pi}_{2CN|k}^{(0)})/n_{0k}$$
$$+ \hat{\pi}_{2N|k}^{(1)}(1 - \hat{\pi}_{2N|k}^{(1)})/n_{1k}]/(\hat{\pi}_{2CN|k}^{(0)} - \hat{\pi}_{2N|k}^{(1)})^2$$
$$+ [\hat{\pi}_{2CA|k}^{(1)}(1 - \hat{\pi}_{2CA|k}^{(1)})/n_{1k} + \hat{\pi}_{2A|k}^{(0)}(1 - \hat{\pi}_{2A|k}^{(0)})/n_{\theta k}]/$$
$$(\hat{\pi}_{2CA|k}^{(1)} - \hat{\pi}_{2A|k}^{(0)})^2 + [\hat{\pi}_{1CN|k}^{(0)}(1 - \hat{\pi}_{1CN|k}^{(0)})/n_{0k}$$

$$+ \hat{\pi}_{1N|k}^{(1)}(1 - \hat{\pi}_{1N|k}^{(1)})/n_{1k}]/(\hat{\pi}_{1CN|k}^{(0)} - \hat{\pi}_{1N|k}^{(1)})^2$$
$$+ 2[\hat{\pi}_{1CA|k}^{(1)}\hat{\pi}_{2N|k}^{(1)}/n_{1k} + \hat{\pi}_{1A|k}^{(0)}\hat{\pi}_{2CN|k}^{(0)}/n_{0k}]/$$
$$[(\hat{\pi}_{1CA|k}^{(1)} - \hat{\pi}_{1A|k}^{(0)})(\hat{\pi}_{2CN|k}^{(0)} - \hat{\pi}_{2N|k}^{(1)})]$$
$$+ 2[\hat{\pi}_{1CA|k}^{(1)}\hat{\pi}_{2CA|k}^{(1)}/n_{1k} + \hat{\pi}_{1A|k}^{(0)}\hat{\pi}_{2A|k}^{(0)}/n_{0k}]/$$
$$[(\hat{\pi}_{1CA|k}^{(1)} - \hat{\pi}_{1A|k}^{(0)})(\hat{\pi}_{2CA|k}^{(1)} - \hat{\pi}_{2A|k}^{(0)})]$$
$$- 2[\hat{\pi}_{1CA|k}^{(1)}\hat{\pi}_{1N|k}^{(1)}/n_{1k} + \hat{\pi}_{1CN|k}^{(0)}\hat{\pi}_{1A|k}^{(0)}/n_{0k}]/$$
$$[(\hat{\pi}_{1CA|k}^{(1)} - \hat{\pi}_{1A|k}^{(0)})(\hat{\pi}_{1CN|k}^{(0)} - \hat{\pi}_{1N|k}^{(1)})]$$
$$- 2[\hat{\pi}_{2CA|k}^{(1)}\hat{\pi}_{2N|k}^{(1)}/n_{1k} + \hat{\pi}_{2A|k}^{(0)}\hat{\pi}_{2CN|k}^{(0)}/n_{0k}]/$$
$$[(\hat{\pi}_{2CA|k}^{(1)} - \hat{\pi}_{2A|k}^{(0)})(\hat{\pi}_{2CN|k}^{(0)} - \hat{\pi}_{2N|k}^{(1)})]$$
$$+ 2[\hat{\pi}_{1N|k}^{(1)}\hat{\pi}_{2N|k}^{(1)}/n_{1k} + \hat{\pi}_{1CN|k}^{(0)}\hat{\pi}_{2CN|k}^{(0)}/n_{0k}]/$$
$$[(\hat{\pi}_{2CN|k}^{(0)} - \hat{\pi}_{2N|k}^{(1)})(\hat{\pi}_{1CN|k}^{(0)} - \hat{\pi}_{1N|k}^{(1)})]$$
$$+ 2[\hat{\pi}_{2CA|k}^{(1)}\hat{\pi}_{1N|k}^{(1)}/n_{1k} + \hat{\pi}_{2A|k}^{(0)}\hat{\pi}_{1CN|k}^{(0)}/n_{0k}]/$$
$$[(\hat{\pi}_{2CA|k}^{(1)} - \hat{\pi}_{2A|k}^{(0)})(\hat{\pi}_{1CN|k}^{(0)} - \hat{\pi}_{1N|k}^{(1)})].$$

An estimated asymptotic variance $\hat{Var}(\hat{\varphi}_{WLS}^{(LOG)})$ of $\hat{\varphi}_{WLS}^{(LOG)}$ can be shown to be given by $1/\sum_k \hat{W}_k^{(WLSLOR)}$. The above results lead us to obtain the following statistic for testing noninferiority,

$$Z = (\hat{\varphi}_{WLS}^{(LOG)} - \log(1 - \varphi_l))\sqrt{\sum_k \hat{W}_k^{(WLSLOR)}}. \qquad (3.19)$$

We will reject $H_0 : \varphi_0 \leq 1 - \varphi_l$ at the α-level and claim that the experimental treatment is noninferior to the standard treatment if the test statistic (3.19), $Z > Z_\alpha$.

3.3   Testing equivalence

When an increase in the patient positive response rate for an experimental treatment (or a new generic drug) can raise the concern of toxicity, we may wish to test equivalence rather than noninferiority with respect to treatment efficacy. As noted for testing noninferiority, each statistic leading to produce a confidence interval for an index can be employed to develop a corresponding test procedure for testing equivalence. We may claim that an experimental treatment is equivalent to a standard treatment with respect to a given index used to measure the relative treatment effect at the α-level if the corresponding $100(1-2\,\alpha)$ % confidence interval for this index is completely contained in the acceptable interval given by clinicians. For brevity, we will present only the test procedures developed in the previous section for assessing noninferiority to accommodate testing equivalence in a stratified RCT with noncompliance in the following subsections.

3.3.1   Using the difference in proportions

When using the PD to measure the relative treatment effect in establishing equivalence, we want to test $H_0 : \Delta_0 \leq -\varepsilon_l$ or $\Delta_0 \geq \varepsilon_u$ versus $H_a : -\varepsilon_l < \Delta_0 < \varepsilon_u$, where ε_l and ε_u (>0) are the pre-determined maximum clinically acceptable lower and upper margins that the experimental drug can be regarded as equivalent to the standard treatment when the inequality $-\varepsilon_l < \Delta_0 < \varepsilon_u$ holds. Using the Intersection-Union test (Casella and Berger, 1990), we will reject the null hypothesis $H_0 : \Delta_0 \leq -\varepsilon_l$ or $\Delta_0 \geq \varepsilon_u$ at the α-level and claim that the two treatments are equivalent if the test statistic $\hat{\Delta}_{WLS}$ (3.8) simultaneously satisfies the following two inequalities:

$$(\hat{\Delta}_{WLS} + \varepsilon_l)\sqrt{\sum_k \hat{W}_k^{(WLSPD)}} > Z_\alpha \text{ and}$$

$$(\hat{\Delta}_{WLS} - \varepsilon_u)\sqrt{\sum_k \hat{W}_k^{(WLSPD)}} < -Z_\alpha. \qquad (3.20)$$

Similarly, when using the test statistic $\hat{\Delta}_{WLS}^{(TR)}$ (3.10) with the $\tanh^{-1}(\hat{\Delta}_k)$ transformation, we will reject the null hypothesis $H_0 : \Delta_0 \leq -\varepsilon_l$ or $\Delta_0 \geq \varepsilon_u$ at the α-level and claim that the two treatments are equivalent if the test statistic $\hat{\Delta}_{WLS}^{(TR)}$ simultaneously satisfies the following two inequalities:

$$[(\hat{\Delta}_{WLS}^{(TR)}) + \tanh^{-1}(\varepsilon_l)]\sqrt{(1 - \hat{\Delta}_{WLS}^{(2)})^2 \sum_k \hat{W}_k^{(WLSPD)}} > Z_\alpha \text{ and}$$

$$[(\hat{\Delta}_{WLS}^{(TR)}) - \tanh^{-1}(\varepsilon_u)]\sqrt{(1 - \hat{\Delta}_{WLS}^{(2)})^2 \sum_k \hat{W}_k^{(WLSPD)}} < -Z_\alpha. \qquad (3.21)$$

Note that when there is only a single one stratum (i.e. $K = 1$), the test procedure (3.21) reduces to the test procedure (2.16) for the case of no stratum.

3.3.2   Using the ratio of proportions

When using the PR to measure the relative treatment effect among compliers in establishing equivalence, we want to test $H_0 : \gamma_0 \leq 1 - \gamma_l$ or $\gamma_0 \geq 1 + \gamma_u$ versus $H_a : 1 - \gamma_l < \gamma_0 < 1 + \gamma_u$ where γ_l and γ_u (> 0) are the pre-determined maximum clinically acceptable lower and upper margins that the experimental drug can be regarded as equivalent to the standard treatment when the inequality $1 - \gamma_l < \gamma_0 < 1 + \gamma_u$ holds. We will reject $H_0 : \gamma_0 \leq 1 - \gamma_l$ or $\gamma_0 \geq 1 + \gamma_u$ at the α-level and claim that two treatments are equivalent if the test statistic $\hat{\gamma}_{WLS}^{(LOG)}$ (3.14) satisfies the following two inequalities:

$$[\hat{\gamma}_{WLS}^{(LOG)} - \log(1 - \gamma_l)]\sqrt{\sum_k \hat{W}_k^{(WLSLPR)}} > Z_\alpha$$

and

$$[\hat{\gamma}_{WLS}^{(LOG)} - \log(1 + \gamma_u)]\sqrt{\sum_k \hat{W}_k^{(WLSLPR)}} < -Z_\alpha. \tag{3.22}$$

When we have only a single one stratum, the test procedure (3.22) reduces to the test procedure (2.17).

3.3.3   Using the odds ratio of proportions

When using the OR to measure the relative treatment effect in establishing equivalence, we want to test $H_0 : \varphi_0 \leq 1 - \varphi_l$ or $\varphi_0 \geq 1 + \varphi_u$ versus $H_a : 1 - \varphi_l < \varphi_0 < 1 + \varphi_u$, where φ_l and φ_u are the pre-determined maximum clinically acceptable lower and upper margins that the experimental treatment can be regarded as equivalent to the standard treatment when the inequality $1 - \varphi_l < \varphi_0 < 1 + \varphi_u$ is true. We will reject $H_0 : \varphi_0 \leq 1 - \varphi_l$ or $\varphi_0 \geq 1 + \varphi_u$ at the α-level if the test statistic

$\hat{\varphi}_{WLS}^{(LOG)}$ (3.18) simultaneously satisfies the following two inequalities:

$$[\hat{\varphi}_{WLS}^{(LOG)} - \log(1 - \varphi_l)]\sqrt{\sum_k \hat{W}_k^{(WLSLOR)}} > Z_\alpha$$

and

$$[\hat{\varphi}_{WLS}^{(LOG)} - \log(1 + \varphi_u)]\sqrt{\sum_k \hat{W}_k^{(WLSLOR)}} < -Z_\alpha. \qquad (3.23)$$

Note that when $K = 1$, the test procedure (3.23) simplifies to the test procedure (2.18).

3.4   Interval estimation

It is well known that when the number of patients in both treatments is large, we may obtain statistical significance in despite of a possibly small difference of no clinical significance between two treatment effects. On the other hand, we may obtain a null test result even for a given difference of clinical importance in two treatment effects if the number of patients in our trial is small. Because an interval estimator can provide us with the information on both the magnitude of the relative treatment effect and the precision of our inference, interval estimation is probably one of the most useful and important tools to summarize clinical findings. We discuss interval estimation of the PD, PR and OR in a stratified RCT with noncompliance in this section.

3.4.1   Estimation of the proportion difference

First, consider use of the WLS point estimator $\hat{\Delta}_{WLS}$ (3.8) and its asymptotic variance $\hat{Var}(\hat{\Delta}_{WLS}) = 1/\sum_k \hat{W}_k^{(WLSPD)}$. When the number of patients n_{gk} assigned to treatment g in each stratum k is large, we obtain an asymptotic $100(1 - \alpha)\%$ confidence interval for the underlying common Δ_0 based on $\hat{\Delta}_{WLS}$ (3.8) as

$$[\max\{\hat{\Delta}_{WLS} - Z_{\alpha/2}/\sqrt{\sum_k \hat{W}_k^{(WLSPD)}}, -1\},$$

$$\min\{\hat{\Delta}_{WLS} + Z_{\alpha/2}/\sqrt{\sum_k \hat{W}_k^{(WLSPD)}}, 1\}], \qquad (3.24)$$

where max{a, b} and min{a, b} denote the maximum and the minimum of values a and b, respectively. This is due to the fact that the range for Δ_0 is subject to $[-1, 1]$. Note that the ranges for $\tanh^{-1}(x)$ and $\tanh(y)$ $(= (e^y - e^{-y})/(e^y + e^{-y}))$ are $-\infty < \tanh^{-1}(x) < \infty$ and $-1 < \tanh(y) < 1$, respectively. Thus, we can avoid using the functions max{a, b} and min{a, b} in (3.24) when employing these transformations. These lead us to obtain the following asymptotic $100 (1 - \alpha) \%$ confidence interval for the underlying common Δ_0 as

$$[\tanh(\hat{\Delta}_{WLS}^{(TR)} - Z_{\alpha/2}/\sqrt{\sum_k \hat{W}_k^{(WLSPD)}(1 - \hat{\Delta}_{WLS}^2)^2}),$$

$$\tanh(\hat{\Delta}_{WLS}^{(TR)} + Z_{\alpha/2}/\sqrt{\sum_k \hat{W}_k^{(WLSPD)}(1 - \hat{\Delta}_{WLS}^2)^2})]. \quad (3.25)$$

Note that the sampling distribution of $\hat{\Delta}_k$ (3.2), a ratio of two random variables, can be skewed. To alleviate this concern in application of interval estimator (3.24), we employ the general idea behind Fieller's Theorem (Casella and Berger, 1990) and define

$$T_k = (\hat{\pi}_{1+|k}^{(1)} - \hat{\pi}_{1+|k}^{(0)}) - \Delta_0(\hat{\pi}_{+CA|k}^{(1)} - \hat{\pi}_{+A|k}^{(0)}). \quad (3.26)$$

Note that the expectation $E(T_k) = 0$ and an asymptotic variance for T_k is (Exercise 3.6):

$$Var(T_k) = [\pi_{1+|k}^{(1)}(1 - \pi_{1+|k}^{(1)}) + \Delta_0^2\pi_{+CA|k}^{(1)}(1 - \pi_{+CA|k}^{(1)})$$
$$- 2\Delta_0(\pi_{1CA|k}^{(1)} - \pi_{1+|k}^{(1)}\pi_{+CA|k}^{(1)})]/n_{1k} + [\pi_{1+|k}^{(0)}(1 - \pi_{1+|k}^{(0)})$$
$$+ \Delta_0^2\pi_{+A|k}^{(0)}(1 - \pi_{+A|k}^{(0)}) - 2\Delta_0(\pi_{1A|k}^{(0)} - \pi_{1+|k}^{(0)}\pi_{+A|k}^{(0)})]/n_{0k}.$$
$$(3.27)$$

This leads us to consider the linear combination $\sum_k W_k^* T_k$, where $W_k^* = 1/Var(T_k)$. We note the expectation $E(\sum_k W_k^* T_k) = 0$. As all n_{gk} are large, we have

$$P(\{(\sum_k \hat{W}_k^* T_k)^2/Var(\sum_k \hat{W}_k^* T_k)\} \leq Z_{\alpha/2}^2) \approx 1 - \alpha,$$

where $\hat{W}_k^* = 1/\hat{Var}(T_k)$ and $\hat{Var}(T_k)$ is the estimated variance by substituting $\hat{\pi}_{rS|k}^{(g)}$ for $\pi_{rS|k}^{(g)}$, $\hat{\pi}_{r+|k}^{(g)}$ for $\pi_{r+|k}^{(g)}$, $\hat{\pi}_{+S|k}^{(g)}$ for $\pi_{+S|k}^{(g)}$, and $\hat{\Delta}_k$ for Δ_0 in $Var(T_k)$ (3.27). Therefore, we obtain the following quadratic equation

(Exercise 3.7):

$$A^* \Delta_0^2 - 2B^* \Delta_0 + C^* \leq 0, \tag{3.28}$$

where

$$A^* = (\sum_k \hat{W}_k^* (\hat{\pi}_{+CA|k}^{(1)} - \hat{\pi}_{+A|k}^{(0)}))^2 - Z_{\alpha/2}^2 \sum_k (\hat{W}_k^*)^2$$
$$\times [\hat{\pi}_{+CA|k}^{(1)} (1 - \hat{\pi}_{+CA|k}^{(1)})/n_{1k} + \hat{\pi}_{+A|k}^{(0)} (1 - \hat{\pi}_{+A|k}^{(0)})/n_{0k}],$$
$$B^* = (\sum_k \hat{W}_k^* (\hat{\pi}_{1+|k}^{(1)} - \hat{\pi}_{1+|k}^{(0)}))(\sum_k \hat{W}_k^* (\hat{\pi}_{+CA|k}^{(1)} - \hat{\pi}_{+A|k}^{(0)}))$$
$$- Z_{\alpha/2}^2 \sum_k (\hat{W}_k^*)^2 [(\hat{\pi}_{1CA|k}^{(1)} - \hat{\pi}_{1+|k}^{(1)} \hat{\pi}_{+CA|k}^{(1)})/n_{1k}$$
$$+ (\hat{\pi}_{1A|k}^{(0)} - \hat{\pi}_{1+|k}^{(0)} \hat{\pi}_{+A|k}^{(0)})/n_{0k}], \text{ and}$$
$$C^* = (\sum_k \hat{W}_k^* (\hat{\pi}_{1+|k}^{(1)} - \hat{\pi}_{1+|k}^{(0)}))^2 - Z_{\alpha/2}^2 \sum_k (\hat{W}_k^*)^2$$
$$\times [\hat{\pi}_{1+|k}^{(1)} (1 - \hat{\pi}_{1+|k}^{(1)})/n_{1k} + \hat{\pi}_{1+|k}^{(0)} (1 - \hat{\pi}_{1+|k}^{(0)})/n_{0k}].$$

When $A^* > 0$ and $(B^*)^2 - A^* C^* > 0$, an asymptotic $100 (1 - \alpha)$ % confidence interval for Δ_0 is given by

$$[\max\{(B^* - \sqrt{(B^*)^2 - A^* C^*})/A^*, -1\},$$
$$\min\{(B^* + \sqrt{(B^*)^2 - A^* C^*})/A^*, 1\}]. \tag{3.29}$$

Following Cochran (1977, p. 23), we can show that the randomization-based variance of T_k under simple random sampling in stratum k is (Exercise 3.8):

$$\hat{Var}_{RB}(T_k) = [(n_{1k} + n_{0k})^2]/[n_{1k} n_{0k} (n_{1k} + n_{0k} - 1)]\{\hat{\pi}_{1+|k}^{(RB)} (1 - \hat{\pi}_{1+|k}^{(RB)})$$
$$+ \hat{\Delta}_k^2 \hat{\pi}_{+1|k}^{(RB)} (1 - \hat{\pi}_{+1|k}^{(RB)}) - 2\hat{\Delta}_k (\hat{\pi}_{11|k}^{(RB)} - \hat{\pi}_{1+|k}^{(RB)} \hat{\pi}_{+1|k}^{(RB)})\}, \tag{3.30}$$

where

$$\hat{\pi}_{r1|k}^{(RB)} = (n_{1k} \hat{\pi}_{rCA|k}^{(1)} + n_{0k} \hat{\pi}_{rA|k}^{(0)})/(n_{1k} + n_{0k}),$$
$$\hat{\pi}_{r0|k}^{(RB)} = (n_{1k} \hat{\pi}_{rN|k}^{(1)} + n_{0k} \hat{\pi}_{rCN|k}^{(0)})/(n_{1k} + n_{0k}),$$
$$\hat{\pi}_{r+|k}^{(RB)} = \sum_t \hat{\pi}_{rt|k}^{(RB)} \quad \text{for} \quad r = 1, 2, \quad \text{and}$$
$$\hat{\pi}_{+t|k}^{(RB)} = \sum_r \hat{\pi}_{rt|k}^{(RB)} \quad \text{for} \quad t = 1, 0.$$

As both n_{gk} are large, we have

$$P(\{(\sum_k \hat{W}_k^{**} T_k)^2 / Var_{DB}(\sum_k \hat{W}_k^{**} T_k)\} \leq Z_{\alpha/2}^2) \approx 1 - \alpha,$$

where $\hat{W}_k^{**} = 1/\hat{Var}_{RB}(T_k)$. Thus, we consider the following quadratic equation:

$$A^{**} \Delta_0^2 - 2\Delta_0 B^{**} + C^{**} \leq 0, \tag{3.31}$$

where

$$A^{**} = (\sum_k \hat{W}_k^{**} (\hat{\pi}_{+CA|k}^{(1)} - \hat{\pi}_{+A|k}^{(0)}))^2 - Z_{\alpha/2}^2 \sum_k (\hat{W}_k^{**})^2 (n_{1k} + n_{0k})^2 /$$
$$[n_{1k} n_{0k} (n_{1k} + n_{0k} - 1)][\hat{\pi}_{+1|k}^{(RB)} (1 - \hat{\pi}_{+1|k}^{(RB)})],$$

$$B^{**} = (\sum_k \hat{W}_k^{**} (\hat{\pi}_{1+|k}^{(1)} - \hat{\pi}_{1+|k}^{(0)})) (\sum_k \hat{W}_k^{**} (\hat{\pi}_{+CA|k}^{(1)} - \hat{\pi}_{+A|k}^{(0)}))$$
$$- Z_{\alpha/2}^2 \sum_k (\hat{W}_k^{**})^2 (n_{1k} + n_{0k})^2 / [n_{1k} n_{0k} (n_{1k} + n_{0k} - 1)]$$
$$\times (\hat{\pi}_{11|k}^{(RB)} - \hat{\pi}_{1+|k}^{(RB)} \hat{\pi}_{+1|k}^{(RB)}),$$

$$C^{**} = (\sum_k \hat{W}_k^{**} (\hat{\pi}_{1+|k}^{(1)} - \hat{\pi}_{1+|k}^{(0)}))^2 - Z_{\alpha/2}^2 \sum_k (\hat{W}_k^{**})^2 (n_{1k} + n_{0k})^2 /$$
$$[n_{1k} n_{0k} (n_{1k} + n_{0k} - 1)][\hat{\pi}_{1+|k}^{(RB)} (1 - \hat{\pi}_{1+|k}^{(RB)})].$$

When $A^{**} > 0$ and $B^{**2} - A^{**} C^{**} > 0$, we obtain an asymptotic 100 $(1 - \alpha)$ % confidence interval for Δ_0 as

$$[\max\{(B^{**} - \sqrt{B^{**2} - A^{**} C^{**}})/A^{**}, -1\},$$
$$\min\{(B^{**} + \sqrt{B^{**2} - A^{**} C^{**}})/A^{**}, 1\}]. \tag{3.32}$$

Following Sato (2001) and Matsuyama (2002), Lui (2008b) assumed a constant risk additive model (see Section 2.6) and discussed interval estimation of the RD for a RCT with noncompliance in stratified sampling. Under the monotonicity assumption and exclusion restriction assumption (for always-takers and never-takers) as assumed here, we can see that all Lui's estimators are, in fact, identical to those presented as above. In other words, there is no need to make such a strong assumption as the constant risk additive model structure for the estimators derived elsewhere (Lui, 2008b) to be valid for use. Lui (2008b) employed Monte Carlo simulation to evaluate the finite-sample performance of (3.24), (3.25), (3.29) and (3.32) and compared these estimators with the interval estimator for the PD proposed by Matsui (2005) in a variety of situations. Because the interval estimator proposed by Matsui (2005) tends to lose accuracy when the underlying common Δ_0 lies away from 0 (Lui, 2008b), we do not include this interval estimator here for brevity. Lui found that the interval estimator (3.32) can perform well with respect to the coverage probability even when the number of patients n_{gk} per treatment is not large, while the other estimators considered here can be slightly liberal when n_{gk} is not large. Lui also found that the interval estimator (3.25) with $\tanh^{-1}(x)$ is likely more precise than the others with respect to the estimated average length when the probability of compliance is moderate or large. When the number of patients n_{gk} per treatment in all strata is large, all interval estimators are essentially equivalent with respect to both the estimated coverage probability and average length; they can all perform well.

Example 3.2   To illustrate the use of interval estimators (3.24), (3.25), (3.29) and (3.32), we consider the mortality data of CHD during a follow-up period of 7 years taken from a multiple risk factor intervention trial (Multiple Risk Factor Intervention Trial Research Group, 1982; Lui, 2008b) in Table 2.3. As noted previously, since smoking is the only risk factor that has been effectively reduced by the intervention, we restrict our attention to the effect of quitting smoking (Mark and Robins, 1993; Sato, 2000; Matsui, 2005). Based on these data, the estimates $\hat{\Delta}_k$ (3.2) for strata ($k =$) 1 and 2 were -0.0097 and -0.0079, respectively. Furthermore, we obtain the WLS estimator $\hat{\Delta}_{WLS}$ (3.8) for Δ_0 to be -0.0089. When applying interval estimators (3.24), (3.25), (3.29) and (3.32) to produce a 95 % confidence interval, we obtain $[-0.046, 0.029]$, $[-0.046, 0.029]$, $[-0.048, 0.030]$, and $[-0.048, 0.030]$, respectively. Since the number of participants assigned to both comparison groups is quite large here, it is really not surprising to see that all these resulting interval estimates are similar to one another. Because all the above confidence intervals contain 0, we conclude that there is no significant evidence at the 5 % level to support that the intervention program of smoking is effective for reducing the mortality of the CHD.

Because the assumption that the PD is constant across strata may seldom be satisfied in practice, the summary estimator for the PD can be of limited use. Thus, when wishing to obtain a summary inference of the relative treatment effect in stratified analysis, we may commonly consider use of the PR and OR rather than the PD.

3.4.2   Estimation of the proportion ratio

Since the PR is often more stable than the PD across centers (or trials) in a multiple-center trial (or meta-analysis) and is easier to clinically interpret than the OR (Sinclair and Bracken, 1994; Walter, 2000), the PR is likely one of the most commonly used summary indices to measure the relative treatment effect in stratified analysis. Note that the WLS point estimator for γ_0 under the homogeneity assumption of the PR for a RCT with noncompliance is given by (Lui and Chang, 2007):

$$\hat{\gamma}_{WLS} = (\sum_k \hat{W}_k^{(WLSLPR)} \hat{\gamma}_k) / \sum_k \hat{W}_k^{(WLSLPR)}, \qquad (3.33)$$

where $\hat{W}_k^{(WLSLPR)} = 1/\hat{Var}(\log(\hat{\gamma}_k))$. Thus, we obtain an asymptotic 100 $(1 - \alpha)\%$ confidence interval for γ_0 based on $\hat{\gamma}_{WLS}$ (3.33) with the logarithmic transformation as given by (Exercise 3.9),

$$[\hat{\gamma}_{WLS} \exp(-Z_{\alpha/2}/\sqrt{\sum_k \hat{W}_k^{(WLSLPR)}}),$$
$$\hat{\gamma}_{WLS} \exp(Z_{\alpha/2}/\sqrt{\sum_k \hat{W}_k^{(WLSLPR)}})]. \qquad (3.34)$$

Note that we may also consider an asymptotic 100 $(1 - \alpha)\%$ confidence interval for γ_0 based on $\hat{\gamma}_{WLS}^{(LOG)}$ (3.14) with the logarithmic transformation,

$$[\exp(\hat{\gamma}_{WLS}^{(LOG)} - Z_{\alpha/2}/\sqrt{\sum_k \hat{W}_k^{(WLSLPR)}}),$$
$$\exp(\hat{\gamma}_{WLS}^{(LOG)} + Z_{\alpha/2}/\sqrt{\sum_k \hat{W}_k^{(WLSLPR)}})]. \qquad (3.35)$$

When the stratum size is not large, interval estimators (3.34) and (3.35) using the WLS approach is expected to lose accuracy. In this case, we often consider use of the following MH type estimator as given by (Sato,

2001; Lui and Chang, 2007),

$$\hat{\gamma}_{MH} = \sum_k W_k^{(MH)}(\hat{\pi}_{1CA|k}^{(1)} - \hat{\pi}_{1A|k}^{(0)}) / \sum_k W_k^{(MH)}(\hat{\pi}_{1CN|k}^{(0)} - \hat{\pi}_{1N|k}^{(1)}),$$
(3.36)

where $W_k^{(MH)} = (n_{1k}n_{0k})/(n_{1k} + n_{0k})$. This leads us to obtain an asymptotic $100(1 - \alpha)\%$ confidence interval for γ_0 based on $\hat{\gamma}_{MH}$ (3.36) with the logarithmic transformation (Exercise 3.10),

$$[\hat{\gamma}_{MH} \exp(-Z_{\alpha/2}(\hat{Var}(\log(\hat{\gamma}_{MH})))^{1/2}),$$
$$\hat{\gamma}_{MH} \exp(Z_{\alpha/2}(\hat{Var}(\log(\hat{\gamma}_{MH})))^{1/2})].$$
(3.37)

where $\hat{Var}(\log(\hat{\gamma}_{MH})) = \hat{Var}(\hat{\gamma}_{MH})/\hat{\gamma}_{MH}^2$, and

$$\hat{Var}(\hat{\gamma}_{MH}) = \sum_k (W_k^{(MH)})^2 \{\hat{\pi}_{1CA|k}^{(1)}(1 - \hat{\pi}_{1CA|k}^{(1)}) - 2\hat{\gamma}_{MH}\hat{\pi}_{1CA|k}^{(1)}\hat{\pi}_{1N|k}^{(1)}$$
$$+ \hat{\gamma}_{MH}^2(\hat{\pi}_{1N|k}^{(1)}(1 - \hat{\pi}_{1N|k}^{(1)}))\}/$$
$$\{n_{1k}[\sum_k W_k^{(MH)}(\hat{\pi}_{1CN|k}^{(0)} - \hat{\pi}_{1N|k}^{(1)})]^2\}$$
$$+ \sum_k (W_k^{(MH)})^2 \{\hat{\pi}_{1A|k}^{(0)}(1 - \hat{\pi}_{1A|k}^{(0)}) - 2\hat{\gamma}_{MH}\hat{\pi}_{1A|k}^{(0)}\hat{\pi}_{1CN|k}^{(0)}$$
$$+ \hat{\gamma}_{MH}^2(\hat{\pi}_{1CN|k}^{(0)}(1 - \hat{\pi}_{1CN|k}^{(0)}))\}/$$
$$\{n_{0k}[\sum_k W_k^{(MH)}(\hat{\pi}_{1CN|k}^{(0)} - \hat{\pi}_{1N|k}^{(1)})]^2\}.$$

Assuming a constant risk multiplicative model (see Section 2.6.2), Lui and Chang (2007) applied various methods to derive several interval estimators for the PR and evaluated their performance in a variety of situations. By contrast, we here employ the principal stratification approach without assuming the structural constant risk model here. Because of the possible loss of efficiency (as noted in Chapter 2), however, Lui and Chang (2007) did not consider any interval estimator with the logarithmic transformation as presented here. When obtaining a summary estimator over strata, however, we put small weights to those estimators $\hat{\gamma}_k$ with large variations in stratified analysis. Thus, the loss of precision due to using the logarithmic transformation in stratified analysis should generally be of less concern especially when we have a few strata.

Example 3.3   To illustrate the use of the WLS point estimator $\hat{\gamma}_{WLS}$ (3.33) and the MH point estimator $\hat{\gamma}_{MH}$ (3.36), as well as interval estimators (3.34), (3.35) and (3.37), we consider the data in Table 2.3

taken from the multiple risk factor intervention trial (Multiple Risk Factor Intervention Trial Research Group, 1982) on reducing the mortality of coronary heart disease (CHD). Based on these data, we obtain the resulting estimates $\hat{\gamma}_{WLS}$ (3.33) and $\hat{\gamma}_{MH}$ (3.36) to be given by 0.559 and 0.561, respectively. When applying interval estimators (3.34), (3.35) and (3.37), we obtain the 95 % confidence intervals to be [0.065, 4.794], [0.065, 4.773] and [0.067, 4.697], respectively. Since these 95 % confidence intervals include the value of 1, there is no significant evidence at the 5 % to support that the intervention of quitting smoking is effective to reduce the mortality of CHD.

3.4.3   Estimation of the odds ratio

Due to its stability of the OR as compared with the PD between trials (Fleiss, 1981), the OR has been used as a summary index to measure the relative treatment effect in meta analysis or a RCT (Tu, 2003). Because the probability of a positive response is often not small in a RCT, a good interval estimator for the PR is probably inappropriate for use if one's interest is the OR, and vice versa. Thus, we discuss interval estimation of the underlying common value φ_0 under a stratified RCT separately.

As the number n_{gk} of patients for all strata is large, the most commonly used point estimator for φ_0 ($= \varphi_1 = \varphi_2 = \cdots = \varphi_K$) is likely the one using the WLS approach,

$$\hat{\varphi}_{WLS} = \sum_{k=1}^{K} \hat{W}_k^{(WLSLOR)} \hat{\varphi}_k / \sum_{k=1}^{K} \hat{W}_k^{(WLSLOR)}, \qquad (3.38)$$

where $\hat{W}_k^{(WLSLOR)} = 1/\hat{Var}(\log(\hat{\varphi}_k))$ is defined in (3.18). Because the sampling distribution for $\hat{\varphi}_k$ can be skewed, we may commonly consider use of the logarithmic transformation to improve the normal approximation of $\hat{\varphi}_k$. This leads us to consider the interval estimator based on $\hat{\varphi}_{WLS}^{(LOG)}$ (3.18). Thus, we obtain an asymptotic $100(1 - \alpha)$ % confidence interval for φ_0 as

$$[\exp(\hat{\varphi}_{WLS}^{(LOG)} - Z_{\alpha/2}/\sqrt{\sum_{k=1}^{K} \hat{W}_k^{(WLSLOR)}}),$$

$$\exp(\hat{\varphi}_{WLS}^{(LOG)} + Z_{\alpha/2}/\sqrt{\sum_{k=1}^{K} \hat{W}_k^{(WLSLOR)}})]. \qquad (3.39)$$

Note that when every patient complies with his/her assigned treatment (i.e. $\pi_{+A|k} = \pi_{+N|k} = 0$ for all strata k) in a RCT, the interval estimator (3.39) reduces to the commonly-used asymptotic interval estimator for the OR in stratified analysis (Fleiss, 1981; Agresti, 1990; Lui, 2004).

Furthermore, when the number n_{gk} of patients is not large, we may also consider the MH type of point estimator for φ_0,

$$\hat{\varphi}_{MH} = U/V, \tag{3.40}$$

where

$$U = \sum_{k=1}^{K} W_k^{(MH)}(\hat{\pi}_{1CA|k}^{(1)} - \hat{\pi}_{1A|k}^{(0)})(\hat{\pi}_{2CN|K}^{(0)} - \hat{\pi}_{2N|k}^{(1)}),$$

$$V = \sum_{k=1}^{K} W_k^{(MH)}(\hat{\pi}_{2CA|k}^{(1)} - \hat{\pi}_{2A|k}^{(0)})(\hat{\pi}_{1CN|K}^{(0)} - \hat{\pi}_{1N|k}^{(1)}), \text{ and}$$

$$W_k^{(MH)} = (n_{1k}n_{0k})/(n_{1k} + n_{0k}).$$

Note that for a RCT with perfect compliance (i.e. $\pi_{+A|k} = \pi_{+N|k} = 0$ and hence $\hat{\pi}_{rS|k}^{(g)} = 0$, $r = 1, 2$, $S = A, N$ for $g = 1, 0$), one can easily see that the estimator $\hat{\varphi}_{MH}$ (3.40) simplifies to the classical MH point estimator for the OR (Agresti, 1990; Fleiss, 1981; Lui, 2004).

Using the delta method (Casella and Berger, 1990; Agresti, 1990), we obtain an estimated asymptotic variance (Lui and Chang, 2009b) for $\log(\hat{\varphi}_{MH})$ as given by (Exercise 3.11).

$$\widehat{Var}(\log(\hat{\varphi}_{MH})) = \{\sum_k (W_k^{(MH)})^2(\hat{\pi}_{2CN|k}^{(0)} - \hat{\pi}_{2N|k}^{(1)})^2[\hat{\pi}_{1CA|k}^{(1)}(1 - \hat{\pi}_{1CA|k}^{(1)})/$$

$$n_{1k} + \hat{\pi}_{1A|k}^{(0)}(1 - \hat{\pi}_{1A|k}^{(0)})/n_{0k}]$$

$$+ \sum_k (W_k^{(MH)})^2(\hat{\pi}_{1CA|k}^{(1)} - \hat{\pi}_{1A|k}^{(0)})^2[\hat{\pi}_{2CN|k}^{(0)}(1 - \hat{\pi}_{2CN|k}^{(0)})/$$

$$n_{0k} + \hat{\pi}_{2N|k}^{(1)}(1 - \hat{\pi}_{2N|k}^{(1)})/n_{1k}]\}/U^2$$

$$+\{\sum_k (W_k^{(MH)})^2(\hat{\pi}_{1CN|k}^{(0)} - \hat{\pi}_{1N|k}^{(1)})^2[\hat{\pi}_{2CA|k}^{(1)}(1 - \hat{\pi}_{2CA|k}^{(1)})/$$

$$n_{1k} + \hat{\pi}_{2A|k}^{(0)}(1 - \hat{\pi}_{2A|k}^{(0)})/n_{0k}]$$

$$+ \sum_k (W_k^{(MH)})^2(\hat{\pi}_{2CA|k}^{(1)} - \hat{\pi}_{2A|k}^{(0)})^2[\hat{\pi}_{1CN|k}^{(0)}(1 - \hat{\pi}_{1CN|k}^{(0)})/$$

$$n_{0k} + \hat{\pi}_{1N|k}^{(1)}(1 - \hat{\pi}_{1N|k}^{(1)})/n_{1k}]\}/V^2$$

$$+ 2\{\sum_k (W_k^{(MH)})^2(\hat{\pi}_{1CA|k}^{(1)} - \hat{\pi}_{1A|k}^{(0)})(\hat{\pi}_{2CN|k}^{(0)} - \hat{\pi}_{2N|k}^{(1)})$$

$$\times [\hat{\pi}_{1CA|k}^{(1)}\hat{\pi}_{2N|k}^{(1)}/n_{1k} + \hat{\pi}_{1A|k}^{(0)}\hat{\pi}_{2CN|k}^{(0)}/n_{0k}]\}/U^2$$

$$+2\{\sum_k (W_k^{(MH)})^2(\hat{\pi}_{2CN|k}^{(0)} - \hat{\pi}_{2N|k}^{(1)})(\hat{\pi}_{1CN|k}^{(0)} - \hat{\pi}_{1N|k}^{(1)})$$

$$\times [\hat{\pi}_{1CA|k}^{(1)}\hat{\pi}_{2CA|k}^{(1)}/n_{1k} + \hat{\pi}_{1A|k}^{(0)}\hat{\pi}_{2A|k}^{(0)}/n_{0k}]\}/(UV)$$

$$-2\{\sum_k (W_k^{(MH)})^2(\hat{\pi}_{2CA|k}^{(1)} - \hat{\pi}_{2A|k}^{(0)})(\hat{\pi}_{2CN|k}^{(0)} - \hat{\pi}_{2N|k}^{(1)})$$

$$\times [\hat{\pi}_{1CA|k}^{(1)}\hat{\pi}_{1N|k}^{(1)}/n_{1k} + \hat{\pi}_{1CN|k}^{(0)}\hat{\pi}_{1A|k}^{(0)}/n_{0k}]\}/(UV)$$

$$-2\{\sum_k (W_k^{(MH)})^2(\hat{\pi}_{1CA|k}^{(1)} - \hat{\pi}_{1A|k}^{(0)})(\hat{\pi}_{1CN|k}^{(0)} - \hat{\pi}_{1N|k}^{(1)})$$

$$\times [\hat{\pi}_{2CA|k}^{(1)}\hat{\pi}_{2N|k}^{(1)}/n_{1k} + \hat{\pi}_{2A|k}^{(0)}\hat{\pi}_{2CN|k}^{(0)}/n_{0k}]\}/(UV)$$

$$+2\{\sum_k (W_k^{(MH)})^2(\hat{\pi}_{1CA|k}^{(1)} - \hat{\pi}_{1A|k}^{(0)})(\hat{\pi}_{2CA|k}^{(1)} - \hat{\pi}_{2A|k}^{(0)})$$

$$\times [\hat{\pi}_{1N|k}^{(1)}\hat{\pi}_{2N|k}^{(1)}/n_{1k} + \hat{\pi}_{1CN|k}^{(0)}\hat{\pi}_{2CN|k}^{(0)}/n_{0k}]\}/(UV)$$

$$+2\{\sum_k (W_k^{(MH)})^2(\hat{\pi}_{2CA|k}^{(1)} - \hat{\pi}_{2A|k}^{(0)})(\hat{\pi}_{1CN|k}^{(0)} - \hat{\pi}_{1N|k}^{(1)})$$

$$\times [\hat{\pi}_{2CA|k}^{(1)}\hat{\pi}_{1N|k}^{(1)}/n_{1k} + \hat{\pi}_{2A|k}^{(0)}\hat{\pi}_{1CN|k}^{(0)}/n_{0k}]\}/V^2.$$

$$(3.41)$$

Thus, on the basis of (3.40) and (3.41), we obtain an asymptotic 100 $(1 - \alpha)$ % confidence interval for φ_0 as

$$[\hat{\varphi}_{MH} \exp(-Z_{\alpha/2}(\hat{Var}(\log(\hat{\varphi}_{MH})))^{1/2}),$$
$$\hat{\varphi}_{MH} \exp(Z_{\alpha/2}(\hat{Var}(\log(\hat{\varphi}_{MH})))^{1/2})]. \qquad (3.42)$$

When the number of strata $K = 1$ (i.e. there are no strata), the interval estimator (3.39) and interval estimator (3.42) are actually identical.

Note that $\hat{\varphi}_{MH}$ (3.40) can be regarded as a ratio estimator. Following Cochran (1977), we may consider use of the following asymptotic variance estimator for $\hat{\varphi}_{MH}$ with respect to the random sampling scheme when the number of strata K is moderate or large,

$$\hat{Var}_{RSS}(\hat{\varphi}_{MH}) = \sum_{k=1}^{K} (W_k^{(MH)})^2[(\hat{\pi}_{1CA|k}^{(1)} - \hat{\pi}_{1A|k}^{(0)})(\hat{\pi}_{2CN|K}^{(0)} - \hat{\pi}_{2N|k}^{(1)})$$
$$- \varphi_0(\hat{\pi}_{2CA|k}^{(1)} - \hat{\pi}_{2A|k}^{(0)})(\hat{\pi}_{1CN|K}^{(0)} - \hat{\pi}_{1N|k}^{(1)})]^2/\{K(K-1)$$
$$[\sum_{k=1}^{K} W_k^{(MH)}(\hat{\pi}_{2CA|k}^{(1)} - \hat{\pi}_{2A|k}^{(0)})(\hat{\pi}_{1CN|K}^{(0)} - \hat{\pi}_{1N|k}^{(1)})/K]^2\}.$$

$$(3.43)$$

On the basis of (3.40) and (3.43), as the number of strata K is moderate or large, we have the probability

$$P((\hat{\varphi}_{MH} - \varphi_0)^2 \leq Z_{\alpha/2}^2 \sum_{k=1}^{K} (\hat{W}_k^{(MH)})^2 [(\hat{\pi}_{1CA|k}^{(1)} - \hat{\pi}_{1A|k}^{(0)})(\hat{\pi}_{2CN|K}^{(0)} - \hat{\pi}_{2N|k}^{(1)})$$
$$- \varphi_0(\hat{\pi}_{2CA|k}^{(1)} - \hat{\pi}_{2A|k}^{(0)})(\hat{\pi}_{1CN|K}^{(0)} - \hat{\pi}_{1N|k}^{(1)})]^2 /$$
$$\{K(K-1)[\sum_{k=1}^{K} \hat{W}_k^{(MH)}(\hat{\pi}_{2CA|k}^{(1)} - \hat{\pi}_{2A|k}^{(0)})$$
$$\times (\hat{\pi}_{1CN|K}^{(0)} - \hat{\pi}_{1N|k}^{(1)})/K]^2\}) \approx 1 - \alpha. \quad (3.44)$$

From equation (3.44), as long as $A^\dagger > 0$ and $B^{\dagger 2} - A^\dagger C^\dagger > 0$, we can obtain an asymptotic $100(1-\alpha)\%$ confidence interval for φ_0 derived from a quadratic equation with respect to random sampling scheme as (Exercise 3.12)

$$[\max\{(B^\dagger - (B^{\dagger 2} - A^\dagger C^\dagger)^{1/2})/A^\dagger, 0\}, \ (B^\dagger + (B^{\dagger 2} - A^\dagger C^\dagger)^{1/2})/A^\dagger],$$
$$(3.45)$$

where

$$A^\dagger = 1 - Z_{\alpha/2}^2 \sum_{k=1}^{K} (W_k^{(MH)})^2 [(\hat{\pi}_{2CA|k}^{(1)} - \hat{\pi}_{2A|k}^{(0)})(\hat{\pi}_{1CN|K}^{(0)} - \hat{\pi}_{1N|k}^{(1)})]^2 /$$
$$\{K(K-1)[\sum_{k=1}^{K} W_k^{(MH)}(\hat{\pi}_{2CA|k}^{(1)} - \hat{\pi}_{2A|k}^{(0)})(\hat{\pi}_{1CN|K}^{(0)} - \hat{\pi}_{1N|k}^{(1)})/K]^2\},$$

$$B^\dagger = \hat{\varphi}_{MH} - Z_{\alpha/2}^2 \sum_{k=1}^{K} (W_k^{(MH)})^2 (\hat{\pi}_{1CA|k}^{(1)} - \hat{\pi}_{1A|k}^{(0)})(\hat{\pi}_{2CN|K}^{(0)} - \hat{\pi}_{2N|k}^{(1)})$$
$$\times (\hat{\pi}_{2CA|k}^{(1)} - \hat{\pi}_{2A|k}^{(0)})(\hat{\pi}_{1CN|K}^{(0)} - \hat{\pi}_{1N|k}^{(1)})/\{K(K-1)$$
$$\times [\sum_{k=1}^{K} W_k^{(MH)}(\hat{\pi}_{2CA|k}^{(1)} - \hat{\pi}_{2A|k}^{(0)})(\hat{\pi}_{1CN|K}^{(0)} - \hat{\pi}_{1N|k}^{(1)})/K]^2\}, \ \text{and}$$

$$C^\dagger = \hat{\varphi}_{MH}^2 - Z_{\alpha/2}^2 \sum_{k=1}^{K} (W_k^{(MH)})^2 [(\hat{\pi}_{1CA|k}^{(1)} - \hat{\pi}_{1A|k}^{(0)})(\hat{\pi}_{2CN|K}^{(0)} - \hat{\pi}_{2N|k}^{(1)})]^2 /$$
$$\{K(K-1)[\sum_{k=1}^{K} W_k^{(MH)}(\hat{\pi}_{2CA|k}^{(1)} - \hat{\pi}_{2A|k}^{(0)})(\hat{\pi}_{1CN|K}^{(0)} - \hat{\pi}_{1N|k}^{(1)})/K]^2\}.$$

Using Monte Carlo simulation, Lui and Chang (2009b) evaluated and compared the performance of five interval estimators for φ_0, including the three interval estimators (3.39), (3.42) and (3.45) presented here. They found that interval estimators (3.39) and (3.42) can perform well and be preferable to the others in a variety of situations. They noted that the interval estimator (3.45) can be of use when the number of strata K is large, but should not be employed when the number of strata K is small or moderate. They further noted that the interval estimator (3.42) based on the MH type estimator can improve the bias of the interval estimator (3.39) based on the WLS estimator, while the latter tends to shift to the left. Note also that the OR changes to 1/OR when 'positive' and 'negative' outcomes are interchanged. Thus, it is desirable that the confidence limits for the OR are invariant with respect to the reciprocal transformation (Casella and Berger, 1990). We can easily see that interval estimators (3.39) and (3.42) possess this desirable invariance property (Exercise 3.13). Furthermore, we can show that when the two distinct real roots of the quadratic equation for the interval estimator (3.45) exist in $(0, \infty)$, this interval estimator also possesses the above desirable invariance property (Exercise 3.14).

Example 3.4   Consider the data (Table 2.3) taken from the multiple risk factor intervention trial (Multiple Risk Factor Intervention Trial Research Group, 1982) on reducing the mortality of CHD. Given these data, we obtain the corresponding point estimates of the underlying common OR φ_0 when using $\hat{\varphi}_{WLS}$ (3.38) and $\hat{\varphi}_{MH}$ (3.40) to be 0.554 and 0.541, respectively. Because there are only two strata formed by the number of cigarettes per day at baseline, the interval estimator (3.45) should not be used here. When applying the interval estimators (3.39) and (3.42) to produce a 95 % confidence interval, we obtain [0.062, 4.910] and [0.059, 4.944], respectively (Lui and Chang, 2009b). Since these interval estimates contain $\varphi_0 = 1$, there is no significant evidence at the 5 % level to support that the intervention program can reduce the risk of CHD death as compared with the control group. Note that because the mortality rate of CHD in the example (Table 2.3) is quite small, as what one expects, both the point and interval estimates for the OR obtained here are similar to those for the PR obtained in Example 3.3. However, this finding on the similarity of the resulting interval estimates for the PR and OR should not generally hold in most RCTs.

3.5   Test homogeneity of index in large strata

If a treatment effect on patient responses varies between strata, as noted previously, we may not wish to do a summary test or obtain a summary estimator of the treatment effect to avoid providing clinicians with a possibly misleading conclusion. Thus, it is crucial that we can justify the homogeneity assumption for the index used to measure the relative treatment effect based on our subjective knowledge before employing any summary statistics discussed in Sections 3.1–3.4. On the other hand, if we have no prior information on whether the homogeneity assumption is reasonable, it may be advisable that we can employ some test procedures to examine this assumption against our data.

Note that the PD, PR, and OR are three distinct indices. Except for the special case of a null relative treatment effect across strata, the homogeneity of any one of these three indices does not generally imply the homogeneity of the other two. Furthermore, because the characteristics of the sampling distributions for test statistics corresponding to these distinct indices can also be quite different, an approach leading to the development of a good test procedure for one index may not necessarily lead to the development of a good test procedure for the other two, and vice versa. Thus, we need to develop procedures for testing homogeneity and evaluate their performance for each index individually.

3.5.1   Testing homogeneity of the proportion difference

When assessing whether the PD is heterogeneous between strata, we want to test $H_0 : \Delta_1 = \Delta_2 = \cdots = \Delta_K$ versus H_a : not all Δ_k are equal. Recall that the PD for the ITT analysis is $\delta_k = \Delta_k \pi_{+C|k}$. The homogeneity of Δ_k will not imply the homogeneity of δ_k if the proportion of compliers $\pi_{+C|k}$ varies between strata. Similarly, the homogeneity of δ_k may not imply the homogeneity of Δ_k in a RCT with noncompliance either. Therefore, if our interest is the treatment efficacy, we cannot directly apply test procedures, which do not account for noncompliance (Lipsitz, Dear and Laird *et al.*, 1998; Lui and Kelly, 2000a), to test $H_0 : \Delta_1 = \Delta_2 = \cdots = \Delta_K$.

Following Fleiss (1981), we may use the following WLS statistic (Lui and Chang, 2008d) based on $\hat{\Delta}_{WLS}$ (3.8) to test $H_0 : \Delta_1 = \Delta_2 = \cdots = \Delta_K$ as the number of patients n_{gk} is large for all strata k,

$$
\begin{aligned}
T_{WLS}^{(HPD)} &= \sum_k \hat{W}_k^{(WLSPD)} (\hat{\Delta}_k - \hat{\Delta}_{WLS})^2 \\
&= \sum_k \hat{W}_k^{(WLSPD)} \hat{\Delta}_k^2 - \left(\sum_k \hat{W}_k^{(WLSPD)} \hat{\Delta}_k \right)^2 / \sum_k \hat{W}_k^{(WLSPD)},
\end{aligned}
$$

$$(3.46)$$

where the summation is over those K' strata for which $\hat{\Delta}_k$ exists. We will reject $H_0 : \Delta_1 = \Delta_2 = \cdots = \Delta_K$ at the α-level if the test statistic (3.46), $T_{WLS}^{(HPD)} > \chi^2_{\alpha, K'-1}$, where $\chi^2_{\alpha, K'-1}$ is the upper $100(\alpha)$th percentile of the chi-squared distribution with $K' - 1$ degrees of freedom.

Note that the $\tanh^{-1}(x) (= \frac{1}{2} \log((1 + x)/(1 - x)))$ transformation has been often suggested to improve the precision when interval estimation on the PD is considered (Edwardes, 1995; Lui, 2002 and 2005). We may consider using this transformation in application of $T_{WLS}^{(HPD)}$ (3.46). This leads us to obtain the following test statistic,

$$
\begin{aligned}
T_{WLSTR}^{(HPD)} = & \{ \sum_k \hat{W}_k^{(WLSPD)}(\tanh^{-1}(\hat{\Delta}_k) \\
& - \sum_k \hat{W}_k^{(WLSPD)} \tanh^{-1}(\hat{\Delta}_k)/\sum_k \hat{W}_k^{(WLSPD)})^2 \}(1 - \hat{\Delta}_{WLS}^2)^2 \\
= & \{ \sum_k \hat{W}_k^{(WLSPD)}(\tanh^{-1}(\hat{\Delta}_k))^2 \\
& - (\sum_k \hat{W}_k^{(WLSPD)} \tanh^{-1}(\hat{\Delta}_k))^2/\sum_k \hat{W}_k^{(WLSLOR)} \}(1 - \hat{\Delta}_{WLS}^2)^2,
\end{aligned}
$$
(3.47)

where the summation is over those K' strata for which $\hat{\Delta}_k$ exists. We will reject $H_0 : \Delta_1 = \Delta_2 = \cdots = \Delta_K$ at the α-level if the test statistic (3.47), $T_{WLSTR}^{(HPD)} > \chi^2_{\alpha, K'-1}$.

Several other test statistics were also developed elsewhere (Lui and Chang, 2008c) for testing the homogeneity of the PD. Because these test statistics are involved with tedious estimation of numerous parameters, we do not present them here for brevity. On the basis of Monte Carlo simulation, Lui and Chang found that test statistic (3.46) can consistently perform well with respect to Type I error, while the test statistic (3.47) seems to be liberal when the mean stratum size per treatment is not large. This inflation of Type I error for the test statistic (3.47) can exacerbate as the number of strata K increases. However, the test statistic (3.47) may still be preferable to test statistic (3.46) when the mean stratum size λ is large (≥ 100) and K is small (≤ 5). When both λ and K are large, test statistics (3.46) and (3.47) are essentially equivalent with respect to power.

Example 3.5   Consider the mortality data of the CHD (Table 2.3) taken from the multiple risk factor intervention trial (Multiple Risk Factor

Intervention Trial Research Group, 1982) on reducing the mortality of CHD. Based on these data, we obtain the MLE $\hat{\Delta}_k$ (3.2) as -0.0097 and -0.0079, respectively. When applying test statistics (3.46) and (3.47), we obtain both p-values to equal 0.963. This suggests that there be no evidence to claim that the underlying Δ_k varies between strata. This finding is certainly consistent with the above result that the resulting estimates $\hat{\Delta}_k$ for the two strata do not differ much from each other.

3.5.2   Testing homogeneity of the proportion ratio

When testing noninferiority (or equivalence) or obtaining a summary estimator for the PR in stratified analysis, as noted before, we assume that the PR is constant across strata. To examine the homogeneity assumption of the PR, we consider testing $H_0 : \gamma_1 = \gamma_2 \cdots = \gamma_K$ versus H_a : not all γ_k are equal. Note that the homogeneity of the PR $\gamma_k^{(ITT)} = \pi_{1+|k}^{(1)}/\pi_{1+|k}^{(0)}$ for the ITT analysis does not imply the homogeneity of γ_k (3.12) for treatment efficacy, and vice versa. Thus, we cannot directly apply the test procedures (Lui and Kelly, 2000b) to test the homogeneity of PR when the treatment efficacy is of our interest.

When the number of patients n_{gk} is large for all strata, we may consider the most commonly used WLS test procedure (Fleiss, 1981),

$$T_{WLS}^{(HPR)} = \sum_k \hat{W}_k^{(WLSPR)} \hat{\gamma}_k^2 - (\sum_k \hat{W}_k^{(WLSPR)} \hat{\gamma}_k)^2 / \sum_k \hat{W}_k^{(WLSPR)}, \tag{3.48}$$

where $\hat{W}_k^{(WLSPR)} = 1/\hat{Var}((\hat{\gamma}_k)) = 1/[\hat{\gamma}_k^2 \hat{Var}(\log(\hat{\gamma}_k))]$ and the summation is over those K' strata for which $\hat{\gamma}_k$ exists. We will reject $H_0 : \gamma_1 = \gamma_2 \cdots = \gamma_K$ at the α-level if the test statistic (3.48), $T_{WLS}^{(HPR)} > \chi_{\alpha, K'-1}^2$. Note that we may also consider using the logarithmic transformation in derivation of the test statistic based on the WLS approach for testing the homogeneity of the PR (Exercise 3.15).

Following Lui and Kelly (2000b), we consider the MH type test statistic accounting for noncompliance when γ_0 is assumed to be known,

$$\sum_k W_k^{(MH2)} [(\hat{\pi}_{1CA|k}^{(1)} - \hat{\pi}_{1A|k}^{(0)}) - \gamma_0(\hat{\pi}_{1CN|k}^{(0)} - \hat{\pi}_{1N|k}^{(1)})]^2, \tag{3.49}$$

where $W_k^{(MH2)} = [n_{1k}n_{0k}/(n_{1k} + n_{0k})]^2$. Under the null hypothesis $H_0 : \gamma_1 = \gamma_2 \cdots = \gamma_K = \gamma_0$, we can estimate the expectation of (3.49) by (Exercise 3.16):

$$\hat{E}(\sum_k W_k^{(MH2)}[(\hat{\pi}_{1CA|k}^{(1)} - \hat{\pi}_{1A|k}^{(0)}) - \gamma_0(\hat{\pi}_{1CN|k}^{(0)} - \hat{\pi}_{1N|k}^{(1)})]^2)$$

$$= \sum_k W_k^{(MH2)}\{[\hat{\pi}_{1CA|k}^{(1)}(1 - \hat{\pi}_{1CA|k}^{(1)})/n_{1k} + \hat{\pi}_{1A|k}^{(0)}(1 - \hat{\pi}_{1A|k}^{(0)})/n_{0k}]$$

$$+ \hat{\gamma}_{MH}^2[\hat{\pi}_{1N|k}^{(1)}(1 - \hat{\pi}_{1N|k}^{(1)})/n_{1k} + \hat{\pi}_{1CN|k}^{(0)}(1 - \hat{\pi}_{1CN|k}^{(0)})/n_{0k}]$$

$$- 2\hat{\gamma}_{MH}[\hat{\pi}_{1CA|k}^{(1)}\hat{\pi}_{1N|k}^{(1)}/n_{1k} + \hat{\pi}_{1CN|k}^{(0)}\hat{\pi}_{1A|k}^{(0)}/n_{0k}]\}, \qquad (3.50)$$

where $\hat{\gamma}_{MH}$ (3.36) is the MH estimator for the underlying common γ_0. Furthermore, we can show that the estimated variance of the test statistic (3.49) is

$$\hat{Var}(\sum_k W_k^{(MH2)}[(\hat{\pi}_{1CA|k}^{(1)} - \hat{\pi}_{1A|k}^{(0)}) - \gamma_0(\hat{\pi}_{1CN|k}^{(0)} - \hat{\pi}_{1N|k}^{(1)})]^2)$$

$$= \sum_k (W_k^{(MH2)})^2 \hat{Var}([(\hat{\pi}_{1CA|k}^{(1)} - \hat{\pi}_{1A|k}^{(0)}) - \gamma_0(\hat{\pi}_{1CN|k}^{(0)} - \hat{\pi}_{1N|k}^{(1)})]^2),$$

$$(3.51)$$

where $\hat{Var}([(\hat{\pi}_{1CA|k}^{(1)} - \hat{\pi}_{1A|k}^{(0)}) - \gamma_0(\hat{\pi}_{1CN|k}^{(0)} - \hat{\pi}_{1N|k}^{(1)})]^2)$ is given in (A.3.13) in the Appendix to this chapter. Because γ_0 in (3.49) is generally unknown, we can substitute the consistent estimator $\hat{\gamma}_{MH}$ (3.36) for γ_0 in (3.49), and obtain the following statistic for testing $H_0 : \gamma_1 = \gamma_2 \cdots = \gamma_K = \gamma_0$,

$$T_{MH}^{(HPR)} = \{\sum_k W_k^{(MH2)}[(\hat{\pi}_{1CA|k}^{(1)} - \hat{\pi}_{1A|k}^{(0)}) - \hat{\gamma}_{MH}(\hat{\pi}_{1CN|k}^{(0)} - \hat{\pi}_{1N|k}^{(1)})]^2$$

$$- \hat{E}(\sum_k W_k^{(MH2)}[(\hat{\pi}_{1CA|k}^{(1)} - \hat{\pi}_{1A|k}^{(0)}) - \gamma_0(\hat{\pi}_{1CN|k}^{(0)} - \hat{\pi}_{1N|k}^{(1)})]^2)\}/$$

$$\{\hat{Var}(\sum_k W_k^{(MH2)}[(\hat{\pi}_{1CA|k}^{(1)} - \hat{\pi}_{1A|k}^{(0)}) - \gamma_0(\hat{\pi}_{1CN|k}^{(0)} - \hat{\pi}_{1N|k}^{(1)})]^2)\}^{1/2}.$$

$$(3.52)$$

As shown in (Exercise 3.19) under the alternative hypothesis in which γ_k varies between strata, the larger the variation of γ_k, the larger is the expectation of the test statistic $\sum_k W_k^{(MH2)}[(\hat{\pi}_{1CA|k}^{(1)} - \hat{\pi}_{1A|k}^{(0)}) - \gamma_0(\hat{\pi}_{1CN|k}^{(0)} - \hat{\pi}_{1N|k}^{(1)})]^2$ (Lui, 2007e). Thus, we will reject H_0 at the α-level if the test statistic (3.52), $T_{MH}^{(HPR)} > Z_\alpha$, where Z_α is the upper $100(\alpha)$th percentile of the standard normal distribution.

Instead of using the weight $W_k^{(MH2)}$ in (3.49), we can consider use of the estimated optimal weight $\hat{W}_k^{(OP)}$, proportional to the reciprocal of the estimated variance $\hat{Var}([(\hat{\pi}_{1CA|k}^{(1)} - \hat{\pi}_{1A|k}^{(0)}) - \gamma_0(\hat{\pi}_{1CN|k}^{(0)} - \hat{\pi}_{1N|k}^{(1)})]^2)$. Thus, we obtain the test statistic

$$
T_{PRV}^{(HPR)} = \{\sum_k \hat{W}_k^{(OP)}[(\hat{\pi}_{1CA|k}^{(1)} - \hat{\pi}_{1A|k}^{(0)}) - \hat{\gamma}_{MH}(\hat{\pi}_{1CN|k}^{(0)} - \hat{\pi}_{1N|k}^{(1)})]^2
$$
$$
- (\sum_k \hat{W}_k^{(OP)} \hat{E}[(\hat{\pi}_{1CA|k}^{(1)} - \hat{\pi}_{1A|k}^{(0)}) - \gamma_0(\hat{\pi}_{1CN|k}^{(0)} - \hat{\pi}_{1N|k}^{(1)})]^2)\}/
$$
$$
\{\sum_k (\hat{W}_k^{(OP)})^2 \hat{Var}([(\hat{\pi}_{1CA|k}^{(1)} - \hat{\pi}_{1A|k}^{(0)}) - \gamma_0(\hat{\pi}_{1CN|k}^{(0)} - \hat{\pi}_{1N|k}^{(1)})]^2)\}^{1/2}.
$$
$$
(3.53)
$$

We will reject $H_0 : \gamma_1 = \gamma_2 \cdots = \gamma_K = \gamma_0$ at the α-level if the test statistic (3.53), $T_{PRV}^{(HPR)} > Z_\alpha$.

Based on Monte Carlo simulations, Lui (2007e) noted that all test statistics $T_{WLS}^{(HPR)}$ (3.48), $T_{MH}^{(HPR)}$ (3.52) and $T_{PRV}^{(HPR)}$ (3.53) tend to be conservative with respect to Type I error when the mean number of patients per treatment in each stratum is not large or when the number of strata is small. When the number of strata is small ($K = 2$), the test statistic $T_{WLS}^{(HPR)}$ (3.48) is probably preferable to the other two with respect to power for a large mean stratum size per treatment, but $T_{PRV}^{(HPR)}$ (3.53) is likely to be the best for a moderate mean stratum size. When the number of strata K is moderate or large (≥ 5), however, the power of test statistic $T_{MH}^{(HPR)}$ (3.52) is generally larger than those of $T_{WLS}^{(HPR)}$ (3.48) and $T_{PRV}^{(HPR)}$ (3.53).

Example 3.5   To illustrate the use of test statistics $T_{WLS}^{(HPR)}$ (3.48), $T_{MH}^{(HPR)}$ (3.52) and $T_{PRV}^{(HPR)}$ (3.53), we consider the data in Table 2.3. We obtain $\hat{\gamma}_k$ (3.13) for the two strata are 0.503 and 0.607, respectively. When applying test statistics $T_{WLS}^{(HPR)}$ (3.48), $T_{MH}^{(HPR)}$ (3.52) and $T_{PRV}^{(HPR)}$ (3.53), we obtain the corresponding p-value to be 0.932, 0.835, and 0.812. All these values suggest that there should be no significant evidence against the null hypothesis $H_0 : \gamma_1 = \gamma_2$ at the 0.05-level. Note that although these large p-values are possibly due to a small difference as shown above in the PR between the two strata, all test statistics presented here can also lack power due to the small number ($K = 2$) of strata.

3.5.3   Test homogeneity of the odds ratio

Before combining the information on a treatment effect based on the OR from various trials (or centers) in meta-analysis (or a multiple-centre trial), it can be advisable to examine the homogeneity assumption of the OR by testing $H_0 : \varphi_1 = \varphi_2 = \cdots = \varphi_K = \varphi_0$ versus $H_a :$ not all φ_k are equal. Note that the homogeneity of $\varphi_k^{(ITT)} (= (\pi_{1+|k}^{(1)} \pi_{2+|k}^{(0)})/(\pi_{2+|k}^{(1)} \pi_{1+|k}^{(0)}))$ discussed in the ITT analysis does not imply the homogeneity of φ_k considered here, and vice versa. Thus, all classical test procedures discussed elsewhere (Lui, 2004) cannot be directly employed if our interest is to test the homogeneity of treatment efficacy (instead of programmatic effectiveness).

When the number of patients n_{gk} is large, we may consider again applying the following WLS statistic to test $H_0 : \varphi_1 = \varphi_2 = \cdots = \varphi_K = \varphi_0$ (Lui and Chang, 2009c),

$$
\begin{aligned}
T_{WLS}^{(HOR)} &= [1/(\hat{\varphi}_{WLS})^2] \sum_k \hat{W}_k^{(WLSLOR)} (\hat{\varphi}_k - \hat{\varphi}_{WLS})^2 \\
&= [1/(\hat{\varphi}_{WLS})^2][\sum_k \hat{W}_k^{(WLSLOR)} (\hat{\varphi}_k)^2 \\
&\quad - (\sum_k \hat{W}_k^{(WLSLOR)} \hat{\varphi}_k)^2 / \sum_k \hat{W}_k^{(WLSLOR)}],
\end{aligned} \quad (3.54)
$$

where the summation is calculated over those strata k for which $\hat{\varphi}_k$ (3.17) exists, $\hat{\varphi}_{WLS} = \sum_{k=1}^K \hat{W}_k^{(WLSLOR)} \hat{\varphi}_k / \sum_{k=1}^K \hat{W}_k^{(WLSLOR)}$ is the WLS estimator of the underlying common value φ_0, and $\hat{W}_k^{(WLSLOR)} = 1/\hat{Var}(\log(\hat{\varphi}_k))$ is defined in (3.18). Under $H_0 : \varphi_1 = \varphi_2 = \cdots = \varphi_K = \varphi_0$, the test statistic $T_{WLS}^{(HOR)}$ (3.54) follows the χ^2- distribution with $(K' - 1)$ degrees of freedom, where K' is equal to the number K of strata less the number of strata for which $\hat{\varphi}_k$ does not exist. Thus, we reject $H_0 : \varphi_1 = \varphi_2 = \cdots = \varphi_K = \varphi_0$ at the α-level if the statistic (3.54), $T_{WLS}^{(HOR)} > \chi^2_{\alpha, K'-1}$.

In application of $T_{WLS}^{(HOR)}$ (3.54), we may also consider use of the logarithmic transformation of $\hat{\varphi}_k$. This leads us to obtain the following test statistic,

$$
\begin{aligned}
T_{LWLS}^{(HOR)} &= \sum_k \hat{W}_k^{(WLSLOR)} (\log(\hat{\varphi}_k) - \hat{\varphi}_{WLS}^{(LOG)})^2 \\
&= \sum_k \hat{W}_k^{(WLSLOR)} [\log(\hat{\varphi}_k)]^2 \\
&\quad - [\sum_k \hat{W}_k^{(WLSLOR)} \log(\hat{\varphi}_k)]^2 / \sum_k \hat{W}_k^{(WLSLOR)}, \quad (3.55)
\end{aligned}
$$

where $\hat{\varphi}_{WLS}^{(LOG)}$ is given in (3.18). Under the null hypothesis $H_0 : \varphi_1 = \varphi_2 = \cdots = \varphi_K = \varphi_0$, the statistic $T_{LWLS}^{(HOR)}$ follows the χ^2- distribution with $(K' - 1)$ degrees of freedom. Thus, we will reject $H_0 : \varphi_1 = \varphi_2 = \cdots = \varphi_K = \varphi_0$ at the α-level if the test statistic (3.55), $T_{LWLS}^{(HOR)} > \chi_{\alpha, K'-1}^2$.

Following Lipsitz *et al.* (1998) and Lui and Kelly (2000a), we may consider applying the Z-transformation of the test statistic $T_{LWLS}^{(HOR)}$ (3.55) when all n_{gk} and K are large. This leads us to obtain the following test statistic,

$$T_{ZLWLS}^{(HOR)} = [T_{LWLS}^{(HOR)} - (K' - 1)]/[2(K' - 1)]^{1/2}. \qquad (3.56)$$

We reject $H_0 : \varphi_1 = \varphi_2 = \cdots = \varphi_K = \varphi_0$ at the α-level if the test statistic (3.56), $T_{ZLWLS}^{(HOR)} > Z_\alpha$.

Because the mean for a chi-squared distribution is proportional to its variance, we may also consider using the squared root transformation of $T_{LWLS}^{(HOR)}$ (3.55) and obtain the following test statistic,

$$T_{SLWLS}^{(HOR)} = \sqrt{2}[\sqrt{T_{LWLS}^{(HOR)}} - \sqrt{(K' - 1)}]. \qquad (3.57)$$

We reject $H_0 : \varphi_1 = \varphi_2 = \cdots = \varphi_K = \varphi_0$ at the α-level if the test statistic (3.57), $T_{SLWLS} > Z_\alpha$.

When approximating a χ^2- random variable by a normal distribution, Fisher (1924) suggested use of the logarithmic transformation. When all n_{gk} and K are large, this leads us to consider the statistic (Lui and Chang, 2009c),

$$T_{LLWLS}^{(HOR)} = \{\log[T_{LWLS}^{(HOR)}/(K' - 1)]/2 + 1/[2(K' - 1)]\}/\sqrt{1/[2(K' - 1)]}. \qquad (3.58)$$

We will reject $H_0 : \varphi_1 = \varphi_2 = \cdots = \varphi_K = \varphi_0$ at the α-level if the test statistic (3.58), $L_{LLWLS}^{(HOR)} > Z_\alpha$.

Based on Monte Carlo simulation, Lui and Chang (2009c) found that the test statistic $T_{WLS}^{(HOR)}$ (3.54) tends to be too liberal for $K \geq 5$, and so does $T_{ZLWLS}^{(HOR)}$ (3.56) for $K \leq 5$. By contrast, test statistics $T_{LWLS}^{(HOR)}$ (3.55), $T_{SLWLS}^{(HOR)}$ (3.57) and $T_{LLWLS}^{(HOR)}$ (3.58) can consistently perform reasonably well with respect to Type I error in a variety of situations. Lui and Chang (2009c) also found that $T_{LWLS}^{(HOR)}$ (3.55) outperforms the others when the number of strata K is small. When K is moderate ($= 10$), $T_{ZLWLS}^{(HOR)}$ (3.56) can be the best. When both K and n_{gk} are large, all test statistics $T_{LWLS}^{(HOR)}$ (3.55), $T_{ZLWLS}^{(HOR)}$ (3.56), $T_{SLWLS}^{(HOR)}$ (3.57) and $T_{LLWLS}^{(HOR)}$ (3.58) are essentially equivalent (Lui and Chang, 2009c).

Example 3.6   To illustrate the use of test statistics $T_{WLS}^{(HOR)}$ (3.54), $T_{LWLS}^{(HOR)}$ (3.55), $T_{ZLWLS}^{(HOR)}$ (3.56), $T_{SLWLS}^{(HOR)}$ (3.57) and $T_{LLWLS}^{(HOR)}$ (3.58), we consider the data in Table 2.3. Given these data, we obtain the MLE $\hat{\varphi}_k$ for stratum 1 and 2 to be 0.498 and 0.602, respectively. When applying $T_{WLS}^{(HOR)}$ (3.54), $T_{LWLS}^{(HOR)}$ (3.55), $T_{ZLWLS}^{(HOR)}$ (3.56), $T_{SLWLS}^{(HOR)}$ (3.57) and $T_{LLWLS}^{(HOR)}$ (3.58), we obtain the p-values as 0.933, 0.932, 0.759, 0.902, and 0.997, respectively. These all suggest that there should be no statistical evidence against the homogeneity of OR between strata formed by the number of cigarettes per day at baseline. Note that the p-value for using T_{ZLWLS} (3.56) is less than those for using the other test statistics. This is consistent with the findings that the test statistic T_{ZLWLS} (3.56) tends to be liberal (Lui and Chang, 2009c) when the number of strata K is small and hence this test statistic should not be used in this particular case.

We note that the power for all test procedures presented here increases as either the number of strata K or the number of patients per treatment increases. When the number of patients per treatment is small, all test statistics presented here can be invalid for use or lack power especially for the case of a small number of strata. Thus, a nonsignificant test result of homogeneity in this case should not be automatically interpreted as an evidence to support that the homogeneity assumption for the underlying index holds. We note further that power decreases as the extent of noncompliance increases. Therefore, it will be essentially important to reduce the rate of noncompliance if we wish to increase power in hypothesis testing or improve precision in interval estimation under a RCT.

Exercises

3.1 Show that the randomization-based variance $\hat{Var}_{RB}(\hat{\pi}_{1+|k}^{(1)} - \hat{\pi}_{1+|k}^{(0)})$ of $\hat{\delta}_k = \hat{\pi}_{1+|k}^{(1)} - \hat{\pi}_{1+|k}^{(0)}$ when there is no difference between two treatments is given by $\{(n_{1k} + n_{0k})^2/[n_{1k}n_{0k}(n_{1k} + n_{0k} - 1)]\}$ $\hat{\bar{\pi}}_{1+|k}^{(p)}(1 - \hat{\bar{\pi}}_{1+|k}^{(p)})$, where $\hat{\bar{\pi}}_{1+|k}^{(p)} = (n_{1k}\hat{\pi}_{1+|k}^{(1)} + n_{0k}\hat{\pi}_{1+|k}^{(0)})/(n_{1k} + n_{0k})$.

3.2 Show that the variance of $\sum_k \hat{W}_k^{(RB)}(\hat{\pi}_{1+|k}^{(1)} - \hat{\pi}_{1+|k}^{(0)})$, where $\hat{W}_k^{(RB)} = 1/\hat{Var}(\hat{\pi}_{1+|k}^{(1)} - \hat{\pi}_{1+|k}^{(0)})$ can be approximately given by $\sum_k \hat{W}_k^{(RB)}$ as n_{gk} are all large.

3.3 Show that an estimated asymptotic variance of $\hat{\Delta}_k$ under $H_0: \Delta_1 = \Delta_2 = \cdots = \Delta_K = 0$ is given by $\hat{Var}(\hat{\Delta}_k|H_0) = (n_{1k} + n_{0k})\hat{\bar{\pi}}_{1+|k}^{(p)}(1 - \hat{\bar{\pi}}_{1+|k}^{(p)})/[(\hat{\pi}_{+CA|k}^{(1)} - \hat{\pi}_{+A|k}^{(0)})^2 n_{1k}n_{0k}]$ (hint: see Equation (2.6)).

3.4 Note that the estimated asymptotic variance of $\hat{\Delta}_{WLS}$ (3.8) can be shown to approximately equal $1/\sum_k \hat{W}_k^{(WLSPD)}$ when n_{gk} are all large.

3.5 Show that when n_{gk} are all large, the estimated asymptotic variance of $\hat{\Delta}_{WLS}^{(TR)}$ (3.10) can be approximately given by $\hat{Var}(\hat{\Delta}_{WLS}^{(TR)}) = 1/[(1 - \hat{\Delta}_{WLS}^2)^2 \sum_k \hat{W}_k^{(WLSPD)}]$.

3.6 Show that the expectation $E(T_k) = 0$, where $T_k = (\hat{\pi}_{1+|k}^{(1)} - \hat{\pi}_{1+|k}^{(0)}) - \Delta_0(\hat{\pi}_{+CA|k}^{(1)} - \hat{\pi}_{+A|k}^{(0)})$ is defined in (3.26), and that the variance $Var(T_k)$ is given in (3.27).

3.7 Show that $\{(\sum_k \hat{W}_k^* T_k)^2/Var(\sum_k \hat{W}_k^* T_k)\} \leq Z_{\alpha/2}^2$ holds if and only if the quadratic equation: $A^*\Delta_0^2 - 2B^*\Delta_0 + C^* \leq 0$ defined in (3.28) holds.

3.8 Show that the randomization-based variance $\hat{Var}_{RB}(T_k)$ of T_k under simple random sampling in stratum k is (3.30).

3.9 Show that an asymptotic $100(1 - \alpha)$ % confidence interval for γ_0 based on the WLS point estimator $\hat{\gamma}_{WLS}$ (3.33) with the logarithmic transformation is given by (3.34).

3.10 Show that an estimated asymptotic variance $\hat{Var}(\hat{\gamma}_{MH})$ is given by

$$\sum_k (W_k^{(MH)})^2\{\hat{\pi}_{1CA|k}^{(1)}(1 - \hat{\pi}_{1CA|k}^{(1)}) - 2\hat{\gamma}_{MH}\hat{\pi}_{1CA|k}^{(1)}\hat{\pi}_{1N|k}^{(1)}$$
$$+ \hat{\gamma}_{MH}^2(\hat{\pi}_{1N|k}^{(1)}(1 - \hat{\pi}_{1N|k}^{(1)}))\}/\{n_{1k}[\sum_k W_k^{(MH)}(\hat{\pi}_{1CN|k}^{(0)} - \hat{\pi}_{1N|k}^{(1)})]^2\}$$

$$+ \sum_k (W_k^{(MH)})^2 \{\hat{\pi}_{1A|k}^{(0)}(1 - \hat{\pi}_{1A|k}^{(0)}) - 2\hat{\gamma}_{MH}\hat{\pi}_{1A|k}^{(0)}\hat{\pi}_{1CN|k}^{(0)}$$
$$+ \hat{\gamma}_{MH}^2(\hat{\pi}_{1CN|k}^{(0)}(1 - \hat{\pi}_{1CN|k}^{(0)}))\}/\{n_{0k}[\sum_k W_k^{(MH)}(\hat{\pi}_{1CN|k}^{(0)} - \hat{\pi}_{1N|k}^{(1)})]^2\}.$$

3.11 On the basis of the delta method, show that an estimated asymptotic variance for the statistic $\log(\hat{\varphi}_{MH})$ with the logarithmic transformation is given by (3.41).

3.12 Show that we can obtain an asymptotic $100\,(1-\alpha)\,\%$ confidence interval for φ_0 as given by $[\max\{(B^\dagger - (B^{\dagger 2} - A^\dagger C^\dagger)^{1/2})/A^\dagger, 0\}, (B^\dagger + (B^{\dagger 2} - A^\dagger C^\dagger)^{1/2})/A^\dagger]$ defined in (3.45).

3.13 Show that interval estimators (3.37) and (3.40) are invariant respect to the reciprocal transformation (Casella and Berger, 1990).

3.14 Show that as long as the two distinct real roots of the quadratic equation for the interval estimator (3.45) exist in $(0, \infty)$, this interval estimator possesses the invariance property with respect to the reciprocal transformation.

3.15 When we employ the logarithmic transformation based on the WLS approach, derive the simple test statistic for testing $H_0: \gamma_1 = \gamma_2 \cdots = \gamma_K = \gamma_0$?

3.16 Under the null hypothesis $H_0: \gamma_1 = \gamma_2 \cdots = \gamma_K = \gamma_0$, show that the expectation of (3.49) is given by

$$E(\sum_k W_k^{(MH2)}[(\hat{\pi}_{1CA|k}^{(1)} - \hat{\pi}_{1A|k}^{(0)}) - \gamma_0(\hat{\pi}_{1CN|k}^{(0)} - \hat{\pi}_{1N|k}^{(1)})]^2)$$
$$= \sum_k W_k^{(MII2)}\{[\pi_{1CA|k}^{(1)}(1 - \pi_{1CA|k}^{(1)})/n_{1k} + \pi_{1A|k}^{(0)}(1 - \pi_{1A|k}^{(0)})/n_{0k}]$$
$$+ \gamma_{MII}^2[\pi_{1N|k}^{(1)}(1 - \pi_{1N|k}^{(1)})/n_{1k} + \pi_{1CN|k}^{(0)}(1 - \pi_{1CN|k}^{(0)})/n_{0k}]$$
$$- 2\hat{\gamma}_{MH}[\hat{\pi}_{1CA|k}^{(1)}\hat{\pi}_{1N|k}^{(1)}/n_{1k} + \hat{\pi}_{1CN|k}^{(0)}\hat{\pi}_{1A|k}^{(0)}/n_{0k}]\}.$$

3.17 Show that the expectation $E(\hat{\Delta}_k^{(ITT)}) = \Delta_k(C_{1k} + C_{0k} - 1)$, where $\hat{\Delta}_k^{(ITT)} = (\hat{\pi}_{1+|k}^{(1)} - \hat{\pi}_{1+|k}^{(0)})$, $C_{1k}(= \pi_{+C|k} + \pi_{+A|k})$ and $C_{0k}(= \pi_{+C|k} + \pi_{+N|k})$ are the probabilities of compliance in stratum k for treatments $g = 1$ and $g = 0$, respectively. In testing the homogeneity of PD for the ITT analysis, we actually test $H_0: \Delta_1^{(ITT)} = \Delta_2^{(ITT)} = \cdots = \Delta_K^{(ITT)}$, where $\Delta_k^{(ITT)}(= \Delta_k(C_{1k} + C_{0k} - 1))$. Show that the equality $\Delta_1^{(ITT)} = \Delta_2^{(ITT)} = \cdots = \Delta_K^{(ITT)}$ does not necessarily imply the equality $\Delta_1 = \Delta_2 = \cdots = \Delta_K = \Delta_0$, and vice versa.

3.18 Consider the simulated data in Table 3.1 (Lui and Chang, 2008c). What are the estimates $\hat{\Delta}_k$ (3.2) of the PD for stratum k, where $k = 1, 2$? When we use test statistics (3.46) and (3.47), what are the p-values for testing the homogeneity of the PD? (Answers: $\hat{\Delta}_1 = 0.253$ and $\hat{\Delta}_2 = 0.072$; p-value 0.002.)

Table 3.1 The simulated relative frequency of patients under stratified sampling in a RCT with noncompliance.

	Assigned treatment					
	$g = 1$			$g = 0$		
Stratum	Received treatment			Received treatment		
1	$g = 1$	$g = 0$	Total	$g = 1$	$g = 0$	Total
	(CA)	(N)		(A)	(CN)	
Positive	0.402	0.042	0.444	0.044	0.215	0.259
Negative	0.466	0.090	0.556	0.094	0.646	0.740
Total	0.868	0.132	1.000	0.138	0.861	1.000
		$n_{11} = 522$			$n_{01} = 520$	

	Assigned treatment					
	$g = 1$			$g = 0$		
Stratum	Received treatment			Received treatment		
2	$g = 1$	$g = 0$	Total	$g = 1$	$g = 0$	Total
	(CA)	(N)		(A)	(CN)	
Positive	0.401	0.080	0.481	0.054	0.377	0.431
Negative	0.429	0.090	0.519	0.077	0.492	0.569
Total	0.830	0.170	1.000	0.131	0.869	1.000
		$n_{12} = 501$			$n_{02} = 520$	

3.19 Show that under the alternative hypothesis in which γ_k varies between strata, the expectation

$$E(\sum_k W_k^{(MH2)}[(\hat{\pi}_{1CA|k}^{(1)} - \hat{\pi}_{1A|k}^{(0)}) - \gamma_0(\hat{\pi}_{1CN|k}^{(0)} - \hat{\pi}_{1N|k}^{(1)})]^2)$$
$$= \sum_k W_k^{(MH2)} Var(\hat{\pi}_{1C|k}^{(1)} - \gamma_0 \hat{\pi}_{1C|k}^{(0)}) + \sum_k W_k^{(MH2)}(\gamma_k - \gamma_0)^2(\pi_{1C|k}^{(0)})^2$$

where $\hat{\pi}_{1C|k}^{(1)} = (\hat{\pi}_{1CA|k}^{(1)} - \hat{\pi}_{1A|k}^{(0)})$ and $\hat{\pi}_{1C|k}^{(0)} = (\hat{\pi}_{1CN|k}^{(0)} - \hat{\pi}_{1N|k}^{(1)})$.
Thus, the larger the variation of γ_k, the larger is the expectation of the test statistic $\sum_k W_k^{(MH2)}[(\hat{\pi}_{1CA|k}^{(1)} - \hat{\pi}_{1A|k}^{(0)}) - \gamma_0(\hat{\pi}_{1CN|k}^{(0)} - \hat{\pi}_{1N|k}^{(1)})]^2$ (Lui, 2007e).

3.20 Consider the data in Table 3.2 simulated for a RCT with 3 strata, in which underlying OR ($\varphi_1 = \varphi_2 = \varphi_3$) equal to 2.

   (a) What are the estimates $\hat{\Delta}_k$ (3.2) of the PD for stratum k, where $k = 1, 2, 3$? (Answers: $\hat{\Delta}_1 = 0.100$, $\hat{\Delta}_2 = 0.213$, $\hat{\Delta}_3 = 0.069$). When we use test statistics (3.46) and (3.47), what are the p-values for testing the homogeneity of the PD? (Answers: 0.005).

   (b) What are the estimates $\hat{\gamma}_k$ (3.13) of the PR for stratum k, where $k = 1, 2, 3$? (Answers: $\hat{\gamma}_1 = 1.941$; $\hat{\gamma}_2 = 1.436$; $\hat{\gamma}_3 = 1.636$). When we use test statistics $T_{WLS}^{(HPR)}$ (3.48), $T_{MH}^{(HPR)}$ (3.52) and $T_{PRV}^{(HPR)}$ (3.53), what are the p-values for testing the homogeneity of the PR? (Answers: 0.427, 0.597 and 0.640).

   (c) What are the estimates $\hat{\varphi}_k$ (3.17) of the PD for stratum k, where $k = 1, 2, 3$? (Answers: $\hat{\varphi}_1 = 2.177$; $\hat{\varphi}_2 = 2.444$; $\hat{\varphi}_3 = 1.778$). When we use test statistics $T_{WLS}^{(HOR)}$ (3.54), $T_{LWLS}^{(HOR)}$ (3.55), $T_{ZLWLS}^{(HOR)}$ (3.56), $T_{SLWLS}^{(HOR)}$ (3.57) and $T_{LLWLS}^{(HOR)}$ (3.58), what are the p-values for testing the homogeneity of the OR? (Answers: 0.556, 0.540, 0.650, 0.667, 0.494.)

   (d) What are the summary estimates of $\hat{\varphi}_{WLS}$ (3.38) and $\hat{\varphi}_{MH}$ (3.40)? (Answers: $\hat{\varphi}_{WLS} = 2.138$ and $\hat{\varphi}_{MH} = 2.133$).

   (e) What are the resulting asymptotic 95 % confidence intervals for φ_0 when we apply interval estimators (3.39) and (3.42)? This exercise illustrates the case in which the underlying OR is homogeneous, but the underlying PD is heterogeneous.

Table 3.2 The simulated relative frequency of patients under stratified sampling in a RCT with noncompliance

	Assigned treatment					
	$g = 1$			$g = 0$		
Stratum 1	Received treatment			Received treatment		
	$g = 1$ (CA)	$g = 0$ (N)	Total	$g = 1$ (A)	$g = 0$ (CN)	Total
Positive	0.199	0.000	0.199	0.034	0.085	0.119
Negative	0.775	0.027	0.802	0.140	0.742	0.882
Total	0.974	0.027	1.000	0.174	0.837	1.000
		$n_{11} = 408$			$n_{01} = 387$	

	Assigned treatment					
	$g = 1$			$g = 0$		
Stratum 2	Received treatment			Received treatment		
	$g = 1$ (CA)	$g = 0$ (N)	Total	$g = 1$ (A)	$g = 0$ (CN)	Total
Positive	0.573	0.017	0.590	0.020	0.402	0.422
negative	0.360	0.050	0.410	0.123	0.455	0.578
Total	0.933	0.067	1.000	0.143	0.857	1.000
		$n_{12} = 361$			$n_{02} = 440$	

	Assigned treatment					
	$g = 1$			$g = 0$		
Stratum 3	Received treatment			Received treatment		
	$g = 1$ (CA)	$g = 0$ (N)	Total	$g = 1$ (A)	$g = 0$ (CN)	Total
Positive	0.175	0.000	0.175	0.000	0.107	0.107
Negative	0.808	0.018	0.826	0.002	0.891	0.893
Total	0.983	0.018	1.000	0.002	0.998	1.000
		$n_{13} = 395$			$n_{03} = 413$	

Appendix

Derivation of the estimated expectation (3.50) and estimated variance (3.51) for the test statistic (3.52) (Lui, 2007e).

Since the expectation $E((\hat{\pi}_{1CA|k}^{(1)} - \hat{\pi}_{1A|k}^{(0)}) - \gamma_0(\hat{\pi}_{1CN|k}^{(0)} - \hat{\pi}_{1N|k}^{(1)})) = 0$ under $H_0 : \gamma_1 = \gamma_2 = \cdots = \gamma_K = \gamma_0$, $E((\hat{\pi}_{1CA|k}^{(1)} - \hat{\pi}_{1A|k}^{(0)}) - \gamma_0(\hat{\pi}_{1CN|k}^{(0)} - \hat{\pi}_{1N|k}^{(1)}))^2$ is actually equal to the variance $Var((\hat{\pi}_{1CA|k}^{(1)} - \hat{\pi}_{1A|k}^{(0)}) - \gamma_0(\hat{\pi}_{1CN|k}^{(0)} - \hat{\pi}_{1N|k}^{(1)}))$, which can be easily shown to be

$$
\begin{aligned}
&[\pi_{1CA|k}^{(1)}(1 - \pi_{1CA|k}^{(1)})/n_{1k} + \pi_{1A|k}^{(0)}(1 - \pi_{1A|k}^{(0)})/n_{0k}] \\
&+ \gamma_0^2[\pi_{1N|k}^{(1)}(1 - \pi_{1N|k}^{(1)})/n_{1k} + \pi_{1CN|k}^{(0)}(1 - \pi_{1CN|k}^{(0)})/n_{0k}] \\
&- 2\gamma_0[\pi_{1CA|k}^{(1)}\pi_{1N|k}^{(1)}/n_{1k} + \pi_{1CN|k}^{(0)}\pi_{1A|k}^{(0)}/n_{0k}].
\end{aligned} \tag{A.3.1}
$$

Thus, we can estimate $E(\sum_k W_k^{(MH2)}[(\hat{\pi}_{1CA|k}^{(1)} - \hat{\pi}_{1A|k}^{(0)}) - \gamma_0(\hat{\pi}_{1CN|k}^{(0)} - \hat{\pi}_{1N|k}^{(1)})]^2)$ by

$$
\begin{aligned}
&\hat{E}(\sum_k W_k^{(MH2)}[(\hat{\pi}_{1CA|k}^{(1)} - \hat{\pi}_{1A|k}^{(0)}) - \gamma_0(\hat{\pi}_{1CN|k}^{(0)} - \hat{\pi}_{1N|k}^{(1)})]^2) \\
&= \sum_k W_k^{(MH2)}\hat{Var}((\hat{\pi}_{1CA|k}^{(1)} - \hat{\pi}_{1A|k}^{(0)}) - \gamma_0(\hat{\pi}_{1CN|k}^{(0)} - \hat{\pi}_{1N|k}^{(1)})).
\end{aligned} \tag{A.3.2}
$$

where $\hat{Var}((\hat{\pi}_{1CA|k}^{(1)} - \hat{\pi}_{1A|k}^{(0)}) - \gamma_0(\hat{\pi}_{1CN|k}^{(0)} - \hat{\pi}_{1N|k}^{(1)}))$ is obtained from (A.3.1) by simply substituting $\hat{\pi}_{1S|k}^{(g)}$ and $\pi_{1S|k}^{(g)}$ ($S = CA$, N for $g = 1$ and $S = CN$, A for $g = 0$) and the MH estimator $\hat{\gamma}_{MH}$ for γ_0, where

$$
\begin{aligned}
\hat{\gamma}_{MH} = &[\sum_k n_{1k}n_{0k}(\hat{\pi}_{1CA|k}^{(1)} - \hat{\pi}_{1A|k}^{(0)})/(n_{1k} + n_{0k})]/ \\
&[\sum_k n_{1k}n_{0k}(\hat{\pi}_{1CN|k}^{(0)} - \hat{\pi}_{1N|k}^{(1)})/(n_{1k} + n_{0k})].
\end{aligned} \tag{A.3.3}
$$

Furthermore, the variance

$$
\begin{aligned}
&Var(\sum_k W_k^{(MH2)}[(\hat{\pi}_{1CA|k}^{(1)} - \hat{\pi}_{1A|k}^{(0)}) - \gamma_0(\hat{\pi}_{1CN|k}^{(0)} - \hat{\pi}_{1N|k}^{(1)})]^2) \\
&= \sum_k (W_k^{(MH2)})^2 Var([(\hat{\pi}_{1CA|k}^{(1)} - \hat{\pi}_{1A|k}^{(0)}) - \gamma_0(\hat{\pi}_{1CN|k}^{(0)} - \hat{\pi}_{1N|k}^{(1)})]^2).
\end{aligned}
$$

Note that the variance

$$
\begin{aligned}
Var&([(\hat{\pi}_{1CA|k}^{(1)} - \hat{\pi}_{1A|k}^{(0)}) - \gamma_0(\hat{\pi}_{1CN|k}^{(0)} - \hat{\pi}_{1N|k}^{(1)})]^2) \\
&= E((\hat{\pi}_{1CA|k}^{(1)} - \hat{\pi}_{1A|k}^{(0)}) - \gamma_0(\hat{\pi}_{1CN|k}^{(0)} - \hat{\pi}_{1N|k}^{(1)}))^4 \\
&\quad - [Var((\hat{\pi}_{1CA|k}^{(1)} - \hat{\pi}_{1A|k}^{(0)}) - \gamma_0(\hat{\pi}_{1CN|k}^{(0)} - \hat{\pi}_{1N|k}^{(1)}))]^2. \quad (A.3.4)
\end{aligned}
$$

Under the null hypothesis $H_0 : \gamma_1 = \gamma_2 = \cdots = \gamma_K = \gamma_0$, we can show that

$$
\begin{aligned}
E&((\hat{\pi}_{1CA|k}^{(1)} - \hat{\pi}_{1A|k}^{(0)}) - \gamma_0(\hat{\pi}_{1CN|k}^{(0)} - \hat{\pi}_{1N|k}^{(1)}))^4 \\
&= E((\hat{\pi}_{1CA|k}^{(1)*} - \hat{\pi}_{1A|k}^{(0)*}) - \gamma_0(\hat{\pi}_{1CN|k}^{(0)*} - \hat{\pi}_{1N|k}^{(1)*}))^4
\end{aligned}
$$

where $\hat{\pi}_{1S|k}^{(g)*} = \hat{\pi}_{1S|k}^{(g)} - \pi_{1S|k}^{(g)}$ ($S = CA, N$ for $g = 1$ and $S = CN, A$ for $g = 0$).

Note that the expectation $E(\hat{\pi}_{1S|k}^{(g)*}) = 0$. Note also that the expectation

$$
\begin{aligned}
E&((\hat{\pi}_{1CA|k}^{(1)*} - \hat{\pi}_{1A|k}^{(0)*}) - \gamma_0(\hat{\pi}_{1CN|k}^{(0)*} - \hat{\pi}_{1N|k}^{(1)*}))^4 \\
&= E((\hat{\pi}_{1CA|k}^{(1)*} + \gamma_0\hat{\pi}_{1N|k}^{(1)*}) - (\hat{\pi}_{1A|k}^{(0)*} + \gamma_0\hat{\pi}_{1CN|k}^{(0)*}))^4 \\
&= E(\hat{\pi}_{1CA|k}^{(1)*} + \gamma_0\hat{\pi}_{1N|k}^{(1)*})^4 + 6E(\hat{\pi}_{1CA|k}^{(1)*} + \gamma_0\hat{\pi}_{1N|k}^{(1)*})^2 \\
&\quad \times E(\hat{\pi}_{1A|k}^{(0)*} + \gamma_0\hat{\pi}_{1CN|k}^{(0)*})^2 + E(\hat{\pi}_{1A|k}^{(0)*} + \gamma_0\hat{\pi}_{1CN|k}^{(0)*})^4. \quad (A.3.5)
\end{aligned}
$$

This is because $E(\hat{\pi}_{1CA|k}^{(1)*} + \gamma_0\hat{\pi}_{1N|k}^{(1)*})^3 E(\hat{\pi}_{1A|k}^{(0)*} + \gamma_0\hat{\pi}_{1CN|k}^{(0)*}) = 0$ and

$$
E(\hat{\pi}_{1CA|k}^{(1)*} + \gamma_0\hat{\pi}_{1N|k}^{(1)*})E(\hat{\pi}_{1A|k}^{(0)*} + \gamma_0\hat{\pi}_{1CN|k}^{(0)*})^3 = 0.
$$

After some algebraic manipulations, we can show that

$$
\begin{aligned}
E(\hat{\pi}_{1CA|k}^{(1)*} + \gamma_0\hat{\pi}_{1N|k}^{(1)*})^4 &= E(\hat{\pi}_{1CA|k}^{(1)*})^4 + 4\gamma_0 E((\hat{\pi}_{1CA|k}^{(1)*})^3\pi_{1N|k}^{(1)*}) \\
&\quad + 6\gamma_0^2 E((\hat{\pi}_{1CA|k}^{(1)*})^2(\pi_{1N|k}^{(1)*})^2) \\
&\quad + 4\gamma_0^3 E((\hat{\pi}_{1CA|k}^{(1)*})(\pi_{1N|k}^{(1)*})^3) + \gamma_0^4 E(\pi_{1N|k}^{(1)*})^4,
\end{aligned}
$$

$$(A.3.6)$$

for $g = 1, 0$, where

$$
\begin{aligned}
E(\hat{\pi}_{1CA|k}^{(1)*})^4 &= \pi_{1CA|k}^{(1)}(1 - \pi_{1CA|k}^{(1)})[1 + 3\pi_{1CA|k}^{(1)} \\
&\quad \times (1 - \pi_{1CA|k}^{(1)})(n_{1k} - 2)]/n_{1k}^3, \quad (A.3.7)
\end{aligned}
$$

$$E((\hat{\pi}_{1CA|k}^{(1)*})^3\hat{\pi}_{1N|k}^{(1)*}) = -\pi_{1CA|k}^{(1)}\pi_{1N|k}^{(1)}[1 + 3\hat{\pi}_{1CA|k}^{(1)}$$
$$\times (1 - \hat{\pi}_{1CA|k}^{(1)})(n_{1k} - 2)]/n_{1k}^3, \qquad (A.3.8)$$

$$E((\hat{\pi}_{1CA|k}^{(1)*})^2(\hat{\pi}_{1N|k}^{(1)*})^2) = \pi_{1CA|k}^{(1)}\pi_{1N|k}^{(1)}\{n_{1k}[(1 - \pi_{1CA|k}^{(1)})(1 - \pi_{1N|k}^{(1)})$$
$$+ 2\pi_{1CA|k}^{(1)}\pi_{1N|k}^{(1)}] - [(1 - 2\pi_{1CA|k}^{(1)})(1 - 2\pi_{1N|k}^{(1)})$$
$$+ 2\pi_{1CA|k}^{(1)}\pi_{1N|k}^{(1)}]\}/n_{1k}^3, \qquad (A.3.9)$$

$$E((\hat{\pi}_{1CA|k}^{(1)*})(\hat{\pi}_{1N|k}^{(1)*})^3) = -\pi_{1CA|k}^{(1)}\pi_{1N|k}^{(1)}[1 + 3\pi_{1N|k}^{(1)}$$
$$\times (1 - \pi_{1N|k}^{(1)})(n_{1k} - 2)]/n_{1k}^3, \qquad (A.3.10)$$

$$E(\hat{\pi}_{1N|k}^{(1)*})^4 = \pi_{1N|k}^{(1)}(1 - \pi_{1N|k}^{(1)})[1 + 3\pi_{1N|k}^{(1)}$$
$$\times (1 - \pi_{1N|k}^{(1)})(n_{1k} - 2)]/n_{1k}^3. \qquad (A.3.11)$$

Based on (A.3.7)–(A.3.11), we can estimate $E(\hat{\pi}_{1CA|k}^{(1)*} + \gamma_0\hat{\pi}_{1N|k}^{(1)*})^4$ (A.3.6) by substituting $\hat{\pi}_{1S|k}^{(1)}$ for $\pi_{1S|k}^{(1)}$ for $S = CA, N$, and the MH estimator $\hat{\gamma}_{MH}$ for γ_0. We denote this resulting estimator by $\hat{E}(\hat{\pi}_{1CA|k}^{(1)*} + \gamma_0\hat{\pi}_{1N|k}^{(1)*})^4$.

Furthermore, we obtain the estimator

$$\hat{E}(\hat{\pi}_{1CA|k}^{(1)*} + \gamma_0\hat{\pi}_{1N|k}^{(1)*})^2 = \hat{\pi}_{1CA|k}^{(1)}(1 - \hat{\pi}_{1CA|k}^{(1)})/n_{1k} + \hat{\gamma}_{MH}^2\hat{\pi}_{1N|k}^{(1)}$$
$$\times (1 - \hat{\pi}_{1N|k}^{(1)})/n_{1k} - 2\hat{\gamma}_{MH}(\hat{\pi}_{1CA|k}^{(1)}\hat{\pi}_{1N|k}^{(1)})/n_{1k}.$$
$$(A.3.12)$$

Following similar arguments, we can obtain the estimated expectation $\hat{E}(\hat{\pi}_{1A|k}^{(0)*} + \gamma_0\hat{\pi}_{1CN|k}^{(0)*})^4$ and $\hat{E}(\hat{\pi}_{1A|k}^{(0)*} + \gamma_0\hat{\pi}_{1CN|k}^{(0)*})^2$. Thus, we can estimate $Var([(\hat{\pi}_{1CA|k}^{(1)} - \hat{\pi}_{1A|k}^{(0)}) - \gamma_0(\hat{\pi}_{1CN|k}^{(0)} - \hat{\pi}_{1N|k}^{(1)})]^2)$ (A.3.4) by

$$\hat{Var}([(\hat{\pi}_{1CA|k}^{(1)} - \hat{\pi}_{1A|k}^{(0)}) - \gamma_0(\hat{\pi}_{1CN|k}^{(0)} - \hat{\pi}_{1N|k}^{(1)})]^2)$$
$$= \hat{E}(\hat{\pi}_{1CA|k}^{(1)*} + \gamma_0\hat{\pi}_{1N|k}^{(1)*})^4 + 6\hat{E}(\hat{\pi}_{1CA|k}^{(1)*} + \gamma_0\hat{\pi}_{1N|k}^{(1)*})^2$$
$$\times \hat{E}(\hat{\pi}_{1A|k}^{(0)*} + \gamma_0\hat{\pi}_{1CN|k}^{(0)*})^2 + \hat{E}(\hat{\pi}_{1A|k}^{(0)*} + \gamma_0\hat{\pi}_{1CN|k}^{(0)*})^4$$
$$- [\hat{Var}((\hat{\pi}_{1CA|k}^{(1)} - \hat{\pi}_{1A|k}^{(0)}) - \gamma_0(\hat{\pi}_{1CN|k}^{(0)} - \hat{\pi}_{1N|k}^{(1)}))]^2. \qquad (A.3.13)$$

4

Randomized clinical trials with noncompliance under cluster sampling

For cost-efficiency, we may commonly employ a cluster randomized trial (CRT), in which clusters of patients rather than individual patients are randomized units (Loey, Vansteelandt and Goetghebeur, 2001). When obtaining a complete list of clusters is much easier than obtaining a complete list of individual subjects or when individual subjects are naturally grouped into clusters, we may also consider use of cluster sampling for administration convenience. For example, consider the CRT studying the effect of vitamin A supplementation on mortality among preschool children in rural Indonesia (Sommer and Zeger, 1991; Sommer, Tarwotjo and Djunaedi *et al.*, 1986). Villages of children (rather than individual children) were randomly assigned to either an experimental group of receiving two large oral doses of vitamin A supplementation or to a control group of receiving no vitamin A supplementation. There were nearly 20 % of children assigned to the experimental group who failed to receive vitamin A supplementation.

The mortality rates between the two groups over a follow-up of 12 months were then compared. Because children within villages tended to live under a similar environment, the survival outcomes between

Binary Data Analysis of Randomized Clinical Trials with Noncompliance, First Edition. Kung-Jong Lui.
© 2011 John Wiley & Sons, Ltd. Published 2011 by John Wiley & Sons, Ltd.

children within villages were probably correlated. In such cases, statistical methods without accounting for the intraclass correlation between survival outcomes on children within villages can be inappropriate. As a second example, consider the flu vaccine trial in which physicians were randomly assigned to an intervention group of receiving computer-generated reminders for flu shots or to a control group of receiving no such reminders (McDonald, Hui and Tierney, 1991; Zhou and Li, 2006). Patients were then classified by the group to which their physicians were assigned. The rates of flu-related hospitalization between two comparison groups over a 3-year period were then compared. This flu vaccine trial involved randomization of an encouragement by physicians rather than by patients. Because patients who were taken care of by the same physician might have similar characteristics, the outcomes of morbidity between patients taken care by the same physician were probably correlated as well. Other examples regarding the use of a CRT to collect data (Dexter, Wolinsky and Gramelspacher et al., 1998; Ialongo, Werthamer and Kellam et al., 1999) and statistical analyses for continuous data under a CRT, including survival, behavior compliance and Bayesian analyses, appeared elsewhere (Loey, Vansteelandt and Goetghebeur, 2001; Jo, Asparouhov and Muthén, 2008; Jo, Asparouhov and Muthén et al., 2008; Frangakis, Rubin and Zhou, 2002). An excellent and systematic discussion, including the usefulness, the limitations and many real-life examples, on cluster randomized trials in health research also appeared elsewhere (Donner and Klar, 2000).

Under the Dirichlet-multinomial model (Bishop, Fienberg and Holland, 1975), we discuss hypothesis testing, interval estimation and sample size calculation under a CRT with noncompliance. We consider testing superiority between two treatments in the presence of noncompliance under a CRT in Section 4.1. We address testing noninferiority in Section 4.2 and testing equivalence in Section 4.3 based on the proportion difference (PD), the proportion ratio (PR), and the odds ratio (OR) used to measure the relative treatment effect for a CRT with noncompliance. We consider interval estimation of the PD, PR and OR with respect to treatment effect under a CRT with noncompliance in Section 4.4. We discuss sample size determination accounting for both noncompliance and the intraclass correlation based on the proposed procedures for testing superiority, noninferiority and equivalence in Section 4.5. Finally, we include an alternative model-free randomization-based approach to do hypothesis testing and interval estimation under a CRT with noncompliance in Section 4.6.

Suppose that we compare an experimental treatment ($g = 1$) with a standard treatment ($g = 0$) under a CRT, in which we randomly assign to treatment g ($g = 1, 0$) n_g clusters, each consisting of $m_i^{(g)}$ ($i = 1, 2, \ldots, n_g$) patients. Note that if the number n_g of clusters is small, the chance of imbalance in (unobserved or observed) covariates will increase between two randomized arms. This may also invalidate the intent-to-treat (ITT) analysis. Thus, we focus our attention on the case in which the number n_g of clusters in both randomized arms is reasonably large in the following discussion. For each patient we define the vector $(d(1), d(0))'$ as the status of his/her potential treatment receipt, and $d(g) = 1$ if the patient assigned to treatment g ($g = 1, 0$) receives the experimental treatment, and $d(g) = 0$, otherwise. On the basis of the vector of the potential treatment-receipt status, our sampling population can be divided into four subpopulations: compliers (C) (i.e. $d(g) = g$ for $g = 1, 0$), never-takers (N) (i.e. $d(g) = 0$ for $g = 1, 0$), always-takers (A) (i.e. $d(g) = 1$ for $g = 1, 0$), and defiers (D) (i.e. $d(g) = 1 - g$ for $g = 1, 0$). As commonly assumed for a randomized trial with noncompliance, we make the stable unit treatment value assumption (SUTVA) and the monotonicity assumption (i.e. $d(1) \geq d(0)$). The former assumes that there is no interference between patients, while the latter assumes that there are no defiers. Note that because patients within clusters are likely to interact with one another, the SUTVA can be potentially violated in a CRT. On the other hand, because patients from the same cluster are randomly assigned to the same treatment, we may reduce the opportunity of treatment contamination between patients. As noted elsewhere (Jo, Asparouhov and Muthén et al., 2008), the concern of unobserved treatment contamination is generally difficult to handle, while the violation of the interaction can be taken into account statistically by modeling resemblance among patients within the same cluster in data analysis. We focus our discussion on the situation in which the patient response r is dichotomous, and $r = 1$ if the patient has a positive response, $= 2$, otherwise. We define the indictor random variable $y_{ij}^{(g)}(r, S)$ (where $r = 1, 2, S = C, A, N$) for patient j ($j = 1, 2, \ldots, m_i^{(g)}$) in cluster

$i(i = 1, 2, \ldots, n_g)$ assigned to treatment g ($= 1$ for experimental, $= 0$ for standard), and $y_{ij}^{(g)}(r, S) = 1$ if the patient has the response r ($= 1, 2$) and the treatment receipt status S ($= C, A,$ and N), and $= 0$, otherwise. Define $m_{rS|i}^{(g)} = \sum_{j=1}^{m_i^{(g)}} y_{ij}^{(g)}(r, S)$, denoting the number of patients falling in the cell with response r and treatment-receipt status S in cluster i assigned to treatment g. Let $p_{rS|i}^{(g)}$ denote the cell probability of a randomly selected patient who has the response r and the treatment receipt status S in cluster i assigned to treatment g ($g = 1, 0$). For clarity, we may use the following table to summarize the notations denoting various cell probabilities in cluster i ($i = 1, 2, \ldots, n_g$) assigned to treatment g ($g = 1, 0$):

Cluster i ($i = 1, 2, \ldots, n_g$) in the assigned treatment g ($g = 1, 0$)

	Compliers	Always-takers	Never-takers
Positive	$p_{1C|i}^{(g)}$	$p_{1A|i}^{(g)}$	$p_{1N|i}^{(g)}$
Negative	$p_{2C|i}^{(g)}$	$p_{2A|i}^{(g)}$	$p_{2N|i}^{(g)}$

The random vector $(m_{1C|i}^{(g)}, m_{1A|i}^{(g)}, m_{1N|i}^{(g)}, m_{2C|i}^{(g)}, m_{2A|i}^{(g)}, m_{2N|i}^{(g)})$ then follows a multinomial distribution with parameters $m_i^{(g)}$ and $(p_{1C|i}^{(g)}, p_{1A|i}^{(g)}, p_{1N|i}^{(g)}, p_{2C|i}^{(g)}, p_{2A|i}^{(g)}, p_{2N|i}^{(g)})$:

$$\frac{m_i^{(g)}!}{\prod_{r=1}^{2} \prod_{S} m_{rS|i}^{(g)}!} \prod_{r=1}^{2} \prod_{S} (p_{rS|i}^{(g)})^{m_{rS|i}^{(g)}} \tag{4.1}$$

where $\sum_{r=1}^{2} \sum_{S} m_{rS|i}^{(g)} = m_i^{(g)}$, $0 < p_{rS|i}^{(g)} < 1$, and $\sum_{r=1}^{2} \sum_{S} p_{rS|i}^{(g)} = 1$. To account for the intraclass correlation between patient responses within clusters (or equivalently, the cell probability of patient responses varies between clusters), we assume that the vector of cell probabilities $(p_{1C|i}^{(g)}, p_{1A|i}^{(g)}, p_{1N|i}^{(g)}, p_{2C|i}^{(g)}, p_{2A|i}^{(g)}, p_{2N|i}^{(g)})$ independently and identically follows the Dirichlet probability density function (Bishop, Fienberg and Holland, 1975) given by

$$\mathcal{D}(\pi_{1C}^{(g)}, \pi_{1A}^{(g)}, \pi_{1N}^{(g)}, \pi_{2C}^{(g)}, \pi_{2A}^{(g)}, \pi_{2N}^{(g)}, T_g) = \Gamma(T_g)/[\prod_{r=1}^{2} \prod_{S} \Gamma(\beta_{rS}^{(g)})]$$

$$\times [\prod_{r=1}^{2} \prod_{S} (p_{rS|i}^{(g)})^{\beta_{rS}^{(g)}-1}] \tag{4.2}$$

where $T_g = \sum_{r=1}^{2} \sum_S \beta_{rS}^{(g)}$ and $\pi_{rS}^{(g)} = \beta_{rS}^{(g)}/T_g > 0$ for $r = 1, 2$, and $S = C, A, N$. This is because the Dirichlet distribution is rich in shapes and is often used to model the categorical data under cluster sampling (Johnson and Kotz, 1970; Lui, 1991, 2000a, 2000b). Note that $E(Y_{ij}^{(g)}(r, S)) = \pi_{rS}^{(g)}$ (Exercise 4.1) for $r = 1, 2$, $g = 1, 0$, and $S = C, A, N$. Note further that the intraclass correlation between responses $Y_{ij}^{(g)}(r, S)$ and $Y_{ij'}^{(g)}(r, S)$ for $j \neq j'$ on two different patients within cluster i assigned to treatment g can be shown to equal $\rho_g = 1/(T_g + 1)$ (Exercise 4.2). In fact, the intraclass correlation $\rho_g = 1/(T_g + 1)$ defined here can be expressed as a kappa-type correlation (Lui, Cumberland and Mayer *et al.*, 1999). Furthermore, we can easily show that the variance $Var(p_{rs|i}^{(g)}) = \pi_{rs}^{(g)}(1 - \pi_{rs}^{(g)})/(T_g + 1)$ (Exercise 4.3). Thus, the larger the value for T_g(or equivalently, the smaller the intraclass correlation ρ_g), the smaller is the variation of the probability $p_{rs|i}^{(g)}$ between clusters. For convenience, we use the notation '+' to represent summation of cell probabilities over that particular subscript. For examples, the parameter $\pi_{+S}^{(g)}$ means $\pi_{1S}^{(g)} + \pi_{2S}^{(g)}$ or $m_+^{(g)}$ means $\sum_{i=1}^{n_g} m_i^{(g)}$ (for $g = 1, 0$). Because of randomization to treatments, we have $\pi_{+S}^{(1)} = \pi_{+S}^{(0)}$ for $S = C, A, N$. We let π_{+S}, which is the proportion of subpopulation S in the sampling population, denote this common value when there is no confusion. Define $\pi_{1|S}^{(g)} = \pi_{1S}^{(g)}/\pi_{+S}$, the conditional probability of a positive response among patients assigned to treatment g in subpopulation S ($S = C, A, N$). Since clusters are randomized to treatments and always-takers (or never-takers) take the same experimental (or standard) treatment regardless of their assigned treatments, we assume the exclusion restriction assumption (Frangakis and Rubin, 1999) that $\pi_{1|A}^{(1)} = \pi_{1|A}^{(0)}(= \pi_{1|A})$ and $\pi_{1|N}^{(1)} = \pi_{1|N}^{(0)}(= \pi_{1|N})$ for always-takers and never-takers to hold. This together with $\pi_{+S}^{(1)} = \pi_{+S}^{(0)} = \pi_{+S}$ for $S = A, N$ implies that $\pi_{1A}^{(1)} = \pi_{1A}^{(0)}(= \pi_{1A})$ and $\pi_{1N}^{(1)} = \pi_{1N}^{(0)}(= \pi_{1N})$. Under the monotonicity assumption, when a patient assigned to the experimental treatment ($g = 1$) receives the standard treatment ($g = 0$), he/she must be a never-taker and hence the frequency $m_{rN|i}^{(1)}$ is observable. However, when a patient assigned to the experimental treatment receives his/her assigned (experimental) treatment, he/she can be either a complier or an always-taker. Thus, what we can observe is the sum of frequencies

$m_{rCA|i}^{(1)} = m_{rC|i}^{(1)} + m_{rA|i}^{(1)}$ instead of the individual frequency $m_{rC|i}^{(1)}$ and $m_{rA|i}^{(1)}$, separately. Similarly, when a patient assigned to the standard treatment receives the experimental treatment, he/she must be an always-taker and hence the frequency $m_{rA|i}^{(0)}$ is observable. However, if a patient assigned to the standard treatment receives his/her assigned (standard) treatment, he/she can be either a complier or a never-taker. Thus, we can observe only the sum of frequencies $m_{rCN|i}^{(0)} = m_{rC|i}^{(0)} + m_{rN|i}^{(0)}$ rather than the individual frequency $m_{rC|i}^{(0)}$ and $m_{rN|i}^{(0)}$. We define $p_{rCA|i}^{(1)} = p_{rC|i}^{(1)} + p_{rA|i}^{(1)}$ and $\pi_{rCA}^{(1)} = \pi_{rC}^{(1)} + \pi_{rA}^{(1)}$ ($r = 1, 2$) for the experimental treatment ($g = 1$). We further define $p_{rCN|i}^{(0)} = p_{rC|i}^{(0)} + p_{rN|i}^{(0)}$ and $\pi_{rCN}^{(0)} = \pi_{rC}^{(0)} + \pi_{rN}^{(0)}$ ($r = 1, 2$) for the standard treatment ($g = 0$). On the basis of the above model assumptions, the observable random vector $(m_{1CA|i}^{(1)}, m_{1N|i}^{(1)}, m_{2CA|i}^{(1)}, m_{2N|i}^{(1)})$ then follows the multinomial distribution with parameters $m_i^{(1)}$ and $(p_{1CA|i}^{(1)}, p_{1N|i}^{(1)}, p_{2CA|i}^{(1)}, p_{2N|i}^{(1)})$, where $(p_{1CA|i}^{(1)}, p_{1N|i}^{(1)}, p_{2CA|i}^{(1)}, p_{2N|i}^{(1)})$ independently and identically follows the Dirichlet probability density function $\mathcal{D}(\pi_{1CA}^{(1)}, \pi_{1N}, \pi_{2CA}^{(1)}, \pi_{2N}, T_1)$. Also, the observable random vector $(m_{1CN|i}^{(0)}, m_{1A|i}^{(0)}, m_{2CN|i}^{(0)}, m_{2A|i}^{(0)})$ follows the multinomial distribution with parameters $m_i^{(0)}$ and $(p_{1CN|i}^{(0)} \cdot p_{1A|i}^{(0)}, p_{2CN|i}^{(0)} \cdot p_{2A|i}^{(0)})$, where $(p_{1CN|i}^{(0)} \cdot p_{1A|i}^{(0)}, p_{2CN|i}^{(0)} \cdot p_{2A|i}^{(0)})$ independently and identically follows the Dirichlet probability density function $\mathcal{D}(\pi_{1CN}^{(0)}, \pi_{1A}, \pi_{2CN}^{(0)}, \pi_{2A}, T_0)$. Define $\hat{\pi}_{rS}^{(g)} = \sum_{i=1}^{n_g} m_{rS|i}^{(g)} / m_+^{(g)}$ for $r = 1,$ 2, $S = CA, N$ for $g = 1$, or $S = CN, A$ for $g = 0$. We can easily show that $\hat{\pi}_{rS}^{(g)}$ is an unbiased consistent estimator of $\pi_{rS}^{(g)}$ with variance (Exercise 4.4):

$$Var(\hat{\pi}_{rS}^{(g)}) = \pi_{rS}^{(g)}(1 - \pi_{rS}^{(g)})f(\underline{m}_g, \rho_g)/m_+^{(g)}, \qquad (4.3)$$

where $f(\underline{m}_g, \rho_g) = \sum_i m_i^{(g)}(1 + (m_i^{(g)} - 1)\rho_g)/m_+^{(g)}$, $\underline{m}_g = (m_1^{(g)}, m_2^{(g)},$ $\dots, m_{n_g}^{(g)})'$, and $m_+^{(g)} = \sum_{i=1}^{n_g} m_i^{(g)}$, as well as covariance

$$Cov(\hat{\pi}_{rS}^{(g)}, \hat{\pi}_{r'S'}^{(g)}) = -\pi_{rS}^{(g)}\pi_{r'S'}^{(g)} f(\underline{m}_g, \rho_g)/m_+^{(g)}, \quad \text{for } r \neq r' \text{ or } S \neq S'. \qquad (4.4)$$

Note that the parameter $f(\underline{m}_g, \rho_g)(\geq 1)$ is often called the variance inflation factor (VIF) due to the intraclass correlation ρ_g between patient responses within clusters. If $\rho_g = 0$, then $f(\underline{m}_g, \rho_g) = 1$. In fact, we can easily show that $f(\underline{m}_g, \rho_g)$ is an increasing function of the intraclass correlation ρ_g (Exercise 4.5). Given the total number of patients $\sum_{i=1}^{n_g} m_i^{(g)} = m_+^{(g)}$ fixed, we can show that the VIF $f(\underline{m}_g, \rho_g)$ is minimized when the cluster size is constant (i.e. $m_i^{(g)} = m_0^{(g)}$) (Exercise 4.6).

4.1   Testing superiority

Recall that under the monotonicity and exclusion restriction assumptions (for always-takers and never-takers), the ITT analysis estimates the PD, $\delta = \pi_{1+}^{(1)} - \pi_{1+}^{(0)} = \Delta \pi_{+C}$, where $\Delta = \pi_{1|C}^{(1)} - \pi_{1|C}^{(0)}$, the difference in the conditional probabilities of a positive response among compliers between two treatments (Chapter 2). Since $\pi_{+C} > 0$, $\delta = 0$ if and only if $\Delta = 0$. Thus, to test the null hypothesis $H_0: \Delta = 0$, we may apply the ITT analysis to test $H_0: \delta = 0$. Define

$$\bar{Y}^{(g)} = \sum_S \sum_{i=1}^{n_g} \sum_{j=1}^{m_i^{(g)}} Y_{ij}^{(g)}(1, S) / m_+^{(g)} = \sum_S \hat{\pi}_{1S}^{(g)} = \hat{\pi}_{1+}^{(g)}, \quad (4.5)$$

where $\bar{Y}^{(g)}$(or $\hat{\pi}_{1+}^{(g)}$) actually represents the proportion of a positive response among patients assigned to treatment g ($= 1$ for experimental, and $= 0$ for standard) despite what treatment they actually receive. Define $\hat{\delta}^{(CL)} = \bar{Y}^{(1)} - \bar{Y}^{(0)} (= \hat{\pi}_{1+}^{(1)} - \hat{\pi}_{1+}^{(0)})$. One can show that the expectation under the above assumptions is (Exercise 4.7):

$$E(\hat{\delta}^{(CL)}) = E(\hat{\pi}_{1+}^{(1)} - \hat{\pi}_{1+}^{(0)}) = \delta \quad (4.6)$$

We can further show that the variance for $\hat{\delta}^{(CL)}$ is given by

$$Var(\hat{\delta}^{(CL)}) = \sum_{g=0}^{1} [\pi_{1+}^{(g)}(1 - \pi_{1+}^{(g)}) f(\underline{m}_g, \rho_g) / m_+^{(g)}] \quad (4.7)$$

Following Light and Margolin (1971) and Rae (1988), we can estimate the intraclass correlation ρ_g by (Exercise 4.8):

$$\hat{\rho}_g = (BMS_g - WMS_g) / [BMS_g + (m_g^* - 1) WMS_g],$$

$$BMS_g = [\sum_{i=1}^{n_g} \sum_{r=1}^{2} \sum_S (m_{rs|i}^{(g)})^2 / m_i^{(g)}$$

$$- \sum_{r=1}^{2} \sum_S (\sum_{i=1}^{n_g} m_{rS|i}^{(g)})^2 / m_+^{(g)}] / [2(n_g - 1)],$$

$$WMS_g = [m_+^{(g)} - \sum_{i=1}^{n_g} \sum_{r=1}^{2} \sum_S (m_{rs|i}^{(g)})^2 / m_i^{(g)}] / [2(m_+^{(g)} - n_g)], \quad (4.8)$$

where $m_g^* = [(m_+^{(g)})^2 - \sum_i (m_i^{(g)})^2]/[(n_g - 1)m_+^{(g)}]$, the summation of S is over CA and N for $g = 1$, and is over CN and A for $g = 0$. The discussion on interval estimation of the intraclass correlation under the Dirichlet-multinomial distribution appears elsewhere (Lui, Cumberland and Mayer et al., 1999). On the basis of $\hat{\rho}_g$(4.8), we can estimate the variance $Var(\hat{\delta}^{(CL)}|H_0)$ under $H_0 : \Delta = 0$ by

$$\hat{Var}(\hat{\delta}^{(CL)}|H_0) = \hat{\pi}_{1+}^{(p)}(1 - \hat{\pi}_{1+}^{(p)})(\sum_{g=0}^{1} f(\underline{m}_g, \hat{\rho}_g)/m_+^{(g)}) \qquad (4.9)$$

where $\hat{\pi}_{1+}^{(p)} = (m_+^{(1)}\hat{\pi}_{1+}^{(1)} + m_+^{(0)}\hat{\pi}_{1+}^{(0)})/(\sum_{g=0}^{1} m_+^{(g)})$ is the pooled estimate of the two proportions of a positive response for the two treatments. On the basis of $\hat{Var}(\hat{\delta}^{(CL)}|H_0)$ (4.9), we may consider the test statistic

$$Z = \hat{\delta}^{(CL)}/\sqrt{\hat{Var}(\hat{\delta}^{(CL)}|H_0)}. \qquad (4.10)$$

We will reject $H_0 : \Delta = 0$ at the α-level if the test statistic (4.10), $Z > Z_{\alpha/2}$ or $Z < -Z_{\alpha/2}$, where Z_α is the upper $100(\alpha)$th percentile of the standard normal distribution. Although our interest is to detect the superiority of the experimental treatment to the standard treatment, as noted in previous chapters, we may wish to do a two-sided test rather than a one-sided test for ethical and safety reasons (Fleiss, 1981). We will claim that the experimental treatment is superior to the standard treatment if the test statistic (4.10), $Z > Z_{\alpha/2}$ holds. Note also that in application of statistic (4.10) for testing superiority, we may also consider using $\tanh^{-1}(x)(= 0.5 \log((1 + x)/(1 - x)))$ transformation (Edwardes, 1995; Lui, 2002). Since the asymptotic variance $Var(\tanh^{-1}(\hat{\delta}^{(CL)})|H_0)$ under $H_0 : \Delta = 0$ is the same as $Var(\hat{\delta}^{(CL)}|H_0)$, we obtain the following test statistic (Lui and Chang, 2011a),

$$Z = \tanh^{-1}(\hat{\delta}^{(CL)})/\sqrt{\hat{Var}(\hat{\delta}^{(CL)}|H_0)}, \qquad (4.11)$$

where $\hat{Var}(\hat{\delta}^{(CL)}|H_0)$ is given in (4.9). If the test statistic (4.11), $Z > Z_{\alpha/2}$ or $Z < -Z_{\alpha/2}$, we will reject $H_0 : \Delta = 0$ at the α- level. In particular, we will claim that the experimental treatment is superior to the standard treatment if the test statistic (4.11), $Z > Z_{\alpha/2}$ holds. Note that as $m_i^{(g)} = 1$ for all $i = 1, 2, \ldots, n_g$ and $g = 1, 0$, the VIF $f(\underline{m}_g, \rho_g)$ reduces to 1 and thereby, test statistics (4.10) and (4.11) reduce to test statistics (2.3) and (2.4), respectively, for the case of no cluster sampling. Note also that $f(\underline{m}_g, \rho_g)$ simplifies to $(1 + (m_0^{(g)} - 1)\rho_g)$ when $m_i^{(g)} = m_0^{(g)}$ for all i. Thus, we can use $1/(1 + (m_0^{(g)} - 1)\rho_g)$ to measure the relative efficiency of a statistic under cluster sampling with a constant cluster size versus its corresponding statistic under multinomial sampling with no clusters. To help readers appreciate that a substantial loss of efficiency can arise for a small intraclass correlation when the underlying cluster size is large, we summarize the values of $1/(1 + (m_0^{(g)} - 1)\rho_g)$ for the intraclass correlation $\rho_g = 0.005, 0.010, 0.20, 0.05, 0.10, 0.20$ and the cluster size $m_0^{(g)} = 5, 10, 20, 50, 100$ in Table 4.1. We can see that when $\rho_g = 0.02$ and $m_0^{(g)} = 100$, the relative efficiency of a statistic under cluster sampling is only 34% of the corresponding statistic under multinomial sampling. In other words, a small intraclass correlation can cause a substantial loss of efficiency for a test statistic when the cluster size is large. Since the information needed for calculation of the VIF $f(\underline{m}_g, \hat{\rho}_g)$ is sometimes unavailable, we may often choose to ignore the cluster effect in data analysis for simplicity, especially when the intraclass correlation is believed to be small. When the underlying cluster size is large, however, it may be advisable to do sensitivity analysis of our findings as a function of the underlying intraclass correlation ρ_g.

Table 4.1   The relative efficiency $(= 1/(1 + (m_0^{(g)} - 1)\rho_g))$ of a test statistic under cluster sampling with constant cluster size $m_0^{(g)}$ versus no cluster sampling.

| ρ_g | $m_0^{(g)} =$ | | | | |
	5	10	20	50	100
0.005	0.980	0.957	0.913	0.803	0.669
0.010	0.962	0.917	0.840	0.671	0.503
0.020	0.926	0.847	0.725	0.505	0.336
0.050	0.833	0.690	0.513	0.290	0.168
0.100	0.714	0.526	0.345	0.169	0.092
0.200	0.556	0.357	0.208	0.093	0.048

Example 4.1   Consider the data in Table 2.1 regarding a CRT studying the effect of vitamin A supplementation on mortality among preschool children in rural Indonesia (Sommer and Zeger, 1991; Sommer, Tarwotjo, Djunaedi *et al.*, 1986). Children who resided in 225 randomly selected villages out of 450 were assigned to the experimental group of receiving two large oral doses of vitamin A, and children who resided in the remaining 225 villages were assigned to a control group of receiving no vitamin A. The randomized units are villages rather than children here. Thus, we may wish to do sensitivity analysis to study the cluster effect due to the intraclass correlation on our previous finding – there was strong evidence that taking vitamin A supplementation could reduce the mortality of preschool children (*Example 2.1*). Given the data in Table 2.1, we have $m_+^{(1)} = 12094$ and $m_+^{(0)} = 11588$, $\hat{\pi}_{1+}^{(1)} = 0.9962$, and $\hat{\pi}_{1+}^{(0)} = 0.9936$. Because we do not have the information on the individual cluster size $m_i^{(g)}$, we assume the cluster size to be constant and hence we replace $m_i^{(g)}$ in VIF $f(\underline{m}_g, \hat{\rho}_g)$ by the average cluster size $\bar{m}^{(g)} = \sum_i m_i^{(g)}/n_g$. We obtain $\bar{m}^{(1)} = 54(\approx 12094/225)$ and $\bar{m}^{(0)} = 52(\approx 11588/225)$. For given a value of $\rho_1 = \rho_0 = \rho$, we obtain the estimated variance $\widehat{Var}(\hat{\delta}^{(CL)}|H_0)(4.9)$ as $0.0051[(1+53\rho)/12094+(1+51\rho)/11588]$. Note that the larger the intraclass correlation ρ, the smaller is the test value $Z = \hat{\delta}^{(CL)}/\sqrt{\widehat{Var}(\hat{\delta}^{(CL)}|H_0)}$ (4.10). Therefore, we may want to find the maximum value ρ such that the inequality: $|Z| \geq 1.96$ can still hold. Based on the above data, we find the maximum value for ρ without changing our previously significant finding (in Example 2.1) at the 5 %-level is approximately 0.02. If the village size $m_i^{(g)}$ varied, this maximum value for ρ could be even smaller than 0.02 to reverse the previously significant testing result (see Exercise 4.6). Thus, we should always be cautious in ignoring clusters under cluster sampling especially when the underlying cluster size is large.

4.2   Testing noninferiority

When it is unethical to have a placebo control and is difficult to beat a standard treatment, we may consider testing the noninferiority of an experimental treatment to the standard treatment with respect to treatment efficacy in establishing the effectiveness of the experimental treatment.

For administrative convenience, as noted before, we sometimes use clusters of patients cared by the same physicians instead of individual patients as randomized units. Also, we may take more than one measurement per patient to increase the reliability of our data when the measurement on patient responses is not reliable (Fleiss, 1981; Lui, 1991, 1997a). The repeated measurements taken from the same patients are likely correlated and form clusters. In this section, we focus discussion on assessing noninferiority based on the PD, PR and OR under a CRT.

4.2.1   Using the difference in proportions

When testing noninferiority based on the PD, we are interested in finding out whether the underlying PD Δ is larger than $-\varepsilon_l$, where $\varepsilon_l(> 0)$ is the maximum acceptable margin such that the experimental drug can be regarded as noninferior to the standard treatment. Because the inequality $\delta > -\varepsilon_l$ does not necessarily imply that $\Delta > -\varepsilon_l$, as noted in Chapter 2, we cannot apply the ITT analysis here to test noninferiority. Recall that the PD $\Delta(= \pi_{1|C}^{(1)} - \pi_{1|C}^{(0)})$ of a positive response among compliers can be re-expressed as $(\pi_{1+}^{(1)} - \pi_{1+}^{(0)})/(\pi_{+CA}^{(1)} - \pi_{+A}^{(0)})$. Thus, we may substitute $\hat{\pi}_{rS}^{(g)}(= \sum_{i=1}^{n_g} m_{rS|i}^{(g)}/m_+^{(g)})$ for $\pi_{rS}^{(g)}(r = 1, 2,$ for $S = CA, N$ when $g = 1$, or for $S = CN, A$ when $g = 0)$ in Δ, and obtain the consistent estimator under cluster sampling,

$$\hat{\Delta}^{(CL)} = (\hat{\pi}_{1+}^{(1)} - \hat{\pi}_{1+}^{(0)})/(\hat{\pi}_{+CA}^{(1)} - \hat{\pi}_{+A}^{(0)}), \qquad (4.12)$$

where $\hat{\pi}_{+CA}^{(1)} = \hat{\pi}_{1CA}^{(1)} + \hat{\pi}_{2CA}^{(1)}$ and $\hat{\pi}_{+A}^{(0)} = \hat{\pi}_{1A}^{(0)} + \hat{\pi}_{2A}^{(0)}$. Note that $\hat{\Delta}^{(CL)}$ (4.12) is actually identical to the estimator $\hat{\Delta}$(2.5) when we ignore clusters and pool data from all clusters together. Because patient responses within clusters are correlated, however, the variance $Var(\hat{\Delta}^{(CL)})$ is different from $Var(\hat{\Delta})$ for $\hat{\Delta}$ (2.5). Using the delta method (Casella and Berger, 1990), we obtain an asymptotic variance estimator of $\hat{\Delta}^{(CL)}$(4.12) as given by (Exercise 4.9):

$$\hat{Var}(\hat{\Delta}^{(CL)}) = \{[\hat{\pi}_{1+}^{(1)}(1 - \hat{\pi}_{1+}^{(1)})f(\underline{m}_1, \hat{\rho}_1)/m_+^{(1)} + \hat{\pi}_{1+}^{(0)}(1 - \hat{\pi}_{1+}^{(0)})$$
$$\times f(\underline{m}_0, \hat{\rho}_0)/m_+^{(0)}] + \hat{\Delta}^2[\hat{\pi}_{+CA}^{(1)}(1 - \hat{\pi}_{+CA}^{(1)})f(\underline{m}_1, \hat{\rho}_1)/m_+^{(1)}$$
$$+ \hat{\pi}_{+A}^{(0)}(1 - \hat{\pi}_{+A}^{(0)})f(\underline{m}_0, \hat{\rho}_0)/m_+^{(0)}] - 2\hat{\Delta}[(\hat{\pi}_{1CA}^{(1)} - \hat{\pi}_{1+}^{(1)}\hat{\pi}_{+CA}^{(1)})$$

$$\times f(\underline{m}_1, \hat{\rho}_1)/m_+^{(1)} + (\hat{\pi}_{1A}^{(0)} - \hat{\pi}_{1+}^{(0)}\hat{\pi}_{+A}^{(0)})f(\underline{m}_0, \hat{\rho}_0)/m_+^{(0)}]\}/$$
$$(\hat{\pi}_{+CA}^{(1)} - \hat{\pi}_{+A}^{(0)})^2. \tag{4.13}$$

We can easily show that $\hat{Var}(\hat{\Delta}^{(CL)})$(4.13) is expected to be larger than the corresponding $\hat{Var}(\hat{\Delta})$(2.6) (with n_g in (2.6) replaced by $m_+^{(g)}$) due to $f(\underline{m}_g, \hat{\rho}_g) \geq 1$ (Exercise 4.10). Thus, when ignoring clusters in analyzing data under cluster sampling, we tend to underestimate the variance of our test statistic, and thereby, our testing results and interval estimates can be liberal. On the basis of (4.12) and (4.13), we obtain the following test statistic with the $\tanh^{-1}(\hat{\Delta}^{(CL)})$ transformation,

$$Z = [\tanh^{-1}(\hat{\Delta}^{(CL)}) + \tanh^{-1}(\varepsilon_l)]/\sqrt{\hat{Var}(\tanh^{-1}(\hat{\Delta}^{(CL)}))}, \tag{4.14}$$

where $\hat{Var}(\tanh^{-1}(\hat{\Delta}^{(CL)})) = \hat{Var}(\hat{\Delta}^{(CL)})/(1 - (\hat{\Delta}^{(CL)})^2)^2$. We will reject $H_0 : \Delta \leq -\varepsilon_l$ at the α-level if the test statistic (4.14), $Z > Z_\alpha$. Note that statistic (4.14) includes statistic (2.7) as a special case when $m_i^{(g)} = 1$ for all i and both g, or when $\rho_g = 0$ for both g. Although the PD is the most commonly used index to measure the relative treatment effect in a RCT, it can be difficult to provide a fixed constant clinically acceptable margin ε_l, which is applicable to all situations. This is partially due to the fact that the range for the PD is $-1 < \Delta < 1$ and a given fixed value ε_l may possess different clinical significance depending on the underlying probabilities of patient responses. Thus, we may often consider use of the PR and OR to measure the relative treatment effect in testing noninferiority.

4.2.2 Using the ratio of proportions

Recall that the PR of a positive response among compliers is defined as $\gamma = \pi_{1|C}^{(1)}/\pi_{1|C}^{(0)} = \pi_{1C}^{(1)}/\pi_{1C}^{(0)}$(2.8). Because $\pi_{1C}^{(1)} = \pi_{1CA}^{(1)} - \pi_{1A}$, an unbiased consistent estimator under cluster sampling for $\pi_{1C}^{(1)}$ is $\hat{\pi}_{1C}^{(1)} = \hat{\pi}_{1CA}^{(1)} - \hat{\pi}_{1A}^{(0)}$, where $\hat{\pi}_{1CA}^{(1)} = \sum_{i=1}^{n_1} m_{1CA|i}^{(1)}/m_+^{(1)}$ and $\hat{\pi}_{1A}^{(0)} = \sum_{i=1}^{n_0} m_{1A|i}^{(0)}/m_+^{(0)}$. Similarly, because $\pi_{1C}^{(0)} = \pi_{1CN}^{(0)} - \pi_{1N}$, an unbiased consistent estimator for $\pi_{1C}^{(0)}$ is $\hat{\pi}_{1C}^{(0)} = \hat{\pi}_{1CN}^{(0)} - \hat{\pi}_{1N}^{(1)}$, where $\hat{\pi}_{1CN}^{(0)} = \sum_{i=1}^{n_0} m_{1CN|i}^{(0)}/m_+^{(0)}$ and $\hat{\pi}_{1N}^{(1)} = \sum_{i=1}^{n_1} m_{1N|i}^{(1)}/m_+^{(1)}$. Therefore, a consistent estimator for γ under cluster sampling is given by

$$\hat{\gamma}^{(CL)} = (\hat{\pi}_{1CA}^{(1)} - \hat{\pi}_{1A}^{(0)})/(\hat{\pi}_{1CN}^{(0)} - \hat{\pi}_{1N}^{(1)}). \qquad (4.15)$$

Furthermore, we can show that an estimated asymptotic variance $\hat{Var}(\log(\hat{\gamma}^{(CL)}))$ for the statistic $\log(\hat{\gamma}^{(CL)})$ using the logarithmic transformation is given by (Exercise 4.11):

$$\hat{Var}(\log(\hat{\gamma}^{(CL)})) = [\hat{\pi}_{1CA}^{(1)}(1 - \hat{\pi}_{1CA}^{(1)})f(\underline{m}_1, \hat{\rho}_1)/m_+^{(1)} + \hat{\pi}_{1A}^{(0)}(1 - \hat{\pi}_{1A}^{(0)})$$
$$\times f(\underline{m}_0, \hat{\rho}_0)/m_+^{(0)}]/(\hat{\pi}_{1CA}^{(1)} - \hat{\pi}_{1A}^{(0)})^2 + [\hat{\pi}_{1N}^{(1)}(1 - \hat{\pi}_{1N}^{(1)})$$
$$\times f(\underline{m}_1, \hat{\rho}_1)/m_+^{(1)} + \hat{\pi}_{1CN}^{(0)}(1 - \hat{\pi}_{1CN}^{(0)})f(\underline{m}_0, \hat{\rho}_0)/m_+^{(0)}]/$$
$$(\hat{\pi}_{1CN}^{(0)} - \hat{\pi}_{1N}^{(1)})^2 - 2[\hat{\pi}_{1CA}^{(1)}\hat{\pi}_{1N}^{(1)}f(\underline{m}_1, \hat{\rho}_1)/m_+^{(1)} + \hat{\pi}_{1CN}^{(0)}$$
$$\times \hat{\pi}_{1A}^{(0)}f(\underline{m}_0, \hat{\rho}_0)/m_+^{(0)}]/[(\hat{\pi}_{1CA}^{(1)} - \hat{\pi}_{1A}^{(0)})(\hat{\pi}_{1CN}^{(0)} - \hat{\pi}_{1N}^{(1)})].$$
$$(4.16)$$

In testing noninferiority based on the PR, we consider testing $H_0 : \gamma \leq 1 - \gamma_l$ versus $H_a : \gamma > 1 - \gamma_l$, where γ_l is the maximum clinically acceptable margin such that the experimental treatment can be regarded as noninferior to the standard treatment when $\gamma > 1 - \gamma_l$. On the basis of (4.15) and (4.16), we obtain the following test statistic,

$$Z = (\log(\hat{\gamma}^{(CL)}) - \log(1 - \gamma_l))/\sqrt{\hat{Var}(\log(\hat{\gamma}^{(CL)}))}. \qquad (4.17)$$

If the test statistic (4.17), $Z > Z_\alpha$, we will reject $H_0 : \gamma \leq 1 - \gamma_l$ at the α-level and claim that the experimental treatment is noninferior to the standard treatment. Because the PR lacks symmetry and the noninferior margin for the PR leads to produce a corresponding noninferior margin on the PD scale against the general guideline in a draft of establishing the effectiveness of a new *H. pylori* regimen of FDA (1997), as noted in Section 2.2.2, we consider use of the OR in establishing noninferiority.

4.2.3   Using the odds ratio of proportions

In testing noninferiority or doing meta-analysis, the OR has been recommended to use due to its stability in values and its use providing a close agreement of the clinically noninferior margin on the difference scale with the general guideline provided by FDA (1997) (Tu, 1998 and 2003; Wang, Chow and Li, 2002; Garrett, 2003). Recall that the OR of a positive response among compliers between the experimental and standard treatments is defined as $\varphi = (\pi_{1C}^{(1)}\pi_{2C}^{(0)})/(\pi_{2C}^{(1)}\pi_{1C}^{(0)})$ (2.12). Thus, we consider the following consistent estimator for φ as given by (Lui and Chang, 2011b)

$$\hat{\varphi}^{(CL)} = [(\hat{\pi}_{1CA}^{(1)} - \hat{\pi}_{1A}^{(0)})(\hat{\pi}_{2CN}^{(0)} - \hat{\pi}_{2N}^{(1)})]/[(\hat{\pi}_{2CA}^{(1)} - \hat{\pi}_{2A}^{(0)})(\hat{\pi}_{1CN}^{(0)} - \hat{\pi}_{1N}^{(1)})].$$
(4.18)

Using the delta method (Agresti, 1990; Lui, 2004), we obtain an estimated asymptotic variance of $\log(\hat{\varphi}^{(CL)})$ with the logarithmic transformation as (Exercise 4.12):

$$
\begin{aligned}
\widehat{Var}(\log(\hat{\varphi}^{(CL)})) = & [\hat{\pi}_{1CA}^{(1)}(1 - \hat{\pi}_{1CA}^{(1)})f(\underline{m}_1, \hat{\rho}_1)/m_+^{(1)} + \hat{\pi}_{1A}^{(0)}(1 - \hat{\pi}_{1A}^{(0)}) \\
& \times f(\underline{m}_0, \hat{\rho}_0)/m_+^{(0)}]/(\hat{\pi}_{1CA}^{(1)} - \hat{\pi}_{1A}^{(0)})^2 + [\hat{\pi}_{2CN}^{(0)}(1 - \hat{\pi}_{2CN}^{(0)}) \\
& \times f(\underline{m}_0, \hat{\rho}_0)/m_+^{(0)} + \hat{\pi}_{2N}^{(1)}(1 - \hat{\pi}_{2N}^{(1)})f(\underline{m}_1, \hat{\rho}_1)/m_+^{(1)}]/ \\
& (\hat{\pi}_{2CN}^{(0)} - \hat{\pi}_{2N}^{(1)})^2 + [\hat{\pi}_{2CA}^{(1)}(1 - \hat{\pi}_{2CA}^{(1)})f(\underline{m}_1, \hat{\rho}_1)/m_+^{(1)} \\
& + \hat{\pi}_{2A}^{(0)}(1 - \hat{\pi}_{2A}^{(0)})f(\underline{m}_0, \hat{\rho}_0)/m_+^{(0)}]/(\hat{\pi}_{2CA}^{(1)} - \hat{\pi}_{2A}^{(0)})^2 \\
& + [\hat{\pi}_{1CN}^{(0)}(1 - \hat{\pi}_{1CN}^{(0)})f(\underline{m}_0, \hat{\rho}_0)/m_+^{(0)} + \hat{\pi}_{1N}^{(1)}(1 - \hat{\pi}_{1N}^{(1)}) \\
& \times f(\underline{m}_1, \hat{\rho}_1)/m_+^{(1)}]/(\hat{\pi}_{1CN}^{(0)} - \hat{\pi}_{1N}^{(1)})^2 + 2[\hat{\pi}_{1CA}^{(1)}\hat{\pi}_{2N}^{(1)} \\
& \times f(\underline{m}_1, \hat{\rho}_1)/m_+^{(1)} + \hat{\pi}_{1A}^{(0)}\hat{\pi}_{2CN}^{(0)}f(\underline{m}_0, \hat{\rho}_0)/m_+^{(0)}]/ \\
& [(\hat{\pi}_{1CA}^{(1)} - \hat{\pi}_{1A}^{(0)})(\hat{\pi}_{2CN}^{(0)} - \hat{\pi}_{2N}^{(1)})] + 2[\hat{\pi}_{1CA}^{(1)}\hat{\pi}_{2CA}^{(1)}f(\underline{m}_1, \hat{\rho}_1)/ \\
& m_+^{(1)} + \hat{\pi}_{1A}^{(0)}\hat{\pi}_{2A}^{(0)}f(\underline{m}_0, \hat{\rho}_0)/m_+^{(0)}]/[(\hat{\pi}_{1CA}^{(1)} - \hat{\pi}_{1A}^{(0)})(\hat{\pi}_{2CA}^{(1)} \\
& - \hat{\pi}_{2A}^{(0)})] - 2[\hat{\pi}_{1CA}^{(1)}\hat{\pi}_{1N}^{(1)}f(\underline{m}_1, \hat{\rho}_1)/m_+^{(1)} + \hat{\pi}_{1CN}^{(0)}\hat{\pi}_{1A}^{(0)} \\
& \times f(\underline{m}_0, \hat{\rho}_0)/m_+^{(0)}]/[(\hat{\pi}_{1CA}^{(1)} - \hat{\pi}_{1A}^{(0)})(\hat{\pi}_{1CN}^{(0)} - \hat{\pi}_{1N}^{(1)})] \\
& - 2[\hat{\pi}_{2CA}^{(1)}\hat{\pi}_{2N}^{(1)}f(\underline{m}_1, \hat{\rho}_1)/m_+^{(1)} + \hat{\pi}_{2A}^{(0)}\hat{\pi}_{2CN}^{(0)}f(\underline{m}_0, \hat{\rho}_0)/ \\
& m_+^{(0)}]/[(\hat{\pi}_{2CA}^{(1)} - \hat{\pi}_{2A}^{(0)})(\hat{\pi}_{2CN}^{(0)} - \hat{\pi}_{2N}^{(1)})] + 2[\hat{\pi}_{1N}^{(1)}\hat{\pi}_{2N}^{(1)} \\
& \times f(\underline{m}_1, \hat{\rho}_1)/m_+^{(1)} + \hat{\pi}_{1CN}^{(0)}\hat{\pi}_{2CN}^{(0)}f(\underline{m}_0, \hat{\rho}_0)/m_+^{(0)}]/ \\
& [(\hat{\pi}_{2CN}^{(0)} - \hat{\pi}_{2N}^{(1)})(\hat{\pi}_{1CN}^{(0)} - \hat{\pi}_{1N}^{(1)})] + 2[\hat{\pi}_{2CA}^{(1)}\hat{\pi}_{1N}^{(1)}f(\underline{m}_1, \hat{\rho}_1)/ \\
& m_+^{(1)} + \hat{\pi}_{2A}^{(0)}\hat{\pi}_{1CN}^{(0)}f(\underline{m}_0, \hat{\rho}_0)/ \\
& m_+^{(0)}]/[(\hat{\pi}_{2CA}^{(1)} - \hat{\pi}_{2A}^{(0)})(\hat{\pi}_{1CN}^{(0)} - \hat{\pi}_{1N}^{(1)})].
\end{aligned}
$$
(4.19)

In detecting noninferiority, we consider testing $H_0 : \varphi \leq 1 - \varphi_l$ versus $H_a : \varphi > 1 - \varphi_l$, where φ_l is the maximum clinically acceptable margin such that the experimental treatment can be regarded as noninferior to the standard treatment when $\varphi > 1 - \varphi_l$. On the basis of (4.18) and (4.19), we may consider the following test statistic,

$$Z = (\log(\hat{\varphi}^{(CL)}) - \log(1 - \varphi_l))/\sqrt{\hat{Var}(\log(\hat{\varphi}^{(CL)}))}. \qquad (4.20)$$

We will reject $H_0 : \varphi \le 1 - \varphi_l$ at the α-level if the test statistic (4.20), $Z > Z_\alpha$, and claim that the experimental treatment is noninferior to the standard treatment.

4.3   Testing equivalence

When an experimental or a new generic drug is developed, we may be interested in establishing equivalence (rather than noninferiority) with respect to therapeutic efficacy between the experimental (or the generic) drug and the standard drug due to the concern of toxicity. We can easily modify the test procedures for testing noninferiority developed in the previous section to test equivalence under a CRT with noncompliance. For reader's information, we briefly outline these test procedures for testing equivalence based on the PD, PR and OR in the presence of noncompliance, while accounting for the intraclass correlation between patient responses under cluster sampling.

4.3.1   Using the difference in proportions

When assessing equivalence based on the PD, we consider testing $H_0 : \Delta \le -\varepsilon_l$ or $\Delta \ge \varepsilon_u$ versus $H_a : -\varepsilon_l < \Delta < \varepsilon_u$, where ε_l and $\varepsilon_u (> 0)$ are the maximum clinically acceptable lower and upper margins that the experimental treatment can be regarded as equivalent to the standard treatment. Using the Intersection-Union test (Casella and Berger, 1990), we will reject the null hypothesis $H_0 : \Delta \le -\varepsilon_l$ or $\Delta \ge \varepsilon_u$ at the α-level and claim that the two treatments are equivalent if the test statistic $\tanh^{-1}(\hat{\Delta}^{(CL)})$ simultaneously satisfies the following two inequalities,

$$(\tanh^{-1}(\hat{\Delta}^{(CL)}) + \tanh^{-1}(\varepsilon_l))/\sqrt{\hat{Var}(\tanh^{-1}(\hat{\Delta}^{(CL)}))} > Z_\alpha$$

$$\text{and } (\tanh^{-1}(\hat{\Delta}^{(CL)}) - \tanh^{-1}(\varepsilon_u))/\sqrt{\hat{Var}(\tanh^{-1}(\hat{\Delta}^{(CL)}))} < -Z_\alpha,$$

$$(4.21)$$

where $\hat{Var}(\tanh^{-1}(\hat{\Delta}^{(CL)})) = \hat{Var}(\hat{\Delta}^{(CL)})/(1 - (\hat{\Delta}^{(CL)})^2)^2$, $\hat{\Delta}^{(CL)}$ and $\hat{Var}(\hat{\Delta}^{(CL)})$ are given in (4.12) and (4.13), respectively.

4.3.2   Using the ratio of proportions

When assessing equivalence based on the PR, we consider testing H_0 : $\gamma \leq 1 - \gamma_l$ or $\gamma \geq 1 + \gamma_u$ versus $H_a : 1 - \gamma_l < \gamma < 1 + \gamma_u$ where γ_l and γ_u (> 0) are the maximum clinically acceptable lower and upper margins that the experimental treatment can be regarded as equivalent to the standard treatment. We will reject $H_0 : \gamma \leq 1 - \gamma_l$ or $\gamma \geq 1 + \gamma_u$ at the α-level and claim that two treatments are equivalent if the test statistic $\log(\hat{\gamma}^{(CL)})$ simultaneously satisfies the following two inequalities,

$$(\log(\hat{\gamma}^{(CL)}) - \log(1 - \gamma_l))/\sqrt{\hat{Var}(\log(\hat{\gamma}^{(CL)}))} > Z_\alpha.$$

$$\text{and } (\log(\hat{\gamma}^{(CL)}) - \log(1 + \gamma_u))/\sqrt{\hat{Var}(\log(\hat{\gamma}^{(CL)}))} < -Z_\alpha, \quad (4.22)$$

where $\hat{\gamma}^{(CL)}$ and $\hat{Var}(\log(\hat{\gamma}^{(CL)}))$ are given in (4.15) and (4.16), respectively.

4.3.3   Using the odds ratio of proportions

When assessing equivalence based on the OR ($\varphi = (\pi_{1|C}^{(1)}\pi_{2|C}^{(0)})/(\pi_{2|C}^{(1)}\pi_{1|C}^{(0)})$), we want to test $H_0 : \varphi \leq 1 - \varphi_l$ or $\varphi \geq 1 + \varphi_u$ versus $H_a : 1 - \varphi_l < \varphi < 1 + \varphi_u$, where φ_l and φ_u are the maximum clinically acceptable lower and upper margins that the experimental treatment can be regarded as equivalent to the standard treatment. Using the Intersection-Union test, we will reject $H_a : 1 - \varphi_l < \varphi < 1 + \varphi_u$ at the α-level if the test statistic $\log(\hat{\varphi}^{(CL)})$ simultaneously satisfies the following two inequalities,

$$(\log(\hat{\varphi}^{(CL)}) - \log(1 - \varphi_l))/\sqrt{\hat{Var}(\log(\hat{\varphi}^{(CL)}))} > Z_\alpha \text{ and}$$

$$(\log(\hat{\varphi}^{(CL)}) - \log(1 + \varphi_u))/\sqrt{\hat{Var}(\log(\hat{\varphi}^{(CL)}))} < -Z_\alpha \quad (4.23)$$

where $\hat{\varphi}^{(CL)}$ and $\hat{Var}(\log(\hat{\varphi}^{(CL)}))$ are given in (4.18) and (4.19), respectively. Note that test procedures (4.21)–(4.23) reduce to test procedures (2.16)–(2.18), respectively, when $m_i^{(g)} = 1$ for all i and g, or $\rho_g = 0$ for

$g = 1, 0$. Note also that if we employ test procedures (2.16)-(2.18) with ignoring clusters under cluster sampling, as noted previously, we tend to underestimate the standard error of our test statistic and hence the actual Type I error for testing superiority, noninferiority, or equivalence is likely larger than the nominal α-level (Exercise 4.13).

4.4 Interval estimation

Under a CRT, using interval estimators without accounting for the intraclass correlation can lose accuracy with respect to the coverage probability (Exercise 4.14), especially when the cluster size $m_i^{(g)}$ is large. Based on the variance estimators derived in this chapter, we can apply various methods discussed in the previous chapters to obtain the corresponding interval estimators for the PD, PR and OR under a CRT. For brevity, we will present only a single one interval estimator for each of these indices under a CRT with noncompliance.

4.4.1 Estimation of the proportion difference

When the number of clusters n_g is large, the sampling distribution for $(\hat{\Delta}^{(CL)} - \Delta)/(\hat{Var}(\hat{\Delta}^{(CL)}))^{1/2}$, where $\hat{\Delta}^{(CL)}$ and $\hat{Var}(\hat{\Delta}^{(CL)})$ are given in (4.12) and (4.13), respectively, is approximately normal. When doing interval estimation of the PD, we may consider use of the $\tanh^{-1}(x)$ transformation to improve the performance of an interval estimator directly based on $\hat{\Delta}^{(CL)}$ and to avoid the parameter constraint on the range $-1 < \Delta < 1$. This leads us to obtain an asymptotic $100(1-\alpha)\%$ confidence interval for $\Delta(=\pi_{1|C}^{(1)} - \pi_{1|C}^{(0)})$ as given by

$$[\tanh(\tanh^{-1}(\hat{\Delta}^{(CL)}) - Z_{\alpha/2}(\hat{Var}(\tanh^{-1}(\hat{\Delta}^{(CL)})))^{1/2}),$$
$$\tanh(\tanh^{-1}(\hat{\Delta}^{(CL)}) + Z_{\alpha/2}(\hat{Var}(\tanh^{-1}(\hat{\Delta}^{(CL)})))^{1/2})] \quad (4.24)$$

where $\hat{Var}(\tanh^{-1}(\hat{\Delta}^{(CL)})) = \hat{Var}(\hat{\Delta}^{(CL)})/(1 - (\hat{\Delta}^{(CL)})^2)^2$. Although the interval estimator (4.24) has a similar form as the interval estimator (2.20), the average length of (4.24) is likely larger than that of (2.20) due to the intraclass correlation between patient responses within clusters, given a fixed total number of studied patients.

Example 4.2 For the purpose of illustration, we consider the hypothetical data in Table 4.2. These data are simulated for comparing an experimental treatment with a standard treatment, each treatment having 30 clusters of various sizes. Because of randomization, say, we assume that the intraclass correlation between the two treatments are equal (i.e. $\rho_1 = \rho_0$) and hence we may use $\hat{\rho} = (m_+^{(1)}\hat{\rho}_1 + m_+^{(0)}\hat{\rho}_0)/(m_+^{(1)} + m_+^{(0)})$ to estimate the common intraclass correlation ρ, where $\hat{\rho}_g$ is given in (4.8). Given the data in Table 4.2, we obtain $\hat{\rho}_0 = 0.106$ and $\hat{\rho}_1 = 0.100$ and thereby, the estimate of the common intraclass correlation is given by $\hat{\rho} = 0.103$. When using the point estimator (4.12) and the interval estimator (4.24), we obtain $\hat{\Delta}^{(CL)} = 0.109$ and an asymptotic 95 % confidence interval for Δ as given by $[-0.007, 0.222]$. Because the lower limit of this resulting interval estimate is below $\Delta = 0$, there is no significant evidence at the 5 % level to claim that the positive rate of patient response in the experimental treatment is higher than that in the standard treatment.

4.4.2   Estimation of the proportion ratio

Note that an interval estimator derived directly based on $\hat{\gamma}^{(CL)}$(4.15) can be inaccurate due to the possible skewness of the sampling distribution for $\hat{\gamma}^{(CL)}$, while an interval estimator derived from $\log(\hat{\gamma}^{(CL)})$ with the logarithmic transformation can be inefficient due to the possible existence of an extremely small estimate of the denominator γ. Thus, using a similar idea as for deriving (2.26), we may obtain an asymptotic $100(1 - \alpha)$ % confidence interval for γ based on an ad hoc procedure as given by

$$[\gamma_l^{(CL)}, \gamma_u^{(CL)}] \tag{4.25}$$

where $\hat{\gamma}^{(CL)}$ and $\hat{Var}(\log(\hat{\gamma}^{(CL)}))$ are given in (4.15) and (4.16),

$$\hat{Var}(\hat{\gamma}^{(CL)}) = (\hat{\gamma}^{(CL)})^2 \, \hat{Var}(\log(\hat{\gamma}^{(CL)})),$$
$$\gamma_l^{(CL)} = I(\hat{\gamma}^{(CL)}, \hat{Var}(\hat{\gamma}^{(CL)})) \max\{\hat{\gamma}^{(CL)} - Z_{\alpha/2}(\hat{Var}(\hat{\gamma}^{(CL)}))^{1/2}, 0\}$$
$$+ (1 - I(\hat{\gamma}^{(CL)}, \hat{Var}(\hat{\gamma}^{(CL)})))\hat{\gamma}^{(CL)}$$
$$\times \exp(-Z_{\alpha/2}(\hat{Var}(\log(\hat{\gamma}^{(CL)})))^{1/2}),$$
$$\gamma_u^{(CL)} = I(\hat{\gamma}^{(CL)}, \hat{Var}(\hat{\gamma}^{(CL)}))(\hat{\gamma}^{(CL)} + Z_{\alpha/2}(\hat{Var}(\hat{\gamma}^{(CL)}))^{1/2})$$
$$+ (1 - I(\hat{\gamma}^{(CL)}, \hat{Var}(\hat{\gamma}^{(CL)})))\hat{\gamma}^{(CL)}$$
$$\times \exp(Z_{\alpha/2}(\hat{Var}(\log(\hat{\gamma}^{(CL)})))^{1/2}),$$

Table 4.2 Simulated data for comparing an experimental treatment with a standard treatment under a CRT with noncompliance, each treatment having 30 clusters of varying sizes.

	The standard treatment ($i = 1, 2, \ldots, 30$)			
$m_{1CN|i}^{(0)}$	$m_{1A|i}^{(0)}$	$m_{2CN|i}^{(0)}$	$m_{2A|i}^{(0)}$	$m_i^{(0)}$
12	0	8	2	22
11	0	8	9	28
7	0	7	7	21
11	0	10	3	24
13	0	12	1	26
5	0	6	2	13
10	0	5	4	19
10	0	7	1	18
15	2	5	0	22
18	0	7	4	29
13	0	1	3	17
9	2	6	0	17
7	0	10	0	17
11	0	7	2	20
6	0	11	8	25
17	0	2	5	24
10	0	2	1	13
11	0	9	2	22
3	1	12	0	16
7	0	21	1	29
9	7	3	4	23
16	0	10	3	29
19	0	2	1	22
11	0	8	0	19
2	0	15	1	18
18	0	1	1	20
4	1	12	2	19
5	1	8	1	15
7	1	6	0	14
9	0	7	5	21

(*Continued*)

Table 4.2   (*Continued*)

	The experimental treatment ($i = 1, 2, \ldots, 30$)			
$m_{1CA|i}^{(1)}$	$m_{1N|i}^{(1)}$	$m_{2CA|i}^{(1)}$	$m_{2N|i}^{(1)}$	$m_i^{(1)}$
13	0	16	0	29
14	0	11	0	25
6	0	9	0	15
8	0	10	1	19
9	3	6	3	21
6	0	9	0	15
7	0	9	5	21
22	0	1	0	23
7	2	4	0	13
13	0	1	3	17
9	0	10	0	19
4	0	9	3	16
15	0	4	0	19
11	0	10	0	21
18	3	4	0	25
14	0	6	0	20
5	0	10	0	15
8	2	6	0	16
6	0	8	0	14
27	0	6	0	33
11	0	7	0	18
17	0	8	1	26
11	0	8	0	19
21	0	5	3	29
9	0	1	3	13
20	0	5	0	25
8	0	7	0	15
8	0	13	0	21
17	0	1	1	19
10	0	12	0	22

and $I(\hat{\gamma}^{(CL)}, \hat{Var}(\hat{\gamma}^{(CL)}))$ is an indicator random variable, and $I(\hat{\gamma}^{(CL)}, \hat{Var}(\hat{\gamma}^{(CL)})) = 1$ if $\hat{\gamma}^{(CL)}(\exp(Z_{\alpha/2}(\hat{Var}(\log(\hat{\gamma}^{(CL)})))^{1/2}) - \exp(-Z_{\alpha/2}(\hat{Var}(\log(\hat{\gamma}^{(CL)})))^{1/2}))$ is larger than or equal to K times the length $((\hat{\gamma}^{(CL)} + Z_{\alpha/2}(\hat{Var}(\hat{\gamma}^{(CL)}))^{1/2}) - \max\{\hat{\gamma}^{(CL)} - Z_{\alpha/2}(\hat{Var}(\hat{\gamma}^{(CL)}))^{1/2}, 0\})$, and $= 0$, otherwise. A brief discussion on the effect of the chosen constant K can be found in Section 2.4.2. We arbitrarily recommend K to be set equal to 2.5 for use in practice.

Example 4.3   To illustrate the use of the interval estimator (4.25) for the PR, we consider use of the simulated data in Table 4.2 as well. When using the point estimator (4.15), we obtain the estimate $\hat{\gamma}^{(CL)} = 1.184$. This suggests that using the experimental treatment tend to increase the rate of positive responses among compliers as compared with the standard treatment by approximately 18 %. When employing interval estimator (4.25), we obtain an asymptotic 95 % confidence interval for γ as given by [0.979, 1.432]. Because this interval estimate contains $\gamma = 1$, there is no significant evidence at the 5 % level to support that using the experimental treatment can improve the positive rate of patient response as compared with using the standard treatment. This null inference is the same as that based on the statistic $\hat{\Delta}^{(CL)}$ for the PD found in Example 4.2.

4.4.3   Estimation of the odds ratio

Since the estimator $\hat{\varphi}^{(CL)}$(4.18) is a ratio of two statistics, its sampling distribution can be skewed. Thus, as for the PR, an interval estimator directly based on $\hat{\varphi}^{(CL)}$ can lose accuracy, while an interval estimator with the logarithmic transformation of $\hat{\varphi}^{(CL)}$ can lose precision. Again, following the same idea as that in derivation of the interval estimator (2.29), we obtain the following asymptotic $100(1 - \alpha)$ % confidence interval for φ as

$$[\varphi_l^{(CL)}, \varphi_u^{(CL)}], \tag{4.26}$$

where $\hat{\varphi}^{(CL)}$ and $\hat{Var}(\log(\hat{\varphi}^{(CL)}))$ are given in (4.18) and (4.19), $\hat{Var}(\hat{\varphi}^{(CL)}) = (\hat{\varphi}^{(CL)})^2 \hat{Var}(\log(\hat{\varphi}^{(CL)}))$,

$$\varphi_l^{(CL)} = I(\hat{\varphi}^{(CL)}, \hat{Var}(\hat{\varphi}^{(CL)})) \max\{\hat{\varphi}^{(CL)} - Z_{\alpha/2}(\hat{Var}(\hat{\varphi}^{(CL)}))^{1/2}, 0\}$$

$$+(1 - I(\hat{\varphi}^{(CL)}, \hat{Var}(\hat{\varphi}^{(CL)})))\hat{\varphi}^{(CL)}$$
$$\times \exp(-Z_{\alpha/2}(\hat{Var}(\log(\hat{\varphi}^{(CL)})))^{1/2}), \text{ and}$$
$$\varphi_u^{(CL)} = I(\hat{\varphi}^{(CL)}, \hat{Var}(\hat{\varphi}^{(CL)}))(\hat{\varphi}^{(CL)} + Z_{\alpha/2}(\hat{Var}(\hat{\varphi}^{(CL)}))^{1/2})$$
$$+(1 - I(\hat{\varphi}^{(CL)}, \hat{Var}(\hat{\varphi}^{(CL)})))\hat{\varphi}^{(CL)}$$
$$\times \exp(Z_{\alpha/2}(\hat{Var}(\log(\hat{\varphi}^{(CL)})))^{1/2}), \text{ and}$$

where $I(\hat{\varphi}^{(CL)}, \hat{Var}(\hat{\varphi}^{(CL)}))$ is an indicator random variable, $I(\hat{\varphi}^{(CL)}, \hat{Var}(\hat{\varphi}^{(CL)}))$ is 1 if $\hat{\varphi}^{(CL)}(\exp(Z_{\alpha/2}(\hat{Var}(\log(\hat{\varphi}^{(CL)})))^{1/2}) - \exp(-Z_{\alpha/2}(\hat{Var}(\log(\hat{\varphi}^{(CL)})))^{1/2}))$ is larger than or equal to 2.5 times $(\hat{\varphi}^{(CL)} + Z_{\alpha/2}(\hat{Var}(\hat{\varphi}^{(CL)}))^{1/2} - \max\{\hat{\varphi}^{(CL)} - Z_{\alpha/2}(\hat{Var}(\hat{\varphi}^{(CL)}))^{1/2}, 0\})$, and $= 0$, otherwise.

Example 4.4   To illustrate the use of the point estimator (4.18) and interval estimator (4.26) for the OR, we again consider the data in Table 4.2. We obtain $\hat{\varphi}^{(CL)} = 1.615$, which is not similar to $\hat{\gamma}^{(CL)} = 1.184$, as obtained for the PR in Example 4.3. This is because the positive rate of patient responses is not really small in the data and hence the OR is expected to be generally different from the PR. When employing the point estimator (4.26), we obtain an asymptotic 95 % confidence interval for φ as given by [0.930, 2.803]. Because this interval estimate contains $\varphi = 1$, there is no significant evidence at the 5 % level to support that the experimental treatment is superior to the standard treatment.

4.5   Sample size determination

An inadequate number of clusters in a CRT can lead us to overlook an important treatment effect. Thus, it is essentially important to find out how large the minimum number of clusters is needed to assure that one has the desired power of detecting the primary goal of our trial. Because a variance estimator without accounting for the intraclass correlation tends to underestimate the variance of test statistics for a CRT, the sample size calculation formulae discussed in Chapter 2 is not appropriate for use under cluster sampling. In this section, we discuss sample size determination for testing superiority, noninferiority and equivalence based on the test procedures developed in Sections 4.1–4.3 under a CRT with noncompliance.

Define $k = n_0/n_1$, the ratio of sample allocation for the number of clusters between the standard and experimental treatments. Given a fixed ratio k of sample allocation, we focus the following discussion on estimating the minimum required number of clusters n_1 from the experimental treatment. The corresponding estimates of the minimum required number of clusters from the standard treatment and the total minimum required number of clusters for the CRT are then given by $n_0 = kn_1$ and $n_T = (k+1)n_1$, respectively.

4.5.1   Sample size calculation for testing superiority

In determination of the minimum required number of clusters, note that the variance formula $Var(\hat{\delta}^{(CL)})(4.7)$ is probably of limited use. This is because the information on the individual cluster size $m_i^{(g)}$ is unlikely available at the design stage in most practically encountered trials. However, note that the VIF $f(\underline{m}_g, \rho_g) (= \sum_i m_i^{(g)}(1 + (m_i^{(g)} - 1) \rho_g)/m_+^{(g)})$ can be rewritten as (Exercise 4.15):

$$g(\bar{m}^{(g)}, (s_m^{(g)})^2, \rho_g) = \{\bar{m}^{(g)} + [(s_m^{(g)})^2 + (\bar{m}^{(g)})^2 - \bar{m}^{(g)}]\rho_g\}/(\bar{m}^{(g)}),$$

$$(4.27)$$

where $\bar{m}^{(g)} = \sum_{i=1}^{n_g} m_i^{(g)}/n_g$, and $(s_m^{(g)})^2 = \sum_{i=1}^{n_g} (m_i^{(g)} - \bar{m}^{(g)})^2/n_g$ are the mean and the variance of cluster sizes $m_i^{(g)}$, respectively. Thus, we can re-express $Var(\hat{\pi}_{1+}^{(g)})$ as

$$\pi_{1+}^{(g)}(1 - \pi_{1+}^{(g)})g(\bar{m}^{(g)}, (s_m^{(g)})^2, \rho_g)/(n_g\bar{m}^{(g)}). \qquad (4.28)$$

When determining $Var(\hat{\pi}_{1+}^{(g)})(4.28)$, we need only the information on the mean $\bar{m}^{(g)}$ and variance $(s_m^{(g)})^2$ of $m_i^{(g)}$ instead of the individual cluster size $m_i^{(g)}$. When $m_i^{(g)} = m_0^{(g)}$ for all i (i.e. constant cluster size), $\bar{m}^{(g)} = m_0^{(g)}$ and $(s_m^{(g)})^2 = 0$. The variance $Var(\hat{\pi}_{1+}^{(g)})$ reduces to

$$Var(\hat{\pi}_{1+}^{(g)}) = \pi_{1+}^{(g)}(1 - \pi_{1+}^{(g)})(1 + (m_0^{(g)} - 1)\rho_g)/(n_g m_0^{(g)}). \qquad (4.29)$$

However, a CRT with a constant cluster size may not often occur in practice. Note that $g(\bar{m}^{(g)}, (s_m^{(g)})^2, \rho_g)$(4.27) is always larger than $\{1 + (\bar{m}^{(g)} - 1)\rho_g\}$ when there is a variation of $m_i^{(g)}$ between clusters (i.e. $(s_m^{(g)})^2 > 0$) in the presence of a positive intraclass correlation (i.e. $\rho_g > 0$). Thus, a commonly used method for calculation of the minimum required sample size by simply multiplying the minimum required sample size calculated for no cluster sampling by the factor $\{1 + (\bar{m}^{(g)} - 1)\rho_g\}$ tends to underestimate the minimum required sample size under cluster sampling when $m_i^{(g)}$ varies substantially between clusters. Note further that when the cluster size $m_i^{(g)}$ is assumed to follow a probability mass function with mean $\mu_m^{(g)}$ and variance $(\sigma_m^{(g)})^2$, we may assume $\mu_m^{(1)} = \mu_m^{(0)} = \mu_m$ and $(\sigma_m^{(1)})^2 = (\sigma_m^{(0)})^2 = \sigma_m^2$ due to randomization. Therefore, we may replace $\bar{m}^{(g)}$ and $(s_m^{(g)})^2$ in $g(\bar{m}^{(g)}, (s_m^{(g)})^2, \rho_g)$(4.27) by μ_m and σ_m^2, respectively. In particular, if the assumed probability mass function for $m_i^{(g)}$ is the truncated Poisson distribution (excluding 0 observation) with parameter λ_m, the VIF $g(\bar{m}^{(g)}, (s_m^{(g)})^2, \rho_g)$ will be approximately equal to $\{1 + \lambda_m \rho_g\}$(instead of $\{1 + (\lambda_m - 1)\rho_g\}$) in this case. Note that as n_g is large, we may further approximate the variance $Var(\hat{\delta}^{(CL)})$(4.7) based on the above results (4.27) and (4.28) by (Exercise 4.16):

$$Var(\hat{\delta}^{(CL)}) \approx V_{ITTPD}^{(CL)}(\pi_{+C}, \pi_{+A}, \pi_{1|C}^{(1)},$$
$$\pi_{1|C}^{(0)}, \pi_{1|A}, \pi_{1|N}, \mu_m, \sigma_m^2, \rho_1, \rho_0, k)/n_1, \qquad (4.30)$$

where

$$V_{ITTPD}^{(CL)}(\pi_{+C}, \pi_{+A}, \pi_{1|C}^{(1)}, \pi_{1|C}^{(0)}, \pi_{1|A}, \pi_{1|N}, \mu_m, \sigma_m^2, \rho_1, \rho_0, k)$$
$$= \pi_{1+}^{(1)}(1 - \pi_{1+}^{(1)})g(\mu_m, \sigma_m^2, \rho_1)/\mu_m + \pi_{1+}^{(0)}(1 - \pi_{1+}^{(0)})g(\mu_m, \sigma_m^2, \rho_0)/(k\mu_m).$$

Furthermore, as the number n_g of clusters in both treatments is large, the variance $Var(\hat{\delta}^{(CL)})$(4.7) under $H_0 : \Delta(= \pi_{1|C}^{(1)} - \pi_{1|C}^{(0)}) = 0$ can be approximated by

$$Var(\hat{\delta}^{(CL)}|H_0) = V_{ITTPD}^{(CL)}(\pi_{+C}, \pi_{+A}, \pi_{1|C}^{(1)}, \pi_{1|C}^{(0)}, \pi_{1|A},$$
$$\pi_{1|N}, \mu_m, \sigma_m^2, \rho_1, \rho_0, k|H_0)/n_1, \qquad (4.31)$$

where $V_{ITTPD}^{(CL)}(\pi_{+C}, \pi_{+A}, \pi_{1|C}^{(1)}, \pi_{1|C}^{(0)}, \pi_{1|A}, \pi_{1|N}, \mu_m, \sigma_m^2, \rho_1, \rho_0, k|H_0) =$
$\bar{\pi}_{1+}^{(p)}(1 - \bar{\pi}_{1+}^{(p)})\{g(\mu_m, \sigma_m^2, \rho_1)/\mu_m + g(\mu_m, \sigma_m^2, \rho_0)/(k\mu_m)\}$, and $\bar{\pi}_{1+}^{(p)} =$
$\pi_{+C}(\pi_{1|C}^{(1)} + k\pi_{1|C}^{(0)})/(k + 1) + \pi_{+A}\pi_{1|A} + \pi_{+N}\pi_{1|N}$. For simplicity in
notation, we denote $V_{ITTPD}^{(CL)}(\pi_{+C}, \pi_{+A}, \pi_{1|C}^{(1)}, \pi_{1|C}^{(0)}, \pi_{1|A}, \pi_{1|N}, \mu_m, \sigma_m^2, \rho_1,$
$\rho_0, k)$ by $V_{ITTPD}^{(CL)}$, and $V_{ITTPD}^{(CL)}(\pi_{+C}, \pi_{+A}, \pi_{1|C}^{(1)}, \pi_{1|C}^{(0)}, \pi_{1|A}, \pi_{1|N}, \mu_m, \sigma_m^2, \rho_1,$
$\rho_0, k|H_0)$ by $V_{ITTPD|H_0}^{(CL)}$. Based on the test statistic (4.11), we obtain
an estimate of the minimum required number of clusters n_1 from the
experimental treatment for a desired power $1 - \beta$ of detecting a given
difference $\Delta_0(= \pi_{1|C}^{(1)} - \pi_{1|C}^{(0)} \neq 0)$ at the α-level (two-sided test) as (Lui
and Chang, 2011a)

$$n_1 = Ceil\{(Z_{\alpha/2}\sqrt{V_{ITTPD|H_0}^{(CL)}} + Z_\beta\sqrt{V_{ITTPD}^{(CL)}}/[1 - (\pi_{+C}\Delta_0)^2])^2/$$
$$[\tanh^{-1}(\pi_{+C}\Delta_0)]^2\}, \tag{4.32}$$

where $Ceil\{x\}$ is the smallest integer $\geq$ x. Note that the above sample
size formula n_1 (4.32) can be shown to be approximately equivalent
to the classical sample size formula for testing equality based on two
independent sample proportions when there are no clusters (i.e. $m_i^{(g)} = 1$
for all i) under perfect compliance (Lui and Chang, 2011a).

To allow readers to easily appreciate the effect due to various parameters on n_1(4.32), we consider equal sample allocation $n_1 = n_0 = n$ (i.e.
$k = 1$) and summarize in Table 4.3 the minimum required number of
clusters n per treatment for testing $H_0 : \Delta = 0$ at the 5 % level for a
desired power of 80 % of detecting $\Delta(= \pi_{1|C}^{(1)} - \pi_{1|C}^{(0)}) = 0.05, 0.20$ in
the situations, in which the cluster size $m_i^{(g)}$ independently follows the
truncated Poisson distribution (excluding 0 observation) with parameters
$\lambda_m =5, 10, 20, 50$; the conditional probability of a positive responses
in various subpopulations: $\underline{\pi}'_{1|S} = (\pi_{1|C}^{(0)}, \pi_{1|A}, \pi_{1|N}) = A, B$, where $A =$
$(0.20, 0.35, 0.25)$, $B = (0.50, 0.20, 0.30)$; the common intraclass cor-
relation for both treatments $\rho(= \rho_1 = \rho_0) = 0.05, 0.10, 0.20$; and the
subpopulation proportions $\underline{\pi}'_S = (\pi_{+C}, \pi_{+A}, \pi_{+N}) = I, II$, where $I =$
$(0.95, 0.03, 0.02)$, and $II = (0.80, 0.15, 0.05)$.

For example, when $\underline{\pi}'_S =I = (0.95, 0.03, 0.02)$, $\Delta = 0.05$, $\rho =0.10$,
$\underline{\pi}'_{1|S} = A = (0.20, 0.35, 0.25)$, and $\lambda_m = 10$, we need to take 246 clusters
per treatment (Table 4.3). We can see that the estimate of the minimum

Table 4.3 The minimum required number of clusters n per treatment calculated for a desired power of 80 % of detecting $\Delta(=\pi_{1|C}^{(1)} - \pi_{1|C}^{(0)}) = 0.05, 0.20$ in testing $H_0 : \Delta = 0$ at the 5 % level in the situations, the cluster size $m_i^{(g)}$ independently follows the truncated Poisson distribution (excluding 0 observation) with parameters $\lambda_m = 5, 10, 20, 50$; the conditional probability of a positive responses in various subpopulations: $\underline{\pi}'_{1|S} = (\pi_{1|C}^{(0)}, \pi_{1|A}, \pi_{1|N}) = $ **A**, **B**, where **A** = (0.20, 0.35, 0.25), **B** = (0.50, 0.20, 0.30); the common intraclass correlation for both treatments $\rho_1 = \rho_0 = \rho = 0.05, 0.10, 0.20$; the underlying difference $\Delta = 0.05, 0.20$; and the subpopulation proportions $\underline{\pi}'_S = (\pi_{+C}, \pi_{+A}, \pi_{+N}) = $ **I**, **II**, where **I** = (0.95, 0.03, 0.02), and **II** = (0.80, 0.15, 0.05).

$\underline{\pi}'_S$	Δ	ρ	$\underline{\pi}'_{1|S}$	$\lambda_m =$	5	10	20	50
I	0.05	0.05	A		308	185	123	86
			B		435	261	174	122
		0.10	A		369	246	185	148
			B		522	348	261	209
		0.20	A		492	369	308	271
			B		696	522	435	383
	0.20	0.05	A		23	14	10	7
			B		27	16	11	8
		0.10	A		28	19	14	11
			B		32	21	16	13
		0.20	A		37	28	23	20
			B		42	32	27	23
II	0.05	0.05	A		454	273	182	127
			B		611	367	245	171
		0.10	A		545	363	273	218
			B		733	489	367	293
		0.20	A		726	545	454	400
			B		977	733	611	537
	0.20	0.05	A		33	20	13	10
			B		38	23	16	11
		0.10	A		39	26	20	16
			B		46	31	23	19
		0.20	A		52	39	33	29
			B		61	46	38	34

required number of clusters increases as either the intraclass correlation ρ increases or the proportion of compliers decreases. For example, when ρ increases from 0.10 to 0.20 in the above case, we need to take a minimum number of 369 clusters per treatment for a desired power 80 % of detecting $\Delta = 0.05$; the percentage of this increase is 50 % (= (369 − 246)/246). Similarly, we can see that an increase in the minimum required number of clusters can be large as the proportion of compliers drops (i.e. pattern I versus pattern II). Therefore, it will be essentially important to minimize the extent of patient noncompliance if we wish to reduce the number of clusters of patients needed for a CRT. We refer readers to the paper (Lui and Chang, 2011a) for a detailed evaluation of the accuracy of sample size formula (4.32) based on Monte Carlos simulations.

Example 4.5   To illustrate the use of n_1 (4.32), we consider the particular situation in which the configuration is determined by the data in Table 2.1 (Lui and Chang, 2011a). Because it is a simple noncompliance trial, in which only patients assigned to the intervention group may have access to taking the vitamin A supplementation, we assume $\pi_{+A} = 0$. Given these data, we obtain the estimates for the subpopulation proportions π_{+C} and π_{+N} to be 0.80 and 0.20, respectively. We further obtain the estimates for $\pi_{1|C}^{(0)}$ and $\pi_{1|N}$ to be 0.996 and 0.986, respectively. We assume that the cluster size $m_i^{(g)}$ follows a truncated Poisson distribution with an approximate mean cluster size $\lambda_m = 52$ ($\approx 23562/450$). Following Fleiss (1981), we may determine the PD Δ of interest through the *OR* and the relation $\Delta = OR\pi_{1|C}^{(0)}/(OR\pi_{1|C}^{(0)} + (1 - \pi_{1|C}^{(0)})) - \pi_{1|C}^{(0)}$. For example, suppose that we are interested in detecting the effect of vitamin A supplementation when the *OR* of survival is as large as 2 for children taking vitamin A supplementation versus those not taking any vitamin A supplementation. Given $OR = 2$ and $\pi_{1|C}^{(0)} = 0.996$, we obtain $\Delta = 0.002$. Note that the data needed for estimating the intraclass correlation between survival outcomes of children within villages are not available here.

There is generally, however, an inverse relation between the cluster size and the extent of the intraclass correlation (Donner and Klar, 2000). The larger the cluster size, the smaller is the intraclass correlation. Thus, for given such a large mean cluster size as 52, the intraclass correlation of survival between children is expected to be small. We arbitrarily consider $\rho = 0.0, 0.01, 0.05,$ and 0.10. These should cover a reasonable range of a small intraclass correlation. Consider use of equal sample allocation (i.e. $k = 1$) in the configuration determined by the above parameter estimates. We obtain the estimates of the minimum required number $n_1(= n_0)$ (4.32) of clusters per treatment for a desired power 80 % in testing $H_0 : \Delta = 0$ at the 5 % level to be 611, 928, 2197, and 3784 for the intraclass correlation $\rho = 0.0, 0.01, 0.05,$ and 0.10, respectively. When the mean cluster size λ_m is as large as 52 considered in this example, the VIF $(= 1 + 52\rho)$ can be large even for a small intraclass correlation ρ. This explains why the estimate of the minimum required number of clusters increases substantially from 611 to 928 when the underlying intraclass correlation ρ increases only from 0 to 0.01.

4.5.2   Sample size calculation for testing noninferiority

We want to estimate the minimum required number of clusters so that one can have an adequate opportunity to detect the noninferiority of an experimental treatment to the standard treatment when it is true. We begin with sample size calculation for testing noninferiority when using the PD to measure the relative treatment effect under a CRT with noncompliance.

4.5.2.1   Using the difference in proportions

As the number n_g of clusters in both treatments is large, the estimated asymptotic variance $\hat{V}ar(\hat{\Delta}^{(CL)})$(4.13), given a fixed ratio of sample allocation $k = n_1/n_0$, is approximately equal to

$$Var(\hat{\Delta}^{(CL)}) = V_{PD}^{(CL)}(\pi_{+C}, \pi_{+A}, \pi_{1|C}^{(0)}, \Delta, \pi_{1|A},$$
$$\pi_{1|N}, \mu_m, \sigma_m^2, \rho_1, \rho_0, k)/n_1, \qquad (4.33)$$

where

$$V_{PD}^{(CL)}(\pi_{+C}, \pi_{+A}, \pi_{1|C}^{(0)}, \Delta, \pi_{1|A}, \pi_{1|N}, \mu_m, \sigma_m^2, \rho_1, \rho_0, k)$$
$$= \{[\pi_{1+}^{(1)}(1 - \pi_{1+}^{(1)})g(\mu_m, \sigma_m^2, \rho_1)/\mu_m + \pi_{1+}^{(0)}(1 - \pi_{1+}^{(0)})g(\mu_m, \sigma_m^2, \rho_0)/$$
$$(k\mu_m)] + \Delta^2[\pi_{+CA}^{(1)}(1 - \pi_{+CA}^{(1)})g(\mu_m, \sigma_m^2, \rho_1)/\mu_m + \pi_{+A}(1 - \pi_{+A})$$

$$\times g(\mu_m, \sigma_m^2, \rho_0)/(k\mu_m)] - 2\Delta[(\pi_{1CA}^{(1)} - \pi_{1+}^{(1)}\pi_{+CA}^{(1)})g(\mu_m, \sigma_m^2, \rho_1)/\mu_m$$
$$+(\pi_{1A} - \pi_{1+}^{(0)}\pi_{+A})g(\mu_m, \sigma_m^2, \rho_0)/(k\mu_m)]\}/(\pi_{+C})^2.$$

Note that given $\{\pi_{+C}, \pi_{+A}, \pi_{1|C}^{(0)}, \Delta, \pi_{1|A}, \pi_{1|N}, \mu_m, \sigma_m^2, \rho_1, \rho_0, k\}$, we can uniquely determine all parameter values needed to calculate $Var(\hat{\Delta}^{(CL)})$(4.33). For example, we can determine $\pi_{1+}^{(1)}$ and $\pi_{1+}^{(0)}$ by $(\pi_{1|C}^{(0)} + \Delta)\pi_{+C} + \pi_{1|A}\pi_{+A} + \pi_{1|N}\pi_{+N}$ and $\pi_{1|C}^{(0)}\pi_{+C} + \pi_{1|A}\pi_{+A} + \pi_{1|N}\pi_{+N}$, respectively. Thus, we may express $Var(\hat{\Delta}^{(CL)})$ as a function of $\{\pi_{+C}, \pi_{+A}, \pi_{1|C}^{(0)}, \Delta, \pi_{1|A}, \pi_{1|N}, \mu_m, \sigma_m^2, \rho_1, \rho_0, k\}$. Furthermore, we can estimate all these parameters: $\pi_{+A}, \pi_{1|C}^{(0)}, \Delta, \pi_{1|A}, \pi_{1|N}, \mu_m, \sigma_m^2, \rho_1$ and ρ_0 by estimators as presented previously based on data in a pilot study when determining the configurations in calculation of the minimum required number of clusters. For simplicity in notation, we denote $V_{PD}^{(CL)}(\pi_{+C}, \pi_{+A}, \pi_{1|C}^{(0)}, \Delta, \pi_{1|A}, \pi_{1|N}, \mu_m, \sigma_m^2, \rho_1, \rho_0, k)$ by $V_{PD}^{(CL)}$. Furthermore, note that an asymptotic variance $Var(\tanh^{-1}(\hat{\Delta}^{(CL)}))$ is given by $Var(\hat{\Delta}^{(CL)})/(1 - \Delta^2)^2$. Based on the test statistic (4.14) and $Var(\hat{\Delta}^{(CL)})$ (4.33), we may obtain an estimate of the minimum required number of clusters n_1 from the experimental treatment for a desired power $(1 - \beta)$ of detecting noninferiority with a given specified value $\Delta_0(> -\varepsilon_l)$ at a nominal α-level as

$$n_1 = Ceil\{((Z_\alpha + Z_\beta)^2 V_{PD}^{(CL)}/[(1 - \Delta_0^2)^2])/(\tanh^{-1}(\varepsilon_l)$$
$$+ \tanh^{-1}(\Delta_0))^2\}. \tag{4.34}$$

When there are no clusters (i.e. $m_i^{(g)} = 1$ for all i and $g = 1, 0$), the sample size formula (4.34) reduces to that (2.33) for the case in which patients are randomized units.

4.5.2.2   Using the ratio of proportions

When the PR is used to measure the relative treatment effect in establishing noninferiority, it is important to obtain an adequate number of clusters so that one has the desired power of detecting noninferiority when the underlying $\gamma_0 > 1 - \gamma_l$. Note that as the number n_g of clusters in both treatments is large, the estimated asymptotic variance $\hat{Var}(\log(\hat{\gamma}^{(CL)}))$ (4.16), given a fixed ratio of sample allocation $k = n_1/n_0$, is approximately equal to

$$Var(\log(\hat{\gamma}^{(CL)})) = V_{LPR}^{(CL)}(\pi_{+C}, \pi_{+A}, \pi_{1|C}^{(0)}, \gamma, \pi_{1|A}, \pi_{1|N},$$
$$\mu_m, \sigma_m^2, \rho_1, \rho_0, k)/n_1,$$

where

$$V_{LPR}^{(CL)}(\pi_{+C}, \pi_{+A}, \pi_{1|C}^{(0)}, \gamma, \pi_{1|A}, \pi_{1|N}, \mu_m, \sigma_m^2, \rho_1, \rho_0, k)$$
$$= [\pi_{1CA}^{(1)}(1 - \pi_{1CA}^{(1)})g(\mu_m, \sigma_m^2, \rho_1)/\mu_m + \pi_{1A}(1 - \pi_{1A})g(\mu_m, \sigma_m^2, \rho_0)/$$
$$(k\mu_m)]/(\pi_{1C}^{(1)})^2 + [\pi_{1N}(1 - \pi_{1N})g(\mu_m, \sigma_m^2, \rho_1)/\mu_m + \pi_{1CN}^{(0)}$$
$$\times(1 - \pi_{1CN}^{(0)})g(\mu_m, \sigma_m^2, \rho_0)/(k\mu_m)]/(\pi_{1C}^{(0)})^2 - 2[\pi_{1CA}^{(1)}\pi_{1N}$$
$$\times g(\mu_m, \sigma_m^2, \rho_1)/\mu_m + \pi_{1CN}^{(0)}\pi_{1A}g(\mu_m, \sigma_m^2, \rho_0)/$$
$$(k\mu_m)]/[(\pi_{1C}^{(1)})(\pi_{1C}^{(0)})]. \tag{4.35}$$

For simplicity, we denote $V_{LPR}^{(CL)}(\pi_{+C}, \pi_{+A}, \pi_{1|C}^{(0)}, \gamma, \pi_{1|A}, \pi_{1|N}, \mu_m, \sigma_m^2,$ $\rho_1, \rho_0, k)$ by $V_{LPR}^{(CL)}$. On the basis of (4.17) and (4.35), we obtain an estimate of the minimum required number n_1 of clusters from the experimental treatment for a desired power $(1-\beta)$ of detecting noninferiority with a given specified value $\gamma_0(> 1 - \gamma_l)$ at a nominal α-level as

$$n_1 = Ceil\{(Z_\alpha + Z_\beta)^2 V_{LPR}^{(CL)}/(\log(\gamma_0) - \log(1 - \gamma_l))^2\}. \tag{4.36}$$

Note that when all the cluster sizes are equal to 1, the sample size formula (4.36) reduces to that (2.35) for the case of no cluster sampling.

4.5.2.3   Using the odds ratio of proportions

When the OR is used to measure the relative treatment effect in establishing noninferiority, we want to obtain an adequate number of clusters to achieve the desired power of detecting noninferiority when the underlying $\varphi_0 > 1 - \varphi_l$. As the number n_g of clusters in both treatments is large, note that the estimated asymptotic variance $\hat{Var}(\log(\hat{\varphi}^{(CL)}))$ (4.19), given a fixed ratio of sample allocation $k = n_1/n_0$, is approximately equal to (Lui and Chang, 2011b):

$$Var(\log(\hat{\varphi}^{(CL)})) = V_{LOR}^{(CL)}(\pi_{+C}, \pi_{+A}, \pi_{1|C}^{(0)}, \varphi, \pi_{1|A},$$
$$\pi_{1|N}, \mu_m, \sigma_m^2, \rho_1, \rho_0, k)/n_1, \tag{4.37}$$

where

$$V_{LOR}^{(CL)}(\pi_{+C}, \pi_{+A}, \pi_{1|C}^{(0)}, \varphi, \pi_{1|A}, \pi_{1|N}, \mu_m, \sigma_m^2, \rho_1, \rho_0, k)$$

$$= [\pi_{1CA}^{(1)}(1 - \pi_{1CA}^{(1)})g(\mu_m, \sigma_m^2, \rho_1)/\mu_m + \pi_{1A}(1 - \pi_{1A})g(\mu_m, \sigma_m^2, \rho_0)/$$
$$(k\mu_m)]/(\pi_{1C}^{(1)})^2 + [\pi_{2N}(1 - \pi_{2N})g(\mu_m, \sigma_m^2, \rho_1)/\mu_m + \pi_{2CN}^{(0)}(1 - \pi_{2CN}^{(0)})$$
$$\times g(\mu_m, \sigma_m^2, \rho_0)/(k\mu_m)]/(\pi_{2C}^{(0)})^2 + [\pi_{2CA}^{(1)}(1 - \pi_{2CA}^{(1)})g(\mu_m, \sigma_m^2, \rho_1)/$$
$$\mu_m + \pi_{2A}(1 - \pi_{2A})g(\mu_m, \sigma_m^2, \rho_0)/(k\mu_m)]/(\pi_{2C}^{(1)})^2 + [\pi_{1N}(1 - \pi_{1N})$$
$$\times g(\mu_m, \sigma_m^2, \rho_1)/\mu_m + \pi_{1CN}^{(0)}(1 - \pi_{1CN}^{(0)})g(\mu_m, \sigma_m^2, \rho_0)/(k\mu_m)]/(\pi_{1C}^{(0)})^2$$
$$+2[\pi_{1CA}^{(1)}\pi_{2N}g(\mu_m, \sigma_m^2, \rho_1)/\mu_m + \pi_{1A}\pi_{2CN}^{(0)}g(\mu_m, \sigma_m^2, \rho_0)/(k\mu_m)]/$$
$$[(\pi_{1C}^{(1)})(\pi_{2C}^{(0)})] + 2[\pi_{1CA}^{(1)}\pi_{2CA}^{(1)}g(\mu_m, \sigma_m^2, \rho_1)/\mu_m + \pi_{1A}\pi_{2A}$$
$$\times g(\mu_m, \sigma_m^2, \rho_0)/(k\mu_m)]/[(\pi_{1C}^{(1)})(\pi_{2C}^{(1)})] - 2[\pi_{1CA}^{(1)}\pi_{1N}g(\mu_m, \sigma_m^2, \rho_1)/$$
$$\mu_m + \pi_{1CN}^{(0)}\pi_{1A}g(\mu_m, \sigma_m^2, \rho_0)/(k\mu_m)]/[(\pi_{1C}^{(1)})(\pi_{1C}^{(0)})]$$
$$-2[\pi_{2CA}^{(1)}\pi_{2N}g(\mu_m, \sigma_m^2, \rho_1)/\mu_m + \pi_{2A}\pi_{2CN}^{(0)}g(\mu_m, \sigma_m^2, \rho_0)/(k\mu_m)]/$$
$$[(\pi_{2C}^{(1)})(\pi_{2C}^{(0)})] + 2[\pi_{1N}\pi_{2N}g(\mu_m, \sigma_m^2, \rho_1)/\mu_m + \pi_{1CN}^{(0)}\pi_{2CN}^{(0)}$$
$$\times g(\mu_m, \sigma_m^2, \rho_0)/(k\mu_m)]/[(\pi_{2C}^{(0)})(\pi_{1C}^{(0)})] + 2[\pi_{2CA}^{(1)}\pi_{1N}g(\mu_m, \sigma_m^2, \rho_1)/$$
$$\mu_m + \pi_{2A}\pi_{1CN}^{(0)}g(\mu_m, \sigma_m^2, \rho_0)/(k\mu_m)]/[(\pi_{2C}^{(1)})(\pi_{1C}^{(0)})].$$

For simplicity in notation, we denote $V_{LOR}^{(CL)}(\pi_{+C}, \pi_{+A}, \pi_{1|C}^{(0)}, \varphi, \pi_{1|A}, \pi_{1|N}, \mu_m, \sigma_m^2, \rho_1, \rho_0, k)$ by $V_{LOR}^{(CL)}$. Therefore, on the basis of (4.20) and (4.37), we obtain an estimate of the minimum required number of clusters n_1 from the experimental treatment for a desired power $1 - \beta$ of detecting noninferiority with a given $\varphi_0(> 1 - \varphi_l)$ as (Lui and Chang, 2011b):

$$n_1 = Ceil\{(Z_\alpha + Z_\beta)^2 V_{LOR}^{(CL)}/(\log(1 - \varphi_l) - \log(\varphi_0))^2\}. \qquad (4.38)$$

When all cluster sizes $m_i^{(g)} = 1$ (for both $g = 1, 0$), the sample size formula (4.38) simplified to (2.37). Furthermore, when here are no noncompliers (i.e. $\pi_{+A} = \pi_{+N} = 0$) in this case, the sample size formula n_1(4.38) further reduces to that obtained elsewhere for perfect compliance with no cluster sampling (Wang, Chow and Li, 2002).

To allow readers to appreciate the effect due to various sources on the required number of clusters, we summarize in Tables 4.4 at the 5 %

Table 4.4 The minimum required number of clusters n_1(4.38) for a desired power of 80 % of detecting noninferiority with $OR = 0.90$, 1.0, 1.1 in testing $H_0 : \varphi \leq 0.80$ at the 0.05-level for the conditional probability of a positive responses $(\pi_{1|C}^{(0)}, \pi_{1|A}, \pi_{1|N}) = (0.50, 0.20, 0.30)$ in the situations, where the subpopulation proportion $\underline{\pi}_S' = (\pi_{+C}, \pi_{+A}, \pi_{+N}) =$ **I, II**, where **I** $= (0.95, 0.03, 0.02)$, and **II** $= (0.80, 0.15, 0.05)$; the common intraclass correlation for both treatments $\rho_1 = \rho_0 = \rho = 0.10$, 0.20; the cluster size $m_i^{(g)}$ independently follows the truncated Poisson distribution (excluding 0 observation) with parameters $\lambda_m = 10, 20, 50$; and the ratio of sample allocation $k = 1, 2, 3, 4$.

$\underline{\pi}_S'$	OR	ρ	λ_m	$k =$	1	2	3	4
I	0.90	0.10	10		790	593	527	494
			20		593	445	395	371
			50		474	356	316	297
		0.20	10		1185	889	790	741
			20		987	741	659	618
			50		869	652	580	544
	1.00	0.10	10		220	165	147	138
			20		165	124	110	104
			50		132	99	88	83
		0.20	10		330	248	220	207
			20		275	207	184	172
			50		242	182	162	152
	1.10	0.10	10		109	82	73	68
			20		82	61	55	51
			50		65	49	44	41
		0.20	10		163	122	109	102
			20		136	102	91	85
			50		120	90	80	75
II	0.90	0.10	10		1095	822	731	685
			20		821	616	548	514
			50		657	493	439	411
		0.20	10		1642	1232	1096	1027
			20		1369	1027	913	856
			50		1204	904	804	753

Table 4.4 (*Continued*)

$\underline{\pi}'_S$	OR	ρ	λ_m	$k =$	1	2	3	4
1.00	0.10	10		307	230	205	192
		20		230	173	154	144
		50		184	138	123	115
	0.20	10		460	345	307	288
		20		384	288	256	240
		50		338	253	225	211
1.10	0.10	10		152	114	102	96
		20		114	86	76	72
		50		92	69	61	58
	0.20	10		228	171	152	143
		20		190	143	127	119
		50		168	126	112	105

level the estimates of the minimum required number of clusters n_1(4.38) from the experimental treatment for a desired power of 80 % of detecting noninferiority with the underlying specified value $OR = 0.90, 1.0, 1.1$ in testing $H_0 : \varphi \le 0.80$ (i.e. $\varphi_l = 0.2$) for the conditional probability of a positive responses $(\pi_{1|C}^{(0)}, \pi_{1|A}, \pi_{1|N}) = (0.50, 0.20, 0.30)$ in the situations, in which the subpopulation proportion $\underline{\pi}'_S = (\pi_{+C}, \pi_{+A}, \pi_{+N})$ $= \mathbf{I}, \mathbf{II}$, where $\mathbf{I} = (0.95, 0.03, 0.02)$, and $\mathbf{II} = (0.80, 0.15, 0.05)$; the common intraclass correlation for both treatments $\rho_1 = \rho_0 = \rho = 0.10$, 0.20; the cluster size $m_i^{(g)}$ independently follows the truncated Poisson distribution (excluding 0 observation) with parameters $\lambda_m = 10, 20, 50$; and the ratio of sample allocation $K = 1, 2, 3, 4$. As shown in Table 4.4, the minimum required number of clusters n_g for testing noninferiority can be quite large especially when the underlying OR is close to the noninferior margin of $1 - \varphi_l = 0.80$. For example, when $\underline{\pi}'_{1|S} = (0.50, 0.20, 0.30), \underline{\pi}'_S = \mathbf{I}, OR = 0.90, \rho = 0.20, \lambda = 10$, and $k = 1$, we obtain $n_1 = n_0 = 1185$. This may cause difficulty in obtaining such a large number of clusters for testing noninferiority in a CRT with noncompliance in practice. However, if the noninferior margin $(= 1 - \varphi_l)$ is chosen to be 0.55 (Senn, 2000), the minimum required number of clusters would reduce to only $n_1 = n_0 = 68$ in this case. Thus, a careful and thoughtful choice of φ_l subject to budget constraints and clinical significance for testing noninferiority is crucial in the design stage (Lui and Chang, 2011b).

4.5.3   Sample size calculation for testing equivalence

Using similar ideas as those presented in Chapter 2, we can easily extend the discussion on sample size calculation for testing equivalence under no cluster sampling to accommodate a CRT when using the PD, PR and OR to measure the relative treatment effect. For brevity, we simply present the formulae without including the details.

4.5.3.1   Using the difference in proportions

Based on the test procedure (4.21), we may obtain an estimate of the minimum required number of clusters from the experimental treatment n_1 for a desired power $(1-\beta)$ of detecting equivalence with a specified Δ_0 (where $-\varepsilon_l < \Delta_0 < \varepsilon_u$) at a nominal α-level as

$$n_1 = Ceil\{((Z_\alpha + Z_\beta)^2 V_{PD}^{(CL)}/[(1 - \Delta_0^2)^2])(\tanh^{-1}(\varepsilon_l) + \tanh^{-1}(\Delta_0))^2\},$$
$$\text{for } -\varepsilon_l < \Delta_0 < 0, \tag{4.39}$$

and

$$n_1 = Ceil\{((Z_\alpha + Z_\beta)^2 V_{PD}^{(CL)}/[(1 - \Delta_0^2)^2])/(\tanh^{-1}(\varepsilon_u) - \tanh^{-1}(\Delta_0))^2\},$$
$$\text{for } 0 < \Delta_0 < \varepsilon_u. \tag{4.40}$$

When $\varepsilon_l = \varepsilon_u$, we obtain an estimate of the minimum required number of clusters from the experimental treatment n_1 for a desired power $(1-\beta)$ of detecting equivalence with a specified $\Delta_0 = 0$ at a nominal α-level as

$$n_1 = Ceil\{((Z_\alpha + Z_{\beta/2})^2 V_{PD}^{(CL)})/(\tanh^{-1}(\varepsilon_u))^2\}. \tag{4.41}$$

Note that the sample size formulae (4.39)–(4.41) reduce to those (2.40), (2.42) and (2.44), respectively, when individual patients are randomized units (i.e. no cluster sampling).

4.5.3.2 Using the ratio of proportions

Based on the test procedure (4.22), we may obtain an estimate of the minimum required number n_1 of clusters from the experimental treatment for a desired power $(1 - \beta)$ of detecting equivalence with a given specified value $1 - \gamma_l < \gamma_0 < 1 + \gamma_u$ at a nominal α-level as

$$n_1 = Ceil\{(Z_\alpha + Z_\beta)^2 V_{LPR}^{(CL)}/(\log(\gamma_0) - \log(1 - \gamma_l))^2\}$$
$$\text{for } 1 - \gamma_l < \gamma_0 < 1, \tag{4.42}$$
$$n_1 = Ceil\{(Z_\alpha + Z_\beta)^2 V_{LPR}^{(CL)}/(\log(\gamma_0) - \log(1 + \gamma_u))^2\}$$
$$\text{for } 1 < \gamma_0 < 1 + \gamma_u, \tag{4.43}$$

and

$$n_1 = Ceil\{(Z_\alpha + Z_{\beta/2})^2 V_{LPR}^{(CL)}/(\log(1 + \gamma_u))^2\} \quad \text{for } \gamma_0 = 1 \text{ and}$$
$$\log(1 + \gamma_u) = -\log(1 - \gamma_l). \tag{4.44}$$

We can easily see that the sample size formulae (4.42)–(4.44) simplify to those (2.46)–(2.48) when $m_i^{(g)} = 1$ for all i and both g.

4.5.3.3 Using the odds ratio of proportions

Based on the test procedure (4.23), we may obtain an estimate of the minimum required number n_1 of clusters from the experimental treatment for a desired power $(1-\beta)$ of detecting equivalence with a given specified value $1 - \varphi_l < \varphi_0 < 1 + \varphi_u$ at a nominal α-level as

$$n_1 = Ceil\{(Z_\alpha + Z_\beta)^2 V_{LOR}^{(CL)}/(\log(\varphi_0) - \log(1 - \varphi_l))^2\}$$
$$\text{for } 1 - \varphi_l < \varphi_0 < 1, \tag{4.45}$$
$$n_1 = Ceil\{(Z_\alpha + Z_\beta)^2 V_{LOR}^{(CL)}/(\log(\varphi_0) - \log(1 + \varphi_u))^2\}$$
$$\text{for } 1 < \varphi_0 < 1 + \varphi_u, \tag{4.46}$$

and

$$n_1 = Ceil\{(Z_\alpha + Z_{\beta/2})^2 V_{LOR}^{(CL)}/(\log(1 + \varphi_u))^2\} \quad \text{for } \varphi_0 = 1 \text{ and}$$
$$\log(1 + \varphi_u) = -\log(1 - \varphi_l). \tag{4.47}$$

Again, the sample size formulae (4.45)–(4.47) include those formulae (2.50)–(2.52) as special cases for $m_i^{(g)} = 1$ for all i. Furthermore, note that when $\pi_{+C} = 1.0$ with no clusters, sample size formulae (4.42)–(4.44) and (4.45)–(4.47) presented here for testing equivalence further reduce to those published elsewhere for perfect compliance (Tu, 1998; Wang, Chow and Li, 2002). Note also that when deriving sample size calculation formulae (4.39) and (4.40) based on the PD, (4.42) and (4.43) based on the PR, as well as (4.45) and (4.46) based on the OR, we need to make, as discussed in Section 2.5.3, an additional approximation of the power function. When the equivalence margins are chosen not to be small or the chosen non-null parameter value of interest is in the neighborhood of the null value, the estimate of the minimum required number of clusters may not be large enough to assure this power approximation to be accurate, and hence all closed-form sample size calculation formulae (4.39), (4.40), (4.42), (4.43), (4.45) and (4.46) may tend to underestimate the minimum required number of clusters. Thus, in these cases, we may wish to employ the resulting estimate calculated by these formulae as an initial estimate and apply the trial-and-error procedure to find the more accurate estimate of the minimum required number of clusters (see the discussion in Section 2.5.3).

4.6   An alternative randomization-based approach

Following Cochran (1977), we can easily show that an estimated asymptotic randomization-based variance for $\hat{\pi}_{1+}^{(g)}$ (4.5) $(=\sum_i m_{1+|i}^{(g)} / \sum_i m_i^{(g)}$, where $m_{1+|i}^{(g)} = \sum_S m_{1S|i}^{(g)})$ is given by (Exercise 4.18):

$$\hat{Var}_{RB}(\hat{\pi}_{1+}^{(g)}) = \sum_{i=1}^{n_g} (m_{1+|i}^{(g)} - \hat{\pi}_{1+}^{(g)} m_i^{(g)})^2 / [n_g(n_g - 1)(\bar{m}^{(g)})^2], \quad (4.48)$$

where $\bar{m}^{(g)} = \sum_{i=1}^{n_g} m_i^{(g)} / n_g$ for $g = 1, 0$. Under $H_0 : \pi_{1+}^{(1)} = \pi_{1+}^{(0)}$, we may further modify $\hat{Var}_{RB}(\hat{\pi}_{1+}^{(g)})$ (4.48) as given by

$$\hat{Var}_{RB}(\hat{\pi}_{1+}^{(g)}|H_0) = \sum_{i=1}^{n_g} (m_{1+|i}^{(g)} - \hat{\pi}_{1+}^{(p)} m_i^{(g)})^2 / [n_g(n_g - 1)(\bar{m}^{(g)})^2], \quad (4.49)$$

where $\hat{\pi}_{1+}^{(p)} = (m_+^{(1)} \hat{\pi}_{1+}^{(1)} + m_+^{(0)} \hat{\pi}_{1+}^{(0)}) / (m_+^{(1)} + m_+^{(0)})$.

Recall that $\delta = 0$ if and only if $\Delta = 0$. Thus, to test superiority, we may employ the statistic $\hat{\delta}^{(CL)} (=\hat{\pi}_{1+}^{(1)} - \hat{\pi}_{1+}^{(0)})$ for the ITT analysis and its asymptotic randomization-based variance to test $H_0 : \delta = 0$. This leads us to consider the following test statistic:

$$Z = \hat{\delta}^{(CL)}/\sqrt{\hat{Var}_{RB}(\hat{\delta}^{(CL)}|H_0)}, \quad (4.50)$$

where $\quad \hat{Var}_{RB}(\hat{\delta}^{(CL)}|H_0) = \hat{Var}_{RB}(\hat{\pi}_{1+}^{(1)}|H_0) + \hat{Var}_{RB}(\hat{\pi}_{1+}^{(0)}|H_0), \quad$ and $\hat{Var}_{RB}(\hat{\pi}_{1+}^{(g)}|H_0)(g = 1, 0)$ is given in (4.49). We will reject $H_0 : \Delta = 0$ at the α-level if the test statistic (4.50), $Z > Z_{\alpha/2}$ or $Z < -Z_{\alpha/2}$. Furthermore, we may claim that the experimental treatment is superior to the standard treatment if Z(4.50) is larger than the critical value $Z_{\alpha/2}$.

To test noninferiority, as noted previously, we can no longer apply the test procedure based on $\hat{\delta}^{(CL)}$ to test $H_0 : \Delta \le -\varepsilon_l$ versus $H_a : \Delta > -\varepsilon_l$. Instead, we consider the following test statistic for a given value ε,

$$T(\varepsilon) = \hat{\pi}_{1+}^{(1)} - \hat{\pi}_{1+}^{(0)} + \varepsilon(\hat{\pi}_{+CA}^{(1)} - \hat{\pi}_{+A}^{(0)}). \quad (4.51)$$

Under $H_a : \Delta > -\varepsilon_l$, the test statistic $T(\varepsilon_l)$ tends to be positive. Thus, we reject $H_0 : \Delta \le -\varepsilon_l$ at the α-level and claim that the experimental treatment is noninferior to the standard treatment if

$$Z = T(\varepsilon_l)/\sqrt{\hat{Var}_{RB}(T(\varepsilon_l))} > Z_\alpha, \quad (4.52)$$

where

$$\hat{Var}_{RB}(T(\varepsilon_l)) = \hat{Var}_{RB}(\hat{\pi}_{1+}^{(1)} - \hat{\pi}_{1+}^{(0)}) + \varepsilon_l^2 \hat{Var}_{RB}(\hat{\pi}_{+CA}^{(1)} - \hat{\pi}_{+A}^{(0)})$$
$$+ 2\varepsilon_l[\hat{Cov}_{RB}(\hat{\pi}_{1+}^{(1)}, \hat{\pi}_{+CA}^{(1)}) + \hat{Cov}_{RB}(\hat{\pi}_{1+}^{(0)}, \hat{\pi}_{+A}^{(0)})],$$

$\hat{Var}_{RB}(\hat{\pi}_{1+}^{(1)} - \hat{\pi}_{1+}^{(0)}) = \hat{Var}_{RB}(\hat{\pi}_{1+}^{(1)}) + \hat{Var}_{RB}(\hat{\pi}_{1+}^{(0)}), \quad$ as $\quad$ well $\quad$ as $\hat{Var}_{RB}(\hat{\pi}_{+CA}^{(1)} - \hat{\pi}_{+A}^{(0)}), \hat{Cov}_{RB}(\hat{\pi}_{1+}^{(1)}, \hat{\pi}_{+CA}^{(1)}), \quad$ and $\quad \hat{Cov}_{RB}(\hat{\pi}_{1+}^{(0)}, \hat{\pi}_{+A}^{(0)}) \quad$ are given in Exercise 4.19.

Similarly, for testing equivalence, we will reject the null hypothesis $H_0 : \Delta \le -\varepsilon_l$ or $\Delta \ge \varepsilon_u$ at the α-level and claim that the two treatments are equivalent if the following two inequalities simultaneously hold:

$$T(\varepsilon_l)/\sqrt{\hat{Var}_{RB}(T(\varepsilon_l))} > Z_\alpha \quad \text{and}$$

$$T(-\varepsilon_u)/\sqrt{\hat{Var}_{RB}(T(-\varepsilon_u))} < -Z_\alpha. \quad (4.53)$$

Based on the randomization-based variance, we can also derive an interval estimator for the PD. Consider $T(-\Delta) = \hat{\pi}_{1+}^{(1)} - \hat{\pi}_{1+}^{(0)} - \Delta(\hat{\pi}_{+CA}^{(1)} - \hat{\pi}_{+A}^{(0)})$. As the number of clusters n_g in both treatments g is large, we may claim that the expectation $E_{RB}(T(-\Delta)) \approx 0$. This follows immediately from the fact that the ratio estimator is asymptotically unbiased (Cochran, 1977). Thus, we have $P((T(-\Delta))^2/\hat{Var}_{RB}(T(-\Delta)) \leq Z_{\alpha/2}^2) \approx 1 - \alpha$ when both n_g are large. This leads us to consider the following quadratic equation in Δ:

$$A_{RB}\Delta^2 - 2B_{RB}\Delta + C_{RB} \leq 0, \tag{4.54}$$

where

$$A_{RB} = (\hat{\pi}_{+CA}^{(1)} - \hat{\pi}_{+A}^{(0)})^2 - Z_{\alpha/2}^2 \hat{Var}_{RB}(\hat{\pi}_{+CA}^{(1)} - \hat{\pi}_{+A}^{(0)})$$

$$B_{RB} = (\hat{\pi}_{1+}^{(1)} - \hat{\pi}_{1+}^{(0)})(\hat{\pi}_{+CA}^{(1)} - \hat{\pi}_{+A}^{(0)}) - Z_{\alpha/2}^2[\hat{Cov}_{RB}(\hat{\pi}_{1+}^{(1)}, \hat{\pi}_{+CA}^{(1)})$$

$$+ \hat{Cov}_{RB}(\hat{\pi}_{1+}^{(0)}, \hat{\pi}_{+A}^{(0)})], \text{ and}$$

$$C_{RB} = (\hat{\pi}_{1+}^{(1)} - \hat{\pi}_{1+}^{(0)})^2 - Z_{\alpha/2}^2 \hat{Var}_{RB}(\hat{\pi}_{1+}^{(1)} - \hat{\pi}_{1+}^{(0)}).$$

If $A_{RB} > 0$ and $(B_{RB})^2 - A_{RB}C_{RB} > 0$, then an asymptotic $100(1-\alpha)\%$ confidence interval based on randomization for Δ would be given by

$$[\max\{(B_{RB} - \sqrt{(B_{RB})^2 - A_{RB}C_{RB}})/A_{RB}, -1\},$$
$$\min\{(B_{RB} + \sqrt{(B_{RB})^2 - A_{RB}C_{RB}})/A_{RB}, 1\}]. \tag{4.55}$$

Example 4.6 To allow us to compare the resulting interval estimates between using the interval estimator (4.24) based on the Dirichlet-multinomial model and the interval estimator (4.55) using the randomization-based variance, we use the same simulated data as presented in Table 4.2. When employing interval estimator (4.55), we obtain the 95 % confidence interval for Δ as $[-0.013, 0.232]$. We can see that this resulting interval estimate is quite similar to the 95 % confidence interval $[-0.007, 0.222]$ obtained by use of (4.24) in Example 4.2. Both interval estimates suggest that there should be no evidence at the 5 % level that the experimental treatment is better than the standard treatment.

We may apply similar ideas as above to develop the randomization-based procedures for testing noninferiority and equivalence with respect to the PR and OR, as well as interval estimators for these indices. Note that we do not need to assume the Dirichlet-multinomial model when deriving the test statistic (4.50), test procedures (4.52) and (4.53), or the interval estimator (4.55). Based on the randomization-based variance estimator as shown here, however, it is not intuitively obvious for us to appreciate the effect due to the intraclass correlation on the inflation of variance for these test statistics. Thus, it is more difficult to do sensitivity analysis as done in Example 4.1 or even derive sample size formulae based on (4.50), (4.52) and (4.53) in terms of meaningful parameters such as the extent of noncompliance, the underlying intraclass correlation and the prior information on the distribution of cluster sizes.

Finally, note that we may randomly assign clusters (grouped by physicians) of patients to receive either an experimental or a standard treatment within each center in a multi-center RCT. Similarly, we may randomly assign classes of students to either an intervention program or a control program within each school in a randomized trial involving a few schools in experimental sociology. To account for the center (or school) effect on the participant response, we may employ similar ideas and approaches as those discussed in Chapter 3 with strata formed by centers (or schools) together with the appropriate variance formulae accounting for the intraclass correlation as presented in this chapter to do stratified analysis under cluster sampling.

Exercises

4.1 Show that under the assumed Dirichlet-multinomial distribution, the expectation $E(Y_{ij}^{(g)}(r, S)) = E(p_{rS|i}^{(g)}) = \pi_{rS}^{(g)}$.

4.2 Show that the intraclass correlation between responses $Y_{ij}^{(g)}(r, S)$ and $Y_{ij'}^{(g)}(r, S)$ for two randomly selected patients $j \neq j'$ in cluster i assigned to treatment g is equal to $\rho_g = 1/(T_g + 1)$.

4.3 Show the variance $Var(p_{rs|i}^{(g)}) = \pi_{rs}^{(g)}(1 - \pi_{rs}^{(g)})/(T_g + 1)$ under the assumed Dirichlet multinomial model. Thus, for a given fixed $\pi_{rs}^{(g)}$, the larger the parameter T_g, the smaller is the variation of $p_{rs|i}^{(g)}$ between clusters.

4.4 To allow readers to easily appreciate the main results of this exercise, we use simplified notations that are different from those in the main context. Suppose that the random vector $(X_{i1}, X_{i2}, \ldots, X_{iL})$(for $i = 1, 2, \ldots, n$) independently and identically follows the multinomial distribution with parameters m_i and $(p_{i1}, p_{i2}, \ldots, p_{iL})$, where $(p_{i1}, p_{i2}, \ldots, p_{iL})$ independently and identically follows the Dirichlet probability density function: D $(\pi_1, \pi_2, \ldots, \pi_L, T)$.

(a) Define $\hat{\pi}_l = \sum_i X_{il} / \sum_i m_i$. Show that the expectation $E(\hat{\pi}_l) = \pi_l$ for $l = 1, 2, \ldots, L$.

(b) Show that the variance is given by $Var(\hat{\pi}_l) = \pi_l(1 - \pi_l) \times f(\underline{m}, \rho)/m_+$, where $m_+ = \sum_i m_i$, $f(\underline{m}, \rho) = \sum_i m_i(1 + (m_i - 1)\rho)/m_+$, $\rho = 1/(T + 1)$, and where $\underline{m} = (m_1, m_2, \ldots, m_n)'$.

(c) Show that the covariance $Cov(\hat{\pi}_l, \hat{\pi}_{l'}) = -\pi_l \pi_{l'} f(\underline{m}, \rho)/m_+$ for $l \neq l'$.

4.5 Show that the variance inflation factor (VIF) $f(\underline{m}_g, \rho_g) = 1$ when $\rho_g = 0$, and that $f(\underline{m}_g, \rho_g)$ is an increasing function of the intraclass correlation ρ_g.

4.6 Show that given $\sum_{i=1}^{n_g} m_i^{(g)} = m_+^{(g)}$ fixed, the VIF $f(\underline{m}^{(g)}, \rho_g) = \sum_i m_i^{(g)}(1 + (m_i^{(g)} - 1)\rho_g)/m_+^{(g)}$ is minimized when the cluster size is constant (i.e. $m_i^{(g)} = m_0^{(g)}$ for all i).

4.7 Show that the expectation $E(\hat{\delta}^{(CL)}) = E(\hat{\pi}_{1+}^{(1)} - \hat{\pi}_{1+}^{(0)}) = \delta$ and the variance $Var(\hat{\delta}^{(CL)})$ is equal to $\sum_{g=0}^{1} [\pi_{1+}^{(g)}(1 - \pi_{1+}^{(g)})f(\underline{m}_g, \rho_g)/m_+^{(g)}]$.

4.8 Define $BMS_g = [\sum_{i=1}^{n_g} \sum_{r=1}^{2} \sum_S (m_{rS|i}^{(g)})^2 / m_i^{(g)} - (\sum_{r=1}^{2} \sum_S (\sum_{i=1}^{n_g} m_{rS|i}^{(g)})^2 / m_+^{(g)}] / [2(n_g - 1)]$, $WMS_g = [m_+^{(g)} - \sum_{i=1}^{n_g} \sum_{r=1}^{2} \sum_S (m_{rS|i}^{(g)})^2 / m_i^{(g)}] / [2(m_+^{(g)} - n_g)]$, $m_g^* = [(m_+^{(g)})^2 - \sum_i (m_i^{(g)})^2] / [(n_g - 1) m_+^{(g)}]$, where the summation of S is over CA and N for $g = 1$, and is over CN and A for $g = 0$.

(a) Show that $E(m_{rS|i}^{(g)})^2 = m_i^{(g)}(m_i^{(g)} - 1)(\pi_{rS}^{(g)})^2 + m_i^{(g)}(m_i^{(g)} - 1) \pi_{rS}^{(g)}(1 - \pi_{rS}^{(g)}) / (T_g + 1) + m_i^{(g)} \pi_{rS}^{(g)}$, and hence show that $(m_+^{(g)} - n_g) E(WMS_g) = [(m_+^{(g)} - n_g) - (m_+^{(g)} - n_g) \sum_{r=1}^{2} \sum_S (\pi_{rS}^{(g)})^2 - (m_+^{(g)} - n_g) \sum_{r=1}^{2} \sum_S \pi_{rS}^{(g)}(1 - \pi_{rS}^{(g)}) / (T_g + 1)] / 2 = [(m_+^{(g)} - n_g) \sum_{r=1}^{2} \sum_S \pi_{rS}^{(g)}(1 - \pi_{rS}^{(g)}) T_g / (T_g + 1)] / 2$. This leads us to have the expectation $E(WMS_g) = [\sum_{r=1}^{2} \sum_S \pi_{rS}^{(g)}(1 - \pi_{rS}^{(g)}) T_g / (T_g + 1)] / 2$.

(b) Show that $E(\sum_{i=1}^{n_g} m_{rS|i}^{(g)})^2 = m_+^{(g)} \pi_{rS}^{(g)}(1 - \pi_{rS}^{(g)}) + \sum_{i=1}^{n_g} m_i^{(g)} \times (m_i^{(g)} - 1) \pi_{rS}^{(g)}(1 - \pi_{rS}^{(g)}) / (T_g + 1) + (m_+^{(g)} \pi_{rS}^{(g)})^2$, and hence show that $E(BMS_g) = [\sum_{r=1}^{2} \sum_S \pi_{rS}^{(g)}(1 - \pi_{rS}^{(g)}) T_g / (T_g + 1) + m_g^* \times \sum_{r=1}^{2} \sum_S \pi_{rS}^{(g)}(1 - \pi_{rS}^{(g)}) / (T_g + 1)] / 2$, where $m_g^* = [(m_+^{(g)})^2 - \sum_i (m_i^{(g)})^2] / [(n_g - 1) m_+^{(g)}]$. Thus, we obtain a consistent estimator for the intraclass correlation for ρ_g as $\hat{\rho}_g = (BMS_g - WMS_g) / [BMS_g + (m_g^* - 1) WMS_g]$.

4.9 Show that an estimated asymptotic variance $\hat{V}ar(\hat{\Delta}^{(CL)})$ of $\hat{\Delta}^{(CL)}$(4.12) is given by (4.13).

4.10 Show that $\hat{V}ar(\hat{\Delta}^{(CL)})$(4.13) is larger than or equal to $\hat{V}ar(\hat{\Delta})$(2.6) due to $f(\underline{m}_g, \hat{\rho}_g) \geq 1$ when we replace n_g in (2.6) by the total number $m_+^{(g)}$ of patients assigned to treatment g.

4.11 Show that an estimated asymptotic variance $\hat{V}ar(\log(\hat{\gamma}^{(CL)}))$ for the statistic $\log(\hat{\gamma}^{(CL)})$ is given in (4.16).

4.12 Show that an estimated asymptotic variance $\hat{V}ar(\log(\hat{\varphi}^{(CL)}))$ for the statistic $\log(\hat{\varphi}^{(CL)})$ is given in (4.19).

4.13 Show that the actual Type I error of test procedures, including statistics for testing superiority, noninferiority, or equivalence, without accounting for the VIF (or equivalently, assuming that the VIF equals 1) will tend to be larger than the nominal α-level under the assumption that the normal approximation for the test statistic is good.

4.14 Assuming that the normal approximation for a test statistic is valid, show that the coverage probability of a $100(1-\alpha)$th % confidence interval without accounting for the intraclass correlation (or equivalently, assuming the VIF to equal 1) tends to be smaller than the desired confidence level.

4.15 Show that the VIF $f(\underline{m}_g, \rho_g)(= \sum_i m_i^{(g)}(1 + (m_i^{(g)} - 1)\rho_g)/m_+^{(g)})$ can be rewritten as $g(\bar{m}^{(g)}, (s_m^{(g)})^2, \rho_g) = \{\bar{m}^{(g)} + [(s_m^{(g)})^2 + (\bar{m}^{(g)})^2 - \bar{m}^{(g)}]\rho_g\}/(\bar{m}^{(g)})$, where $\bar{m}^{(g)} = \sum_{i=1}^{n_g} m_i^{(g)}/n_g$, and $(s_m^{(g)})^2 = \sum_{i=1}^{n_g} (m_i^{(g)} - \bar{m}^{(g)})^2/n_g$.

4.16 Show that we can approximate variance $Var(\hat{\delta}^{(CL)})$ (4.7) by $Var(\hat{\delta}^{(CL)}) \approx V_{ITTPD}^{(CL)}(\pi_{+C}, \pi_{+A}, \pi_{1|C}^{(1)}, \pi_{1|C}^{(0)}, \pi_{1|A}, \pi_{1|N}, \mu_m, \sigma_m^2, \rho_1, \rho_0, k)/n_1$, where $V_{ITTPD}^{(CL)}(\pi_{+C}, \pi_{+A}, \pi_{1|C}^{(1)}, \pi_{1|C}^{(0)}, \pi_{1|A}, \pi_{1|N}, \mu_m, \sigma_m^2, \rho_1, \rho_0, k) = \pi_{1+}^{(1)}(1 - \pi_{1+}^{(1)})g(\mu_m, \sigma_m^2, \rho_1)/\mu_m + \pi_{1+}^{(0)}(1 - \pi_{1+}^{(0)})g(\mu_m, \sigma_m^2, \rho_0)/(k\mu_m)$, where μ_m and σ_m^2 are the mean and variance of the cluster size $m_i^{(g)}$ for the two treatments under comparison.

4.17 Suppose that if X_1 and X_2 are mutually independent, and X_i ($i = 1, 2$) has the gamma probability density function: $f_{X_i}(x_i) = x_i^{\alpha_i-1}e^{-x_i}/\Gamma(\alpha_i)$, the random variable $Y_1 = X_1/(X_1 + X_2)$ follows the beta probability density function: $f_{Y_1}(y_1) = \Gamma(\alpha_1 + \alpha_2)y_1^{\alpha_1-1}(1 - y_1)^{\alpha_2-1}/[\Gamma(\alpha_1)\Gamma(\alpha_2)]$. Show that if $X_1, X_2, \ldots, X_n$ are mutually independent, and X_i ($i = 1, 2, \ldots, n$) has the gamma probability density function: $f_{X_i}(x_i) = x_i^{\alpha_i-1}e^{-x_i}/\Gamma(\alpha_i)$, where $\alpha_i > 0$, the random variables $Y_i = X_i/\sum_i X_i$ ($i = 1, 2, \ldots, n$) will have the joint Dirichlet probability density: $\Gamma(\sum_i \alpha_i)\prod_i y_i^{\alpha_i-1}/\prod_i \Gamma(\alpha_i)$, $0 < y_i < 1$, and $\sum_i y_i = 1$. We can use the above results to generate the desired Dirichlet density distribution when applying the random number generators for the gamma probability density function available in SAS (1990).

4.18 Show that an asymptotic variance estimator for $\hat{\pi}_{1+}^{(g)}$ (4.5) based on randomization is given by (4.48) (hint: $\hat{\pi}_{1+}^{(g)}$ can be viewed as a ratio estimator discussed in Cochran (1977)).

4.19 Applying the randomization-based variance formula for the ratio estimator discussed in Cochran (1977), derive the following variance and covariance estimators:

(a) $$\hat{Var}_{RB}(\hat{\pi}_{+CA}^{(1)} - \hat{\pi}_{+A}^{(0)}) = \hat{Var}_{RB}(\hat{\pi}_{+CA}^{(1)}) + \hat{Var}_{RB}(\hat{\pi}_{+A}^{(0)}),$$

where $\hat{Var}_{RB}(\hat{\pi}_{+CA}^{(1)}) = \sum_{i=1}^{n_1} (m_{+CA|i}^{(1)} - \hat{\pi}_{+CA}^{(1)} m_i^{(1)})^2 / $
$[n_1(n_1 - 1)(\bar{m}^{(1)})^2],$

and

$$\hat{Var}_{RB}(\hat{\pi}_{+A}^{(0)}) = \sum_{i=1}^{n_0} (m_{+A|i}^{(0)} - \hat{\pi}_{+A}^{(0)} m_i^{(0)})^2 / $$
$[n_0(n_0 - 1)(\bar{m}^{(0)})^2];$

(b) $$\hat{Cov}_{RB}(\hat{\pi}_{1+}^{(1)}, \hat{\pi}_{+CA}^{(1)}) = \hat{Var}_{RB}(\hat{\pi}_{1CA}^{(1)}) + \hat{Cov}_{RB}(\hat{\pi}_{1CA}^{(1)}, \hat{\pi}_{2CA}^{(1)})$$
$$+ \hat{Cov}_{RB}(\hat{\pi}_{1CA}^{(1)}, \hat{\pi}_{1N}^{(1)}) + \hat{Cov}_{RB}(\hat{\pi}_{2CA}^{(1)}, \hat{\pi}_{1N}^{(1)}),$$

where

$$\hat{Var}_{RB}(\hat{\pi}_{1CA}^{(1)}) = \sum_{i=1}^{n_1} (m_{1CA|i}^{(1)} - \hat{\pi}_{1CA}^{(1)} m_i^{(1)})^2 / $$
$[n_1(n_1 - 1)(\bar{m}^{(1)})^2], \hat{Cov}_{RB}(\hat{\pi}_{1CA}^{(1)}, \hat{\pi}_{2CA}^{(1)}) = \sum_{i=1}^{n_1} (m_{1CA|i}^{(1)}$
$- \hat{\pi}_{1CA}^{(1)} m_i^{(1)})(m_{2CA|i}^{(1)} - \hat{\pi}_{2CA}^{(1)} m_i^{(1)}) / [n_1(n_1 - 1)(\bar{m}^{(1)})^2],$
$\hat{Cov}_{RB}(\hat{\pi}_{1N}^{(1)}, \hat{\pi}_{1CA}^{(1)}) = \sum_{i=1}^{n_1} (m_{1N|i}^{(1)} - \hat{\pi}_{1N}^{(1)} m_i^{(1)})(m_{1CA|i}^{(1)}$
$- \hat{\pi}_{1CA}^{(1)} m_i^{(1)}) / [n_1(n_1 - 1)(\bar{m}^{(1)})^2], \hat{Cov}_{RB}(\hat{\pi}_{1N}^{(1)}, \hat{\pi}_{2CA}^{(1)})$
$= \sum_{i=1}^{n_1} (m_{1N|i}^{(1)} - \hat{\pi}_{1N}^{(1)} m_i^{(1)})(m_{2CA|i}^{(1)} - \hat{\pi}_{2CA}^{(1)} m_i^{(1)}) / $
$[n_1(n_1 - 1)(\bar{m}^{(1)})^2].$

Thus, we have

$$\hat{Cov}_{RB}(\hat{\pi}_{1+}^{(1)}, \hat{\pi}_{+CA}^{(1)}) = \sum_{i=1}^{n_1} (m_{1+|i}^{(1)} - \hat{\pi}_{1+}^{(1)} m_i^{(1)})(m_{+CA|i}^{(1)}$$
$$- \hat{\pi}_{+CA}^{(1)} m_i^{(1)}) / [n_1(n_1 - 1)(\bar{m}^{(1)})^2].$$

(c) $$\hat{Cov}_{RB}(\hat{\pi}_{1+}^{(0)}, \hat{\pi}_{+A}^{(0)}) = \hat{Var}_{RB}(\hat{\pi}_{1A}^{(0)}) + \hat{Cov}_{RB}(\hat{\pi}_{1CN}^{(0)}, \hat{\pi}_{1A}^{(0)})$$
$$+ \hat{Cov}_{RB}(\hat{\pi}_{1A}^{(0)}, \hat{\pi}_{2A}^{(0)}) + \hat{Cov}_{RB}(\hat{\pi}_{1CN}^{(0)}, \hat{\pi}_{2A}^{(0)}),$$

where

$$\hat{Var}_{RB}(\hat{\pi}_{1A}^{(0)}) = \sum_{i=1}^{n_0} (m_{1A|i}^{(0)} - \hat{\pi}_{1A}^{(0)} m_i^{(0)})^2 / $$
$[n_0(n_0 - 1)(\bar{m}^{(0)})^2], \hat{Cov}_{RB}(\hat{\pi}_{1CN}^{(0)}, \hat{\pi}_{1A}^{(0)})$
$= \sum_{i=1}^{n_0} (m_{1CN|i}^{(0)} - \hat{\pi}_{1CN}^{(0)} m_i^{(0)})(m_{1A|i}^{(0)} - \hat{\pi}_{1A}^{(0)} m_i^{(0)}) / $

$$[n_0(n_0 - 1)(\bar{m}^{(0)})^2], \ \hat{C}ov_{RB}(\hat{\pi}_{1A}^{(0)}, \hat{\pi}_{2A}^{(0)})$$

$$= \sum_{i=1}^{n_0} (m_{1A|i}^{(0)} - \hat{\pi}_{1A}^{(0)} m_i^{(0)})(m_{2A|i}^{(0)} - \hat{\pi}_{2A}^{(0)} m_i^{(0)})/$$

$$[n_0(n_0 - 1)(\bar{m}^{(0)})^2], \ \hat{C}ov_{RB}(\hat{\pi}_{1CN}^{(0)}, \hat{\pi}_{2A}^{(0)})$$

$$= \sum_{i=1}^{n_0} (m_{1CN|i}^{(0)} - \hat{\pi}_{1CN}^{(0)} m_i^{(0)})(m_{2A|i}^{(0)} - \hat{\pi}_{2A}^{(0)} m_i^{(0)})/$$

$$[n_0(n_0 - 1)(\bar{m}^{(0)})^2].$$

Thus, we have

$$\hat{C}ov_{RB}(\hat{\pi}_{1+}^{(0)}, \hat{\pi}_{+A}^{(0)}) = \sum_{i=1}^{n_0} (m_{1+|i}^{(0)} - \hat{\pi}_{1+}^{(0)} m_i^{(0)})(m_{+A|i}^{(0)} - \hat{\pi}_{+A}^{(0)} m_i^{(0)})/$$

$$[n_0(n_0 - 1)(\bar{m}^{(0)})^2].$$

Appendix

The following program is used to produce the minimum required number
of clusters presented in Table 4.3 for testing superiority in a CRT with
noncompliance.

```
data step1;
*** We assume that the cluster size follows the Poisson distribution;
 array fn(w1) fnx1-fnx4;
 za=1.96;
 zb=0.842;
 nsimul=10000;
 do pattern=1 to 2; ** subpopulation distribution;
  if pattern= 1 then do;
   psc=0.95; psa=0.03; psn=0.02; *** distribution of compliers always-
takers and never-takers;
 end;
 if pattern = 2 then do;
 psc=0.80; psa=0.15; psn=0.05;
 end;
do delta=0.05,0.10,0.20; *** desired difference to be detected;
do rho=0.05,0.10,0.20; *** intraclass correlation;
do rprob=1 to 2; ** conditional prob of positive response;
          ** for different subpopulations in the standard treatment;
 if rprob =1 then do;
 rpc=0.20; rpa=0.35; rpn=0.25;
 end;
 if rprob = 2 then do;
 rpc=0.50; rpa=0.20; rpn=0.30;
 end;
do msize=5,10,20,50; *** mean cluster size;
pi0=psc*(rpc+rpc+delta)/2+psa*rpa+psn*rpn;
s0=2*pi0*(1-pi0)*(1+msize*rho)/msize;
pi1=psc*rpc+psa*rpa+psn*rpn;
pi2=psc*(rpc+delta)+psa*rpa+psn*rpn;
s1=(pi1*(1-pi1)+pi2*(1-pi2))*(1+msize*rho)/msize;
n=ceil((za*sqrt(s0)+zb*sqrt(s1)/(1-(delta*psc)**2))**2/((0.5*log
((1+delta*psc)/(1-delta*psc)))**2));
if msize eq 5 then w1=1;
if msize eq 10 then w1=2;
if msize eq 20 then w1=3;
if msize eq 50 then w1=4;
fn=n;
if msize eq 50 then
 put pattern 1-5 delta 6-10 2 rho 11-15 2 rprob 16-20 fnx1 26-35 fnx2
36-45 fnx3 46-55 fnx4 56-65;
 end; ** end of do mmsize;
 end; ** end of do rprob;
 end; ** end of do rho;
```

```
end; ** do delta;
end; ** do pattern;
```

The following program is used to produce the minimum required number of clusters presented in Table 4.4 for testing noninferiority based on the OR in a CRT with noncompliance.

```
data step1;
*** We assume that the cluster size follows the Poisson distribution;
 array fn(w1) fnx1-fnx4;
 za=probit(0.95);
 zb=probit(0.80);
 ldellow=log(0.80);
 do rprob=1; ** conditional probability of a positive response;
        ** for different subpopulation in the standard treatment;
   if rprob = 1 then do;
   rpc=0.50; rpa=0.20; rpn=0.30;
   end;
 do pattern=1,2; ** subpopulation distribution;
   if pattern= 1 then do;
   psc=0.95; psa=0.03; psn=0.02;
   end;
   if pattern = 2 then do;
   psc=0.80; psa=0.15; psn=0.05;
   end;
do or=0.90,1.0,1.1;
do rho=0.10,0.20;
do msize=10,20,50;
do sratio=1,2,3,4; ** ratio of sample allocation;
   rpce=or*rpc/(1+(or-1)*rpc);
   pi1cae=psc*rpce+psa*rpa;
   pi2cae=psc*(1-rpce)+psa*(1-rpa);
   pi1ne=psn*rpn;
   pi2ne=psn*(1-rpn);
   pi1cns=psc*rpc+psn*rpn;
   pi2cns=psc*(1-rpc)+psn*(1-rpn);
   pi1as=psa*rpa;
   pi2as=psa*(1-rpa);
   vinf=(1+msize*rho);
   s1=(pi1cae*(1-pi1cae)*vinf/msize+pi1as*(1-
pi1as)*vinf/(sratio*msize))/(pi1cae-pi1as)**2;
   s2=(pi2ne*(1-pi2ne)*vinf/msize+pi2cns*(1-
pi2cns)*vinf/(sratio*msize))/(pi2cns-pi2ne)**2;
   s3=(pi2cae*(1-pi2cae)*vinf/msize+pi2as*(1-
pi2as)*vinf/(sratio*msize))/(pi2cae-pi2as)**2;
   s4=(pi1ne*(1-pi1ne)*vinf/msize+pi1cns*(1-
pi1cns)*vinf/(sratio*msize))/(pi1cns-pi1ne)**2;

s12=(pi1cae*pi2ne*vinf/msize+pi1as*pi2cns*vinf/(sratio*msize))/((pi1cae
-pi1as)*(pi2cns-pi2ne));
```

```
s13=(pi1cae*pi2cae*vinf/msize+pi1as*pi2as*vinf/(sratio*msize))/((pi1cae
-pi1as)*(pi2cae-pi2as));

s14=(pi1cae*pi1ne*vinf/msize+pi1cns*pi1as*vinf/(sratio*msize))/((pi1cae
-pi1as)*(pi1cns-pi1ne));

s23=(pi2cae*pi2ne*vinf/msize+pi2as*pi2cns*vinf/(sratio*msize))/((pi2cae
-pi2as)*(pi2cns-pi2ne));

s24=(pi1ne*pi2ne*vinf/msize+pi1cns*pi2cns*vinf/(sratio*msize))/((pi2cns
-pi2ne)*(pi1cns-pi1ne));

s34=(pi2cae*pi1ne*vinf/msize+pi2as*pi1cns*vinf/(sratio*msize))/((pi2cae
-pi2as)*(pi1cns-pi1ne));
  svar=s1+s2+s3+s4+2*s12+2*s13-2*s14-2*s23+2*s24+2*s34;
  n1s=ceil((za+zb)**2*svar/((ldellow-log(or))**2));
  n1=n1s; ** number of clusters needed from the experimental group;
 if sratio eq 1 then w1=1;
 if sratio eq 2 then w1=2;
 if sratio eq 3 then w1=3;
 if sratio eq 4 then w1=4;
 fn=n1;
 if sratio eq 4 then
 put pattern 1-5 or 6-10 2 rho 11-15 2 msize 21-25 fnx1 26-35 fnx2 36-
45 fnx3 46-55 fnx4 56-65;
 end; ** end of do sratio;
 end; ** end of do msize;
 end; ** end of do rho;
 end; ** do or;
 end; ** do pattern;
 end; ** do rprob;
```

5

Randomized clinical trials with both noncompliance and subsequent missing outcomes

It is not uncommon to encounter a randomized clinical trial (RCT), in which there are patients who do not comply with their assigned treatments (Sato, 2000, 2001; Matsuyama, 2002; Jo, 2002; Matsui, 2005; Barnard, Frangakis and Hill *et al.*, 2003) and/or have subsequent missing outcomes (Frangakis and Rubin, 1999; Zhou and Li, 2006; Mealli and Rubin, 2002; Mealli, Imbens and Ferro *et al.*, 2004; O'Malley and Normand, 2005; Little and Yau, 1998; Baker and Kramer, 2005). Noncompliance can occur due to a previously negative experience of taking a treatment (Lui, 2007b) or a change of patient's mind to accept a treatment after randomization (Walter, Guyatt and Montori *et al.*, 2006), while subsequent missing outcomes may arise from patient's withdrawal or loss to follow up especially for a RCT with a long duration (Frangakis and Rubin, 1999). For studying certain treatments, such as a trial of taking a flu vaccine (McDonald, Hui and Tierney, 1992) or an investigation of quitting cigarette smoking (Multiple Risk Factor Interventional Trial Research Group, 1982), the traditional RCT, in which participants are randomized to receive or not to receive the treatment, is inapplicable due to ethical concerns. The randomized

Binary Data Analysis of Randomized Clinical Trials with Noncompliance, First Edition. Kung-Jong Lui.
© 2011 John Wiley & Sons, Ltd. Published 2011 by John Wiley & Sons, Ltd.

encouragement design (RED), in which participants are randomized to receive or not to receive an encouragement for the use of a treatment, is often suggested.

However, because participants may decide to receive a treatment or drop out from a trial despite whether they receive an encouragement or not, both noncompliance and missing outcomes can commonly occur in a RED. For example, consider the flu vaccine trial in which physicians were randomly assigned to either an intervention group of receiving computer-generated reminders for flu shots or to a control group of receiving no such reminders (Zhou and Li, 2006). Patients were then classified by the group to which their physicians were assigned (Table 5.1). The risks of morbidity between two comparison groups over a 3-year period in an academic primary care practice were then compared. Note that a physician assigned to the intervention group of receiving a reminder might not give a patient flu shots if the physician felt on the basis of the individual patient information that the patient was not at the risk of flu. As seen from Table 5.1, approximately 79 % of patients in the intervention group did not receive flu shots.

On the other hand, a physician assigned to the control group might still give a patient flu shots if the physician believed that the particular patient was at the high risk of flu. This may explain why there were approximately 14 % (Table 5.1) of patients who received vaccine in the control group. Furthermore, there were approximately 38 % to 39 % of patients whose outcomes of flu-related hospitalization were missing in both assigned groups. Because missing outcomes do not generally occur completely at random, the commonly-used intent-to-treat (ITT) analysis for testing the null treatment effect conditional upon the observed data of patients with known outcomes can be inappropriate (Frangakis and Rubin, 1999). Furthermore, to avoid the loss of power in detecting a treatment effect of interest, it is important to incorporate both noncompliance and subsequent missing outcomes into sample size calculation in designing a RCT. Note that use of such a naïve traditional adjustment method for missing data as dividing the resulting sample size calculated with assuming all patients with known outcomes by the probability of nonmissing outcome can produce a misleading result (Skalski, 1992; Lui, 1994; Lui and Chang, 2008a). Note also that when the outcome is continuous rather than dichotomous as focused here, the discussion

Table 5.1   The observed frequency and the observed proportion in percentage (in parenthesis) of flu-related hospitalization over a 3-year period between the intervention group of receiving computer-generated reminders for flu shot and the control group of receiving no such reminders.

| | Intervention group of receiving reminders | | | Control group of receiving no reminders | | |
| | Flu vaccine | | | Flu vaccine | | |
	Yes	No	Total	Yes	No	Total
Hospitalization Yes	20 (1.51)	47 (3.54)	67 (5.05)	16 (1.24)	49 (3.80)	65 (5.04)
No	256 (19.28)	499 (37.58)	755 (56.85)	143 (11.09)	573 (44.42)	716 (55.50)
Unknown	9 (0.68)	497 (37.42)	506 (38.10)	17 (1.32)	492 (38.14)	509 (39.46)
Total	285 (21.46)	1043 (78.54)	1328 (100)	176 (13.64)	1114 (86.36)	1290 (100)

on estimation of the treatment effect in the presence of noncompliance and subsequent missing outcomes can be found elsewhere (O'Malley and Normand, 2005; Yau and Little, 2001; Barnard, Frangakis and Hill *et al.*, 2003).

In analysis of binary data for a RCT with noncompliance and subsequent missing outcomes, one of the main challenging issues is that the underlying parameters are not uniquely identifiable without imposing additional parameter constraints beyond those discussed in Chapter 2 for the case with noncompliance only. As noted elsewhere (Mealli and Rubin, 2002), however, there are no universally appropriate assumptions in simultaneously modeling noncompliance and subsequent missing outcomes. The most plausible assumptions of imposing parameter constraints are generally specific to each particular RCT. Because they have been assumed and discussed in many places (Frangakis and Rubin, 1999; Zhou and Li, 2006; Mealli and Rubin, 2002; Mealli, Imbens and Ferro *et al.*, 2004; Lui and Chang, 2008a, 2008b, 2010), we focus our attention on studying treatment efficacy under the compound exclusion restriction assumption and latent ignorability. To estimate the treatment efficacy, we also make the common assumptions for a RCT with noncompliance, including the stable unit treatment value assumption (SUTVA) and the monotonicity assumption. We discuss testing superiority between two treatments for a RCT with noncompliance and subsequent missing outcomes in Section 5.1. We address testing noninferiority in Section 5.2 and testing equivalence in Section 5.3 when using the proportion difference (PD), the proportion ratio (PR) and the odds ratio (OR) to measure the relative treatment effect in the presence of both noncompliance and subsequent missing outcomes. We discuss interval estimation of the PD, PR, and OR for a RCT with noncompliance and subsequent missing outcomes in Section 5.4. We derive in Section 5.5 sample size formulae based on the test procedures presented here for testing superiority, noninferiority, and equivalence discussed in Sections 5.1–5.3. We provide in Section 5.6 readers with an alternative model, which assumes observations missing at random (MAR) (Little and Rubin, 2002), as well as derive the corresponding maximum likelihood estimator (MLE) for the PD, PR and OR and their asymptotic variances. Readers can then apply these results to do hypothesis testing, interval estimation, sample size determination, and evaluate the robustness of estimators derived from assuming the compound exclusion restriction model under the alternative MAR model. We also include the modified Frangakis and Rubin's model considered by Mealli, Imbens and Ferro *et al.* (2004) and show the corresponding MLE of PD, PR and OR in exercises. Since none of the above models is really testable, however, we may determine in practice the relatively preferable model based on the resulting parameter estimates against what we believe from our best subjective knowledge in a given RCT (Mealli and Rubin, 2002).

Suppose that we randomly assign patients to either the experimental ($g = 1$) treatment or the standard (or placebo) ($g = 0$) treatment. Following Angrist, Imbens and Rubin (1996), we define for each patient the vector $(d(1), d(0))'$ as the status of his/her potential treatment receipt, and $d(g) = 1$ if the patient assigned to treatment g receives the experimental treatment, and $d(g) = 0$, otherwise. Thus, our sampling population can be divided into four subpopulations: compliers (i.e. $d(g) = g$ for $g = 1, 0$), never-takers (i.e. $d(g) = 0$ for $g = 1, 0$), always-takers (i.e. $d(g) = 1$ for $g = 1, 0$), and defiers (i.e. $d(g) = 1 - g$ for $g = 1, 0$). As assumed in most RCTs with noncompliance (Angrist, Imbens and Rubin, 1996; Li and Frangakis, 2005; Zhou and Li, 2006), we make the SUTVA and the monotonicity assumption (i.e. $d(1) \geq d(0)$). The former is to assume that there is no interference between participated patients, while the latter is to assume that there are no defiers. Under the monotonicity assumption, when a patient assigned to the experimental treatment ($g = 1$) receives the standard treatment ($g = 0$), he/she must be a never-taker. Similarly, when a patient assigned to the standard treatment receives the experimental treatment, he/she must be an always-taker. However, when a patient assigned to the experimental treatment receives his/her assigned (experimental) treatment, he/she can be either a complier or an always-taker. Also, if a patient assigned to the standard treatment receives his/her assigned (standard) treatment, he/she can be either a complier or a never-taker. For the assigned treatment g ($g = 1, 0$), let $\pi_{1S}^{(g)}$ denote the cell probability of a randomly selected patient who has a positive response and falls in category $S : S = C$ for compliers, $= A$ for always-takers, and $= N$ for never-takers.

Furthermore, let $\pi_{2S}^{(g)}$ denote the corresponding cell probability of a negative response and a treatment-received status S for a randomly selected patient assigned to treatment g. We use '+' notation to designate summation of cell probabilities over that particular subscript. For example, the parameter $\pi_{+S}^{(g)}$ represents $\pi_{1S}^{(g)} + \pi_{2S}^{(g)}$, which denotes the proportion of subpopulation S in the assigned treatment g. Because of random assignment, we may assume that $\pi_{+S}^{(1)} = \pi_{+S}^{(0)} = \pi_{+S}$, where π_{+S} denotes the proportion of subpopulation S (where $S = C, A, N$) in the sampling population. Define $\pi_{1|S}^{(g)} = \pi_{1S}^{(g)}/\pi_{+S}$, the conditional probability of a positive response among subpopulation S ($S = C, A, N$) in the assigned treatment g ($g = 1, 0$). Because patients are randomly assigned to one of the two treatments and patients who are always-takers (or never-takers) will take the same experimental (or standard) treatment regardless of their assigned treatments, the exclusion restriction assumption that $\pi_{1|A}^{(1)} = \pi_{1|A}^{(0)}$ for always-takers and $\pi_{1|N}^{(1)} = \pi_{1|N}^{(0)}$ for never-takers (Angrist et al., 1996; Frangakis and Rubin, 1999) is likely to hold in a double-blind trial, especially when noncompliance occurs soon after assignment (Frangakis and Baker, 2001). These together with $\pi_{+S}^{(1)} = \pi_{+S}^{(0)} = \pi_{+S}$ ($S = C, A, N$) imply that $\pi_{rA}^{(1)} = \pi_{rA}^{(0)}$ and $\pi_{rN}^{(1)} = \pi_{rN}^{(0)}$ for $r = 1, 2$. When there is no confusion, we denote $\pi_{rA}^{(g)}$ and $\pi_{rN}^{(g)}$ by π_{rA} and π_{rN}, respectively. Due to the refusal or loss to follow-up, we may come across some patients with missing outcomes (Frangakis and Rubin, 1999). Furthermore, these missing outcomes may occur not completely at random and depend on both the underlying characteristics of patients S, $S = C, N, A$ and the actual treatment receipt $d(g)(= 1$ for experimental, and $= 0$ for standard).

Given an assigned treatment g and the characteristics S of a patient, we can uniquely determine the treatment receipt $d(g)$. For example, by definition, when $g = 1$ and $S = C$, $d(g)$ must be 1, or when $g = 0$ and $S = C$, $d(g)$ must be 0. Following Frangakis and Rubin (1999), we assume that the probability of nonmissing outcomes depends on only the characteristics S and the actual treatment receipt $d(g)$. We let $\eta_S^{(g)}$ denote the probability of obtaining a nonmissing outcome for a randomly selected patient from the assigned treatment g with characteristics S. Because patients with $S = A$ (or N) would have received the same treatment regardless of their assigned treatments, by assumption, we have $\eta_A^{(1)} = \eta_A^{(0)}(= \eta_A)$ and $\eta_N^{(1)} = \eta_N^{(0)}(= \eta_N)$. The above assumptions that $\pi_{1|S}^{(1)} = \pi_{1|S}^{(0)}$ and $\eta_S^{(1)} = \eta_S^{(0)}(= \eta_S)$ for $S = A, N$, are called the 'compound exclusion restriction assumption for always-takers and never-takers' defined and discussed elsewhere (Zhou and Li, 2006; Frangakis and Rubin, 1999). Given the latent subpopulation S, we further assume that the nonmissing outcome and the patient response are conditionally independent; this is called the latent ignorability (Frangakis and Rubin, 1999; Zhou and Li, 2006). On the basis of the above assumptions, we may summarize the latent probability structure for the observed data of patients assigned to the experimental treatment by use of the following table:

Assigned experimental treatment ($g = 1$)

Treatment received		Experimental	Control	
		Compliers and always-takers (CA)	Never-takers (N)	Total
Outcome	Positive	$\eta_C^{(1)}\pi_{1C}^{(1)} + \eta_A\pi_{1A}$	$\eta_N\pi_{1N}$	$\eta_C^{(1)}\pi_{1C}^{(1)} + \eta_A\pi_{1A}$ $+ \eta_N\pi_{1N}$
	Negative	$\eta_C^{(1)}\pi_{2C}^{(1)} + \eta_A\pi_{2A}$	$\eta_N\pi_{2N}$	$\eta_C^{(1)}\pi_{2C}^{(1)} + \eta_A\pi_{2A}$ $+ \eta_N\pi_{2N}$
	Unknown	$(1 - \eta_C^{(1)})\pi_{+C}$ $+ (1 - \eta_A)\pi_{+A}$	$(1 - \eta_N)\pi_{+N}$	$(1 - \eta_C^{(1)})\pi_{+C}$ $+ (1 - \eta_A)\pi_{+A}$ $+ (1 - \eta_N)\pi_{+N}$
	Total	$\pi_{+C} + \pi_{+A}$	π_{+N}	1.0

For example, the probability for a randomly selected patient who has received the assigned experimental treatment and a known positive response is given by $\eta_C^{(1)}\pi_{1C}^{(1)} + \eta_A\pi_{1A}$. As a second example, the probability for a randomly selected patient who has received the assigned (experimental) treatment and had an unknown outcome is $(1 - \eta_C^{(1)})\pi_{+C} + (1 - \eta_A)\pi_{+A}$. Similarly, we may summarize the latent probability structure for the observed data of patients assigned to the standard (or placebo) treatment by use of the following table:

Assigned standard treatment or placebo ($g = 0$)

Treatment received	Control	Experimental	
	Compliers and never-takers (CN)	Always-takers (A)	Total
Outcome Positive	$\eta_C^{(0)}\pi_{1C}^{(0)} + \eta_N\pi_{1N}$	$\eta_A\pi_{1A}$	$\eta_C^{(0)}\pi_{1C}^{(0)} + \eta_N\pi_{1N}$ $+ \eta_A\pi_{1A}$
Negative	$\eta_C^{(0)}\pi_{2C}^{(0)} + \eta_N\pi_{2N}$	$\eta_A\pi_{2A}$	$\eta_C^{(0)}\pi_{2C}^{(0)} + \eta_N\pi_{2N}$ $+ \eta_A\pi_{2A}$
Unknown	$(1 - \eta_C^{(0)})\pi_{+C}$ $+ (1 - \eta_N)\pi_{+N}$	$(1 - \eta_A)\pi_{+A}$	$(1 - \eta_C^{(0)})\pi_{+C}$ $+ (1 - \eta_N)\pi_{+N}$ $+ (1 - \eta_A)\pi_{+A}$
Total	$\pi_{+C} + \pi_{+N}$	π_{+A}	1.0

For convenience in the following discussion, let $E_{rS}^{(g)}$ ($r = 1, 2, 3$, and $S = CA, N$ for $g = 1$, or $S = CN, A$ for $g = 0$) denote the corresponding cell probability for row r and column S in the assigned treatment g. For examples, the parameter $E_{rCA}^{(1)}$ represents $\eta_C^{(1)}\pi_{rC}^{(1)} + \eta_A\pi_{rA}$ for $r = 1, 2$, and the parameter $E_{3CA}^{(1)}$ represents $(1 - \eta_C^{(1)})\pi_{+C} + (1 - \eta_A)\pi_{+A}$. Thus, we have the marginal probabilities: $E_{+CA}^{(1)} = \pi_{+C} + \pi_{+A}$ and $E_{+N}^{(1)} = \pi_{+N}$ in the experimental treatment, while we have the marginal probabilities: $E_{+CN}^{(0)} = \pi_{+C} + \pi_{+N}$ and $E_{+A}^{(0)} = \pi_{+A}$ in the standard treatment. We further have $E_{r+}^{(g)} = \eta_C^{(g)}\pi_{rC}^{(g)} + \eta_N\pi_{rN} + \eta_A\pi_{rA}$ for $g = 1, 0$ and $r = 1, 2$, and $E_{3+}^{(g)} = (1 - \eta_C^{(g)})\pi_{+C} + (1 - \eta_A)\pi_{+A} + (1 - \eta_N)\pi_{+N}$. Recall that the PD in the probability of a positive response among compliers between two treatments is defined as $\Delta = \pi_{1|C}^{(1)} - \pi_{1|C}^{(0)}$ (2.1). Therefore, we can re-express Δ(2.1) in terms of probabilities $E_{rS}^{(g)}$ and $\eta_C^{(g)}$ defined here as

$$\Delta = (E_{1CA}^{(1)} - E_{1A}^{(0)})/[\eta_C^{(1)}(1 - E_{+N}^{(1)} - E_{+A}^{(0)})]$$
$$- (E_{1CN}^{(0)} - E_{1N}^{(1)})/[\eta_C^{(0)}(1 - E_{+N}^{(1)} - E_{+A}^{(0)})]. \tag{5.1}$$

Suppose that we randomly assign n_g patients to receive the experimental ($g = 1$) and standard ($g = 0$) treatments, respectively. Let $n_{rS}^{(g)}$ ($r = 1, 2, 3$, and $S = CA, N$ for $g = 1$ or $S = CN, A$ for $g = 0$) denote the number of patients falling in the cell with the probability $E_{rS}^{(g)}$ in the assigned treatment g. The random frequencies $\{n_{rS}^{(1)} | r = 1, 2, 3, \text{ and } S = CA, N\}$ for the assigned treatment $g = 1$ then follow the multinomial distribution with parameters n_1 and $\{E_{rS}^{(1)} | r = 1, 2, 3, \text{ and } S = CA, N\}$, while the random frequencies $\{n_{rS}^{(0)} | r = 1, 2, 3, S = CN, A\}$ for the assigned treatment $g = 0$ follow the multinomial distribution with parameters n_0 and $\{E_{rS}^{(0)} | r = 1, 2, 3, \text{ and } S = CN, A\}$. Note that the model assumed here is a saturated model (Exercise 5.1). Thus, the MLE of $E_{rS}^{(g)}$ is then $\hat{E}_{rS}^{(g)} = n_{rS}^{(g)} / n_g$. Note also that $\eta_C^{(1)} = (E_{(2)CA}^{(1)} - E_{(2)A}^{(0)}) / \pi_{+C}$, where $\pi_{+C} = (1 - E_{+N}^{(1)} - E_{+A}^{(0)})$, $E_{(2)CA}^{(1)} = E_{1CA}^{(1)} + E_{2CA}^{(1)}$, and $E_{(2)A}^{(0)} = E_{1A}^{(0)} + E_{2A}^{(0)}$. By the functional invariance property of the MLE (Casella and Berger, 1990), the MLE for $\eta_C^{(1)}$ is $\hat{\eta}_C^{(1)} = (\hat{E}_{(2)CA}^{(1)} - \hat{E}_{(2)A}^{(0)}) / \hat{\pi}_{+C}$, where $\hat{\pi}_{+C} = (1 - \hat{E}_{+N}^{(1)} - \hat{E}_{+A}^{(0)})$, $\hat{E}_{(2)CA}^{(1)} = \hat{E}_{1CA}^{(1)} + \hat{E}_{2CA}^{(1)}$, and $\hat{E}_{(2)A}^{(0)} = \hat{E}_{1A}^{(0)} + \hat{E}_{2A}^{(0)}$. Similarly, the MLE for $\eta_C^{(0)}$ is $\hat{\eta}_C^{(0)} = (\hat{E}_{(2)CN}^{(0)} - \hat{E}_{(2)N}^{(1)}) / \hat{\pi}_{+C}$, where $\hat{E}_{(2)CN}^{(0)} = \hat{E}_{1CN}^{(0)} + \hat{E}_{2CN}^{(0)}$ and $\hat{E}_{(2)N}^{(1)} = \hat{E}_{1N}^{(1)} + \hat{E}_{2N}^{(1)}$. Therefore, we obtain the MLE for $\pi_{1|C}^{(1)}$ and $\pi_{1|C}^{(0)}$ as given by $\hat{\pi}_{1|C}^{(1)} = (\hat{E}_{1CA}^{(1)} - \hat{E}_{1A}^{(0)}) / [\hat{\eta}_C^{(1)} (1 - \hat{E}_{+N}^{(1)} - \hat{E}_{+A}^{(0)})] = (\hat{E}_{1CA}^{(1)} - \hat{E}_{1A}^{(0)}) / (\hat{E}_{(2)CA}^{(1)} - \hat{E}_{(2)A}^{(0)})$ and $\hat{\pi}_{1|C}^{(0)} = (\hat{E}_{1CN}^{(0)} - \hat{E}_{1N}^{(1)}) / [\hat{\eta}_C^{(0)} (1 - \hat{E}_{+N}^{(1)} - \hat{E}_{+A}^{(0)})] = (\hat{E}_{1CN}^{(0)} - \hat{E}_{1N}^{(1)}) / (\hat{E}_{(2)CN}^{(0)} - \hat{E}_{(2)N}^{(1)})$, respectively.

5.1   Testing superiority

When a new experimental treatment is developed, we may first want to find out whether the treatment efficacy of the experimental treatment is larger than that of the standard treatment (or placebo). For safety and ethical reasons (Fleiss, 1981, p. 29), however, we do a two-sided test (rather than a one-sided test) and consider testing $H_0 : \Delta = 0$ versus $H_a : \Delta \neq 0$. When rejecting the null hypothesis $H_0 : \Delta = 0$ at a given small nominal α-level, we will claim that the experimental treatment is superior to the standard treatment (or placebo) if the probability of a positive response in the former is larger than that in the latter. Conditional upon patients with known outcomes, the ITT analysis is a consistent estimator of $E_{1+}^{(1)}/E_{(2)+}^{(1)} - E_{1+}^{(0)}/E_{(2)+}^{(0)}$, where $E_{(2)+}^{(g)} = \eta_C^{(g)}\pi_{+C} + \eta_N\pi_{+N} + \eta_A\pi_{+A}$ for $g = 1, 0$. We can easily show that $E_{1+}^{(1)}/E_{(2)+}^{(1)} - E_{1+}^{(0)}/E_{(2)+}^{(0)}$ is generally not equal to 0 even under $H_0 : \Delta = 0$ (Exercise 5.2). Thus, we can no longer apply the ITT analysis conditional upon patients with known outcomes to test $H_0 : \Delta = 0$ in the presence of subsequent missing outcomes under the compound exclusion restriction assumption for always-takers and never-takers (Frangakis and Rubin, 1999).

By the functional invariance of the MLE (Casella and Berger, 1990), we obtain the MLE for Δ (5.1) in the presence of subsequent missing outcomes as

$$\hat{\Delta}^{(MI)} = (\hat{E}_{1CA}^{(1)} - \hat{E}_{1A}^{(0)})/(\hat{E}_{(2)CA}^{(1)} - \hat{E}_{(2)A}^{(0)})$$

$$- (\hat{E}_{1CN}^{(0)} - \hat{E}_{1N}^{(1)})/(\hat{E}_{(2)CN}^{(0)} - \hat{E}_{(2)N}^{(1)}). \qquad (5.2)$$

Note that when there are no patients with missing outcomes (i.e. $\eta_C^{(1)} = \eta_C^{(0)} = \eta_N = \eta_A = 1$), the MLE $\hat{\Delta}^{(MI)}$ (5.2) can be shown to reduce to $\hat{\Delta}$ (2.5) for the case of no missing data (Exercise 5.3). Using the delta method, we can show that the asymptotic variance $Var(\hat{\Delta}^{(MI)})$ for the MLE $\hat{\Delta}^{(MI)}$ (5.2) is given by (Exercise 5.4):

$$Var(\hat{\Delta}^{(MI)}) = \{E_{1CA}^{(1)}(1 - E_{1CA}^{(1)})/n_1 + E_{1A}^{(0)}(1 - E_{1A}^{(0)})/n_0 + (\pi_{1|C}^{(1)})^2$$

$$\times [E_{(2)CA}^{(1)}(1 - E_{(2)CA}^{(1)})/n_1 + E_{(2)A}^{(0)}(1 - E_{(2)A}^{(0)})/n_0] - 2\pi_{1|C}^{(1)}$$

$$\times [(E_{1CA}^{(1)} - E_{1CA}^{(1)}E_{(2)CA}^{(1)})/n_1 + (E_{1A}^{(0)} - E_{1A}^{(0)}E_{(2)A}^{(0)})/n_0]\}/(E_{(2)CA}^{(1)} - \hat{E}_{(2)A}^{(0)})^2$$

$$+ \{E_{1N}^{(1)}(1 - E_{1N}^{(1)})/n_1 + E_{1CN}^{(0)}(1 - E_{1CN}^{(0)})/n_0 + (\pi_{1|C}^{(0)})^2[E_{(2)N}^{(1)}(1 - E_{(2)N}^{(1)})/n_1$$

$$+ E_{(2)CN}^{(0)}(1 - E_{(2)CN}^{(0)})/n_0] - 2\pi_{1|C}^{(0)}[(E_{1N}^{(1)} - E_{1N}^{(1)}E_{(2)N}^{(1)})/n_1$$

$$+ (E_{1CN}^{(0)} - E_{1CN}^{(0)}E_{(2)CN}^{(0)})/n_0]\}/(E_{(2)CN}^{(0)} - E_{(2)N}^{(1)})^2 - 2\{(E_{1CA}^{(1)}E_{1N}^{(1)}/n_1$$

$$+ E_{1A}^{(0)}E_{1CN}^{(0)}/n_0) - \pi_{1|C}^{(0)}(E_{1CA}^{(1)}E_{(2)N}^{(1)}/n_1 + E_{1A}^{(0)}E_{(2)CN}^{(0)}/n_0)$$

$$- \pi_{1|C}^{(1)}(E_{(2)CA}^{(1)}E_{1N}^{(1)}/n_1 + E_{(2)A}^{(0)}E_{1CN}^{(0)}/n_0) + \pi_{1|C}^{(1)}\pi_{1|C}^{(0)}(E_{(2)CA}^{(1)}E_{(2)N}^{(1)}/n_1$$

$$+ E_{(2)A}^{(0)}E_{(2)CN}^{(0)}/n_0)\}/[(E_{(2)CA}^{(1)} - E_{(2)A}^{(0)})(E_{(2)CN}^{(0)} - E_{(2)N}^{(1)})]. \qquad (5.3)$$

We may simply substitute $\hat{E}_{rS}^{(g)}$ for $E_{rS}^{(g)}$, $\hat{E}_{(2)S}^{(g)}$ for $E_{(2)S}^{(g)}$, and $\hat{\pi}_{1|C}^{(g)}$ for $\pi_{1|C}^{(g)}$ in $Var(\hat{\Delta}^{(MI)})$ (5.3) to obtain the estimated variance $\hat{Var}(\hat{\Delta}^{(MI)})$.

Furthermore, using the delta method, we obtain the asymptotic variance $Var(\tanh^{-1}(\hat{\Delta}^{(MI)})) = Var(\hat{\Delta}^{MI})/(1 - \Delta^2)^2$. When the number n_g of patients in both treatments g is large, we may consider the following test statistic with the $\tanh^{-1}(X)$ transformation to test $H_0 : \Delta = 0$ versus $H_a : \Delta \neq 0$. We will reject H_0 at the α-level if the test statistic (Lui and Chang, 2008a):

$$\tanh^{-1}(\hat{\Delta}^{(MI)})/\sqrt{\hat{Var}(\hat{\Delta}^{(MI)})} > Z_{\alpha/2} \text{ or } \tanh^{-1}(\hat{\Delta}^{(MI)})/\sqrt{\hat{Var}(\hat{\Delta}^{(MI)})} < -Z_{\alpha/2},$$

(5.4)

where Z_α is the upper $100(\alpha)th$ percentile of the standard normal distribution.

Furthermore, we will claim that the experimental treatment is superior to the standard treatment if $\tanh^{-1}(\hat{\Delta}^{(MI)})/\sqrt{\hat{Var}(\hat{\Delta}^{(MI)})} > Z_{\alpha/2}$ holds. Based on Monte Carlo simulation, Lui and Chang (2008a) noted that the test procedure (5.4) can perform well with respect to Type I error in a variety of situations. Note that under $H_0 : \Delta = 0$ (or equivalently, $\pi_{1|C}^{(1)} = \pi_{1|C}^{(0)}$), we may also substitute $\hat{E}_{rS}^{(g)}$ for $E_{rS}^{(g)}$, $\hat{E}_{(2)S}^{(g)}$ for $E_{(2)S}^{(g)}$, and the pooled estimator $\hat{\tilde{\pi}}_{1|C}^{(p)} = (n_1\hat{\pi}_{1|C}^{(1)} + n_0\hat{\pi}_{1|C}^{(0)})/(n_1 + n_0)$ for both $\pi_{1|C}^{(1)}$ and $\pi_{1|C}^{(0)}$ in $Var(\hat{\Delta}^{(MI)})$ (5.3) when employing the test procedure (5.4).

Example 5.1   To improve flu outcomes, flu vaccination has been annually recommended for elderly people and persons at high risk of influenza. Because it is unethical to randomize flu shots to high-risk adult patients, the traditional RCT has been rarely carried out to assess the efficacy of a flu vaccine. To alleviate this ethical concern, McDonald, Hui and Tierney (1991) employed the RED, in which physicians were randomly assigned to either the experimental group of receiving a computer-generated reminder for giving their patients flu vaccine or the control group of receiving no such a reminder. The patients were then classified by the group to which the physicians were assigned. The risks of morbidity on patients between two comparison groups were then compared in an academic primary care practice. We summarize the frequencies of patients with flu-related hospitalization according to the receipt of reminders and the status of flu shots in Table 5.1. Because we do not have the information on clusters of patients cared by the same physicians, we ignore clusters and assume individual patients as randomization units for the purpose of illustration only. As noted in Chapter 4, the test result without accounting for the intraclass correlation between patients within clusters is likely to be liberal here. Given these data, we obtain the MLE $\hat{\Delta}^{(MI)}$ and its estimated asymptotic standard error $\hat{SD}(\hat{\Delta}^{(MI)})(= \sqrt{\hat{Var}(\hat{\Delta}^{(MI)})})$ to be -0.005 and 0.114, respectively. When applying the test statistic $\tanh^{-1}(\hat{\Delta}^{(MI)})/\sqrt{\hat{Var}(\hat{\Delta}^{(MI)})}$ to test $H_0 : \Delta = 0$, we obtain the p-value to be 0.964. The actual p-value can be even larger than this if we account for the intraclass correlation between patient outcomes of flu-related hospitalization within physicians. Thus, there is no evidence that the flu shot can reduce the risk of flu-related hospitalization.

5.2   Testing noninferiority

When a generic drug has fewer side effects, lower cost, or is more convenient to administer than a standard drug, we may consider use of the former as a substitute for the latter if one can demonstrate that the generic drug is noninferior to the standard drug with respect to treatment efficacy. In this section, we discuss testing noninferiority when using the PD, PR and OR to measure the relative treatment efficacy in the presence of both noncompliance and subsequent missing outcomes.

5.2.1   Using the difference in proportions

We consider first testing $H_0 : \Delta \leq -\varepsilon_l$ versus $H_a : \Delta > -\varepsilon_l$, where $\varepsilon_l(> 0)$ is the maximum acceptable margin such that the experimental drug can be regarded as noninferior to the standard treatment when $\pi_{1|C}^{(1)} > \pi_{1|C}^{(0)} - \varepsilon_l$. On the basis of $\hat{\Delta}^{(MI)}$ (5.2) and $\hat{Var}(\hat{\Delta}^{(MI)})$ obtained from (5.3) with substituting $\hat{E}_{rS}^{(g)}$ for $E_{rS}^{(g)}$, $\hat{E}_{(2)S}^{(g)}$ for $E_{(2)S}^{(g)}$, and $\hat{\pi}_{1|C}^{(g)}$ for $\pi_{1|C}^{(g)}$, we may consider the test statistic with the $\tanh^{-1}(x)$ transformation:

$$Z = [\tanh^{-1}(\hat{\Delta}^{(MI)}) + \tanh^{-1}(\varepsilon_l)]/\sqrt{\hat{Var}(\tanh^{-1}(\hat{\Delta}^{(MI)}))}, \qquad (5.5)$$

where $\hat{Var}(\tanh^{-1}(\hat{\Delta}^{(MI)})) = \hat{Var}(\hat{\Delta}^{(MI)})/(1 - (\hat{\Delta}^{(MI)})^2)^2$. We will reject $H_0 : \Delta \leq -\varepsilon_l$ at the α-level if the test statistic (5.5), $Z > Z_\alpha$.

5.2.2 Using the ratio of proportions

Recall that the PR, representing the ratio of conditional probabilities of a positive response among compliers between the experimental and standard treatments, is defined as $\gamma = \pi_{1|C}^{(1)}/\pi_{1|C}^{(0)} = \pi_{1C}^{(1)}/\pi_{1C}^{(0)}$ (2.8). In terms of cell probabilities $E_{rS}^{(g)}$'s and $\eta_C^{(g)}$ defined in the above tables, we can re-express γ as

$$\gamma = [(E_{1CA}^{(1)} - E_{1A}^{(0)})/\eta_C^{(1)}]/[(E_{1CN}^{(0)} - E_{1N}^{(1)})/\eta_C^{(0)}]. \tag{5.6}$$

Substituting $\hat{E}_{rS}^{(g)}$ for $E_{rS}^{(g)}$ and $\hat{\eta}_C^{(g)}$ for $\eta_C^{(g)}$ in (5.6), we obtain the MLE for the PR as given by (Lui and Chang, 2008b)

$$\hat{\gamma}^{(MI)} = [(\hat{E}_{1CA}^{(1)} - \hat{E}_{1A}^{(0)})/\hat{\eta}_C^{(1)}]/[(\hat{E}_{1CN}^{(0)} - \hat{E}_{1N}^{(1)})/\hat{\eta}_C^{(0)}] = [(\hat{E}_{(2)CN}^{(0)} - \hat{E}_{(2)N}^{(1)})$$
$$\times (\hat{E}_{1CA}^{(1)} - \hat{E}_{1A}^{(0)})]/[(\hat{E}_{(2)CA}^{(1)} - \hat{E}_{(2)A}^{(0)})(\hat{E}_{1CN}^{(0)} - \hat{E}_{1N}^{(1)})]. \tag{5.7}$$

Using the delta method, we obtain the asymptotic variance $Var(\log(\hat{\gamma}^{(MI)}))$ for $\hat{\gamma}^{(MI)}$ (5.7) with the logarithmic transformation as given by (Exercise 5.5):

$$Var(\log(\hat{\gamma}^{(MI)})) = [E_{(2)CN}^{(0)}(1 - E_{(2)CN}^{(0)})/n_0 + E_{(2)N}^{(1)}(1 - E_{(2)N}^{(1)})/n_1]/$$
$$(E_{(2)CN}^{(0)} - E_{(2)N}^{(1)})^2 + [E_{1CA}^{(1)}(1 - E_{1CA}^{(1)})/n_1 + E_{1A}^{(0)}(1 - E_{1A}^{(0)})/n_0]/$$
$$(E_{1CA}^{(1)} - E_{1A}^{(0)})^2 + [E_{(2)CA}^{(1)}(1 - E_{(2)CA}^{(1)})/n_1 + E_{(2)A}^{(0)}(1 - E_{(2)A}^{(0)})/n_0]/$$
$$(E_{(2)CA}^{(1)} - E_{(2)A}^{(0)})^2 + [E_{1CN}^{(0)}(1 - E_{1CN}^{(0)})/n_0 + E_{1N}^{(1)}(1 - E_{1N}^{(1)})/n_1]/$$
$$(E_{1CN}^{(0)} - E_{1N}^{(1)})^2 + 2[E_{(2)CN}^{(0)}E_{1A}^{(0)}/n_0 + E_{(2)N}^{(1)}E_{1CA}^{(1)}/n_1]/[(E_{(2)CN}^{(0)}$$
$$- E_{(2)N}^{(1)})(E_{1CA}^{(1)} - E_{1A}^{(0)})] - 2[E_{(2)CN}^{(0)}E_{(2)A}^{(0)}/n_0 + E_{(2)N}^{(1)}E_{(2)CA}^{(1)}/n_1]/$$
$$[(E_{(2)CN}^{(0)} - E_{(2)N}^{(1)})(E_{(2)CA}^{(1)} - E_{(2)A}^{(0)})] - 2[(E_{1CN}^{(0)} - E_{1CN}^{(0)}E_{(2)CN}^{(0)})/n_0$$
$$+ (E_{1N}^{(1)} - E_{1N}^{(1)}E_{(2)N}^{(1)})/n_1]/[(E_{(2)CN}^{(0)} - E_{(2)N}^{(1)})(E_{1CN}^{(0)} - E_{1N}^{(1)})]$$
$$- 2[(E_{1CA}^{(1)} - E_{1CA}^{(1)}E_{(2)CA}^{(1)})/n_1 + (E_{1A}^{(0)} - E_{1A}^{(0)}E_{(2)A}^{(0)})/n_0]/[(E_{1CA}^{(1)} - E_{1A}^{(0)})$$
$$\times (E_{(2)CA}^{(1)} - E_{(2)A}^{(0)})] - 2(E_{1CA}^{(1)}E_{1N}^{(1)}/n_1 + E_{1A}^{(0)}E_{1CN}^{(0)}/n_0)/[(E_{1CA}^{(1)} - E_{1A}^{(0)})$$
$$\times (E_{1CN}^{(0)} - E_{1N}^{(1)})] + 2(E_{(2)CA}^{(1)}E_{1N}^{(1)}/n_1 + E_{(2)A}^{(0)}E_{1CN}^{(0)}/n_0)/$$
$$[(E_{(2)CA}^{(1)} - E_{(2)A}^{(0)})(E_{1CN}^{(0)} - E_{1N}^{(1)})]. \tag{5.8}$$

We can obtain the estimate $\hat{Var}(\log(\hat{\gamma}^{(MI)}))$ by simply substituting $\hat{E}_{rS}^{(g)}$ for $E_{rS}^{(g)}$ and $\hat{E}_{(2)S}^{(g)}$ for $E_{(2)S}^{(g)}$ in $Var(\log(\hat{\gamma}^{(MI)}))$ (5.8).

To establish the noninferiority of an experimental to a standard treatment, we consider testing $H_0 : \gamma \leq 1 - \gamma_l$ versus $H_a : \gamma > 1 - \gamma_l$, where γ_l is the maximum clinically acceptable margin such that the experimental treatment can be regarded as noninferior to the standard treatment when $\gamma > 1 - \gamma_l$. When rejecting $H_0 : \gamma \leq 1 - \gamma_l$ at the α-level, we claim that the experimental treatment is noninferior to the standard treatment. On the basis of $\hat{\gamma}^{(MI)}$ (5.7) and $\widehat{Var}(\log(\hat{\gamma}^{(MI)}))$, we obtain the following test statistic (Lui and Chang, 2008b),

$$Z = (\log(\hat{\gamma}^{(MI)}) - \log(1 - \gamma_l))/\sqrt{\widehat{Var}(\log(\hat{\gamma}^{(MI)}))}. \qquad (5.9)$$

We reject $H_0 : \gamma \leq 1 - \gamma_l$ at the α-level when the test statistic (5.9), $Z > Z_\alpha$. As noted in Chapter 2, however, using the PR to measure the relative treatment effect in establishing noninferiority can contradict the general guideline in a draft of establishing the effectiveness of a new *H. pylori* regimen that the corresponding noninferior margin ε_l on the PD scale (FDA, 1997) should get small when the underlying response rates become large and close to 1. Thus, Garrett (2003) contended that the OR should be the most rational index to measure the relative treatment effect when establishing noninferiority or equivalence.

5.2.3   Using the odds ratio of proportions

Since the determination of a fixed clinically acceptable margin on the PD scale can be sometimes difficult and the choice of a fixed clinically acceptable margin on the PR scale may deviate from the general guideline of the FDA (1997), we may consider use of the OR to measure the relative treatment effect in establishing noninferiority or equivalence (Tu, 1998 and 2003; Wang, Chow and Li, 2002; Garrett, 2003). Recall that the OR of the conditional probabilities of a positive response among compliers between the experimental and standard treatments is defined as $\varphi = (\pi_{1C}^{(1)}\pi_{2C}^{(0)})/(\pi_{2C}^{(1)}\pi_{1C}^{(0)})$ (2.12). In terms of $E_{rS}^{(g)}$'s, we can re-express φ as

$$\varphi = [(E_{1CA}^{(1)} - E_{1A}^{(0)})(E_{2CN}^{(0)} - E_{2N}^{(1)})]/[(E_{2CA}^{(1)} - E_{2A}^{(0)})(E_{1CN}^{(0)} - E_{1N}^{(1)})].$$
$$(5.10)$$

Substituting $\hat{E}_{rS}^{(g)}$ for $E_{rS}^{(g)}$ in (5.10), we obtain the MLE for φ as (Lui and Chang, 2010),

$$\hat{\varphi}^{(MI)} = [(\hat{E}_{1CA}^{(1)} - \hat{E}_{1A}^{(0)})(\hat{E}_{2CN}^{(0)} - \hat{E}_{2N}^{(1)})]/[(\hat{E}_{2CA}^{(1)} - \hat{E}_{2A}^{(0)})(\hat{E}_{1CN}^{(0)} - \hat{E}_{1N}^{(1)})].$$

(5.11)

Using the delta method (Agresti, 1990), we obtain an estimated asymptotic variance for the test statistic $\log(\hat{\varphi}^{(MI)})$ using the logarithmic transformation as given by (Exercise 5.6):

$$
\begin{aligned}
Var(\log(\hat{\varphi}^{(MI)})) &= [E_{1CA}^{(1)}(1 - E_{1CA}^{(1)})/n_1 + E_{1A}^{(0)}(1 - E_{1A}^{(0)})/n_0]/ \\
&\quad (E_{1CA}^{(1)} - E_{1A}^{(0)})^2 + [E_{2CN}^{(0)}(1 - E_{2CN}^{(0)})/n_0 + E_{2N}^{(1)}(1 - E_{2N}^{(1)})/n_1]/ \\
&\quad (E_{2CN}^{(0)} - E_{2N}^{(1)})^2 + [E_{2CA}^{(1)}(1 - E_{2CA}^{(1)})/n_1 + E_{2A}^{(0)}(1 - E_{2A}^{(0)})/n_0]/ \\
&\quad (E_{2CA}^{(1)} - E_{2A}^{(0)})^2 + [E_{1CN}^{(0)}(1 - E_{1CN}^{(0)})/n_0 + E_{1N}^{(1)}(1 - E_{1N}^{(1)})/n_1]/ \\
&\quad (E_{1CN}^{(0)} - E_{1N}^{(1)})^2 + 2[E_{1CA}^{(1)}E_{2N}^{(1)}/n_1 + E_{1A}^{(0)}E_{2CN}^{(0)}/n_0]/[(E_{1CA}^{(1)} - E_{1A}^{(0)}) \\
&\quad \times (E_{2CN}^{(0)} - E_{2N}^{(1)})] + 2[E_{1CA}^{(1)}E_{2CA}^{(1)}/n_1 + E_{1A}^{(0)}E_{2A}^{(0)}/n_0]/[(E_{1CA}^{(1)} - E_{1A}^{(0)}) \\
&\quad \times (E_{2CA}^{(1)} - E_{2A}^{(0)})] - 2[E_{1CA}^{(1)}E_{1N}^{(1)}/n_1 + E_{1CN}^{(0)}E_{1A}^{(0)}/n_0]/[(E_{1CA}^{(1)} - E_{1A}^{(0)}) \\
&\quad \times (E_{1CN}^{(0)} - E_{1N}^{(1)})] - 2[E_{2CA}^{(1)}E_{2N}^{(1)}/n_1 + E_{2A}^{(0)}E_{2CN}^{(0)}/n_0]/[(E_{2CA}^{(1)} - E_{2A}^{(0)}) \\
&\quad \times (E_{2CN}^{(0)} - E_{2N}^{(1)})] + 2[E_{1N}^{(1)}E_{2N}^{(1)}/n_1 + E_{1CN}^{(0)}E_{2CN}^{(0)}/n_0]/[(E_{2CN}^{(0)} - E_{2N}^{(1)}) \\
&\quad \times (E_{1CN}^{(0)} - E_{1N}^{(1)})] + 2[E_{2CA}^{(1)}E_{1N}^{(1)}/n_1 + E_{2A}^{(0)}E_{1CN}^{(0)}/n_0]/ \\
&\quad [(E_{2CA}^{(1)} - E_{2A}^{(0)})(E_{1CN}^{(0)} - E_{1N}^{(1)})].
\end{aligned}
$$

(5.12)

We can substitute $\hat{E}_{rS}^{(g)}$ for $E_{rS}^{(g)}$ in (5.12) to obtain $\hat{Var}(\log(\hat{\varphi}^{(MI)}))$. Consider testing $H_0 : \varphi \leq 1 - \varphi_l$ versus $H_a : \varphi > 1 - \varphi_l$, where φ_l is the maximum clinically acceptable margin such that the experimental treatment can be regarded as noninferior to the standard treatment when $\varphi > 1 - \varphi_l$. On the basis of $\hat{\varphi}^{(MI)}$ (5.11) and $\hat{Var}(\log(\hat{\varphi}^{(MI)}))$, we consider the following test statistic:

$$Z = (\log(\hat{\varphi}^{(MI)}) - \log(1 - \varphi_l))/\sqrt{\hat{Var}(\log(\hat{\varphi}^{(MI)}))}.$$

(5.13)

If the test statistic (5.13), $Z > Z_\alpha$, we will reject $H_0 : \varphi \leq 1 - \varphi_l$ at the α-level and claim that the experimental treatment is noninferior to the standard treatment.

5.3   Testing equivalence

When a generic drug is developed, we may wish to investigate whether the therapeutic efficacy of the generic drug is equivalent to that of the standard drug (Dunnett and Gent, 1977; Westlake, 1979; Hauck and Anderson, 1984 and 1986; Liu and Chow, 1992). A significant decrease in the response rate of using an experimental drug as compared with the standard treatment is certainly not desirable, while a substantial increase in the response rate of using the former may raise the concern that the experimental treatment can be more toxic than the standard treatment. Thus, we may wish to consider testing equivalence rather than noninferiority. However, if the outcome of interest is mortality, we may always want to test noninferiority instead of equivalence. This is because death is most likely regarded as being more serious than the concern of any other side effects due to toxicity. In this section, we discuss testing equivalence for using the PD, PR and OR to measure the relative treatment effect for a RCT with noncompliance and subsequent missing outcomes.

5.3.1   Using the difference in proportions

When using the PD ($\Delta = \pi_{1|C}^{(1)} - \pi_{1|C}^{(0)}$) to measure the relative treatment effect in establishing equivalence, we want to test $H_0 : \Delta \leq -\varepsilon_l$ or $\Delta \geq \varepsilon_u$ versus $H_a : -\varepsilon_l < \Delta < \varepsilon_u$, where ε_l and ε_u (>0) are the maximum clinically acceptable lower and upper margins that the experimental drug can be regarded as equivalent to the standard treatment. Using the Intersection-Union test (Casella and Berger, 1990), we will reject the null hypothesis $H_0 : \Delta \leq -\varepsilon_l$ or $\Delta \geq \varepsilon_u$ at the α-level and claim that the two treatments are equivalent if the test statistic $\tanh^{-1}(\hat{\Delta}^{(MI)})$ simultaneously satisfies the following two inequalities:

$$(\tanh^{-1}(\hat{\Delta}^{(MI)}) + \tanh^{-1}(\varepsilon_l))/\sqrt{\hat{Var}(\tanh^{-1}(\hat{\Delta}^{(MI)}))} > Z_\alpha,$$

$$\text{and} \quad (\tanh^{-1}(\hat{\Delta}^{(MI)}) - \tanh^{-1}(\varepsilon_u))/\sqrt{\hat{Var}(\tanh^{-1}(\hat{\Delta}^{(MI)}))} < -Z_\alpha,$$

$$(5.14)$$

where $\hat{Var}(\tanh^{-1}(\hat{\Delta}^{(MI)})) = \hat{Var}(\hat{\Delta}^{(MI)})/(1 - (\hat{\Delta}^{(MI)^2})^2$, $\hat{\Delta}^{(MI)}$ is given by (5.2) and $\hat{Var}(\hat{\Delta}^{(MI)})$ is obtained from (5.3) with substituting $\hat{E}_{rS}^{(g)}$ for $E_{rS}^{(g)}$, $\hat{E}_{(2)S}^{(g)}$ for $E_{(2)S}^{(g)}$, and $\hat{\pi}_{1|C}^{(g)}$ for $\pi_{1|C}^{(g)}$, respectively.

5.3.2   Using the ratio of proportions

When using the PR ($\gamma = \pi_{1|C}^{(1)}/\pi_{1|C}^{(0)}$) to measure the relative treatment effect in establishing equivalence, we want to test $H_0 : \gamma \le 1 - \gamma_l$ or $\gamma \ge 1 + \gamma_u$ versus $H_a : 1 - \gamma_l < \gamma < 1 + \gamma_u$ where γ_l and γ_u (> 0) are the maximum clinically acceptable lower and upper margins that the experimental drug can be regarded as equivalent to the standard treatment when the inequality $1 - \gamma_l < \gamma < 1 + \gamma_u$ holds. We will reject $H_0 : \gamma \le 1 - \gamma_l$ or $\gamma \ge 1 + \gamma_u$ at the α-level and claim that two treatments are equivalent if the test statistic $\log(\hat{\gamma}^{(MI)})$ simultaneously satisfies the following two inequalities:

$$(\log(\hat{\gamma}^{(MI)}) - \log(1 - \gamma_l))/\sqrt{\hat{Var}(\log(\hat{\gamma}^{(MI)}))} > Z_\alpha,$$

$$\text{and}\quad (\log(\hat{\gamma}^{(MI)}) - \log(1 + \gamma_u))/\sqrt{\hat{Var}(\log(\hat{\gamma}^{(MI)}))} < -Z_\alpha, \quad (5.15)$$

where $\hat{\gamma}^{(MI)}$ is given (5.7) and $\hat{Var}(\log(\hat{\gamma}^{(MI)}))$ is obtained from (5.8) with substituting $\hat{E}_{rS}^{(g)}$ for $E_{rS}^{(g)}$ and $\hat{E}_{(2)S}^{(g)}$ for $E_{(2)S}^{(g)}$, respectively. Since using the PR to measure the relative treatment effect in establishing equivalence may not, as noted previously, produce on the PD scale the acceptable margins that follow along with the general philosophy in a draft of FDA (1997). Thus, we may consider use of the OR to measure the relative treatment effect in establishing equivalence.

5.3.3   Using the odds ratio of proportions

When using the OR ($\varphi = (\pi_{1|C}^{(1)}\pi_{2|C}^{(0)})/(\pi_{2|C}^{(1)}\pi_{1|C}^{(0)})$) to measure the relative treatment effect in establishing equivalence, we want to test $H_0 : \varphi \le 1 - \varphi_l$ or $\varphi \ge 1 + \varphi_u$ versus $H_a : 1 - \varphi_l < \varphi < 1 + \varphi_u$, where φ_l and φ_u are the maximum clinically acceptable lower and upper margins that the experimental treatment can be regarded as equivalent to the standard treatment when the inequality $1 - \varphi_l < \varphi < 1 + \varphi_u$ is true. Using the Intersection-Union test, we reject $H_a : 1 - \varphi_l < \varphi < 1 + \varphi_u$ at the

α-level when the following two inequalities simultaneously hold:

$$(\log(\hat{\varphi}^{(MI)}) - \log(1 - \varphi_l))/\sqrt{\hat{Var}(\log(\hat{\varphi}^{(MI)}))} > Z_\alpha,$$

$$\text{and} \quad (\log(\hat{\varphi}^{(MI)}) - \log(1 + \varphi_u))/\sqrt{\hat{Var}(\log(\hat{\varphi}^{(MI)}))} < -Z_\alpha, \quad (5.16)$$

where $\hat{\varphi}^{(MI)}$ is given in (5.11) and $\hat{Var}(\log(\hat{\varphi}^{(MI)}))$ is given in (5.12) with substituting $\hat{E}_{rS}^{(g)}$ for $E_{rS}^{(g)}$, respectively.

Note that test procedures (5.14)–(5.16) reduce to the test procedures (2.16)–(2.18), respectively, when there are no patients with subsequent missing outcome.

5.4   Interval estimation

Due to its usefulness in conveying the information on both the accuracy and precision of our inference, an interval estimator for an index used to measure the relative treatment effect is the most commonly used statistical tool to report clinical findings. Note that we can also determine whether two treatments are therapeutically equivalent by simply claiming that two treatments are equivalent at the α-level if the corresponding $100(1\text{-}2\alpha)$ % confidence interval is completely contained in the pre-determined acceptable range. In the following section, we discuss interval estimation of the PD, PR and OR when they are used to measure the relative treatment effect for a RCT in the presence of noncompliance and subsequent missing outcomes in the following section.

5.4.1   Estimation of the proportion difference

Note that all methods considered in Section 2.4.1 of Chapter 2 for the PD can be used to produce an interval estimator for $\Delta(= \pi_{1|C}^{(1)} - \pi_{1|C}^{(0)})$ here. For brevity, we present only the interval estimator with the $\tanh^{-1}(x)$ transformation. On the basis of $\hat{\Delta}^{(MI)}$ (5.2) and $Var(\hat{\Delta}^{(MI)})$ (5.3) with substituting $\hat{E}_{rS}^{(g)}$ for $E_{rS}^{(g)}$, $\hat{E}_{(2)S}^{(g)}$ for $E_{(2)S}^{(g)}$, and $\hat{\pi}_{1|C}^{(g)}$ for $\pi_{1|C}^{(g)}$, respectively, we obtain an asymptotic $100(1-\alpha)$ % confidence interval for Δ as given by

$$[\tanh(\tanh^{-1}(\hat{\Delta}^{(MI)}) - Z_{\alpha./2}(\hat{Var}(\tanh^{-1}(\hat{\Delta}^{(MI)})))^{1/2}),$$
$$\tanh(\tanh^{-1}(\hat{\Delta}^{(MI)}) + Z_{\alpha./2}(\hat{Var}(\tanh^{-1}(\hat{\Delta}^{(MI)})))^{1/2})], \quad (5.17)$$

where $\hat{Var}(\tanh^{-1}(\hat{\Delta}^{(MI)})) = \hat{Var}(\hat{\Delta}^{(MI)})/(1 - (\hat{\Delta}^{(MI)})^2)^2$.   Using   the
$\tanh^{-1}(x)$ transformation can not only avoid the consideration of the
parameter constraint $-1 < \Delta < 1$, but also improve the precision of
the interval estimator for the PD.

Example 5.2   Consider the RED of flu vaccination trial in Table 5.1.
When estimating the PD of flu-related hospitalization among compliers
between vaccination and nonvaccination, we obtain the MLE $\hat{\Delta}^{(MI)}$ (5.2)
to be -0.005. When applying interval estimators (5.17), we obtain the
95 % confidence intervals to be $[-0.225, 0.215]$, that covers 0. Thus,
there is no evidence to support that the flu vaccination can reduce the risk
of the flu-related hospitalization at the 5 % level. Also, we can see that
the above resulting interval estimate is relatively wide. This can be due
to the fact that there is large percentage of patients with noncompliance
and/or missing outcomes in Table 5.1. Furthermore, if we choose the pre-
determined margins $\varepsilon_l = \varepsilon_u = 0.20$ for testing equivalence, because the
above 95 % confidence interval is not contained in $[-0.20, 0.20]$, we
cannot conclude that the effect on the risk of flu-related hospitalization
is equivalent between the vaccinated and nonvaccinated groups at the
2.5 % (rather than the 5 %) level.

5.4.2   Estimation of the proportion ratio

On the basis of $\hat{\gamma}^{(MI)}$ (5.7) and $\hat{Var}(\log(\hat{\gamma}^{(MI)}))$ obtained from (5.8) with
substituting $\hat{E}_{rS}^{(g)}$ for $E_{rS}^{(g)}$ and $\hat{E}_{(r)S}^{(g)}$ for $E_{(r)S}^{(g)}$, we may obtain an asymptotic
$100(1 - \alpha)$ percent confidence interval for γ using Wald's statistic as

$$[\max\{\hat{\gamma}^{(MI)} - Z_{\alpha/2}(\hat{Var}(\hat{\gamma}^{(MI)}))^{1/2}, 0\}, \hat{\gamma}^{(MI)} + Z_{\alpha/2}(\hat{Var}(\hat{\gamma}^{(MI)}))^{1/2}],$$

(5.18)

where $\hat{Var}(\hat{\gamma}^{(MI)}) = (\hat{\gamma}^{(MI)})^2 \hat{Var}(\log(\hat{\gamma}^{(MI)}))$. Note that because the sampling distribution of $\hat{\gamma}^{(MI)}$ (5.7) can be skewed, we may consider use of
the logarithmic transformation to improve the normal approximation.
On the basis of $\hat{\gamma}^{(MI)}$ (5.7) and $\hat{Var}(\log(\hat{\gamma}^{(MI)}))$, we obtain an asymptotic
$100(1 - \alpha) \%$ confidence interval for γ with the logarithmic transformation as

$$[\hat{\gamma}^{(MI)} \exp(-Z_{\alpha/2}(\hat{Var}(\log(\hat{\gamma}^{(MI)})))^{1/2}), \hat{\gamma}^{(MI)} \exp(Z_{\alpha/2}(\hat{Var}(\log(\hat{\gamma}^{(MI)})))^{1/2})].$$

(5.19)

Note that using the interval estimator (5.19) can sometimes, as noted in Chapter 2, cause a loss of precision. Following the same idea as that used for deriving the interval estimator (2.26), we define the indicator random variable $I(\hat{\gamma}^{(MI)}, \hat{Var}(\hat{\gamma}^{(MI)}))$ to be 1 if the length $\hat{\gamma}^{(MI)}(\exp(Z_{\alpha/2}(\hat{Var}(\log(\hat{\gamma}^{(MI)})))^{1/2}) - \exp(-Z_{\alpha/2}(\hat{Var}(\log(\hat{\gamma}^{(MI)})))^{1/2}))$ of using the interval estimator (5.19) is larger than or equal to K times the length $(\hat{\gamma}^{(MI)} + Z_{\alpha/2}(\hat{Var}(\hat{\gamma}^{(MI)}))^{1/2} - \max\{\hat{\gamma}^{(MI)} - Z_{\alpha/2}(\hat{Var}(\hat{\gamma}^{(MI)}))^{1/2}, 0\})$ of using the interval estimator (5.18), and 0, otherwise. Thus, we obtain an asymptotic $100(1 - \alpha)\%$ confidence interval for γ as

$$[\gamma_l^{(MI)}, \ \gamma_u^{(MI)}], \tag{5.20}$$

where

$$\gamma_l^{(MI)} = I(\hat{\gamma}^{(MI)}, \hat{Var}(\hat{\gamma}^{(MI)})) \max\{\hat{\gamma}^{(MI)} - Z_{\alpha/2}(\hat{Var}(\hat{\gamma}^{(MI)}))^{1/2}, 0\}$$
$$+ (1 - I(\hat{\gamma}^{(MI)}, \hat{Var}(\hat{\gamma}^{(MI)})))\hat{\gamma}^{(MI)} \exp(-Z_{\alpha/2}(\hat{Var}(\log(\hat{\gamma}^{(MI)})))^{1/2}),$$

and

$$\gamma_u^{(MI)} = I(\hat{\gamma}^{(MI)}, \hat{Var}(\hat{\gamma}^{(MI)}))(\hat{\gamma}^{(MI)} + Z_{\alpha/2}(\hat{Var}(\hat{\gamma}^{(MI)}))^{1/2})$$
$$+ (1 - I(\hat{\gamma}^{(MI)}, \hat{Var}(\hat{\gamma}^{(MI)})))\hat{\gamma}^{(MI)} \exp(Z_{\alpha/2}(\hat{Var}(\log(\hat{\gamma}^{(MI)})))^{1/2}).$$

When using the interval estimator (5.20), we may set the constant K to equal 2.5 based on some relevant empirical evaluations (Lui, 2007a) for other situations.

Example 5.3 Based on the data in Table 5.1 studying the flu-rated hospitalization rate, we obtain the MLE $\hat{\gamma}^{(MI)}$ (5.7) to be 0.861. When applying interval estimators (5.18)–(5.20), we obtain the 95 % confidence intervals to be [0.000, 5.488], [0.004, 177.695] and [0.000, 5.488], respectively. Since these resulting interval estimates all cover 1, there is no evidence to support that that taking the flu vaccination can reduce the flu-related hospitalization rate. This example also illustrates the case in which the interval estimator (5.19) using the logarithmic transformation may sometimes cause a substantial loss of precision.

5.4.3 Estimation of the odds ratio

On the basis of $\hat{\varphi}^{(MI)}$ (5.11) and $\hat{Var}(\log(\hat{\varphi}^{(MI)}))$ obtained from (5.12) by substituting $\hat{E}_{rS}^{(g)}$ for $E_{rS}^{(g)}$, we may obtain an asymptotic $100(1-\alpha)\%$ confidence interval for φ using Wald's statistic as (Lui and Chang, 2010),

$$[\max\{\hat{\varphi}^{(MI)} - Z_{\alpha/2}(\hat{Var}(\hat{\varphi}^{(MI)}))^{1/2}, 0\}, \ \hat{\varphi}^{(MI)} + Z_{\alpha/2}(\hat{Var}(\hat{\varphi}^{(MI)}))^{1/2}].$$
(5.21)

where $\hat{Var}(\hat{\varphi}^{(MI)}) = (\hat{\varphi}^{(MI)})^2 \hat{Var}(\log(\hat{\varphi}^{(MI)}))$. Since the sampling distribution of $\hat{\varphi}^{(MI)}$ (5.11) can be skewed, the interval estimator (5.21) may not perform well, especially when the number of patients in a trial is not large. Thus, we may consider use of the logarithmic transformation to improve the normal approximation of $\hat{\varphi}^{(MI)}$. This leads us to obtain the following asymptotic $100(1-\alpha)\%$ confidence interval for φ with the logarithmic transformation as

$$[\hat{\varphi}^{(MI)} \exp(-Z_{\alpha/2}(\hat{Var}(\log(\hat{\varphi}^{(MI)})))^{1/2}),$$
$$\hat{\varphi}^{(MI)} \exp(Z_{\alpha/2}(\hat{Var}(\log(\hat{\varphi}^{(MI)})))^{1/2})].$$
(5.22)

When every patient complies with his/her assigned treatment and has known outcome (i.e. $\pi_{+A} = \pi_{+N} = 0$ and $\eta_C^{(1)} = \eta_C^{(0)} = \eta_A = \eta_N = 1$) in a RCT, the interval estimator (5.22) reduces to the most commonly used asymptotic interval estimator for the OR using the logarithmic transformation published elsewhere (Fleiss, 1981; Lui, 2004). Although use of the logarithmic transformation may improve the coverage probability of a confidence interval for the OR, it can sometimes cause a loss of precision. To alleviate the possible loss of accuracy in use of (5.21) and the possible loss of precision in use of (5.22), we may consider use of a similar ad hoc procedure as for deriving (5.20) by combining (5.21) and (5.22). We define the indicator random variable $I(\hat{\varphi}^{(MI)}, \hat{Var}(\hat{\varphi}^{(MI)}))$ to be 1 if the length $\hat{\varphi}^{(MI)}(\exp(Z_{\alpha/2}(\hat{Var}(\log(\hat{\varphi}^{(MI)})))^{1/2}) - \exp(-Z_{\alpha/2}(\hat{Var}(\log(\hat{\varphi}^{(MI)})))^{1/2}))$ of (5.22) is larger than or equal to K times of the length $(\hat{\varphi}^{(MI)} + Z_{\alpha/2}(\hat{Var}(\hat{\varphi}^{(MI)}))^{1/2} - \max\{\hat{\varphi}^{(MI)} - Z_{\alpha/2}(\hat{Var}(\hat{\varphi}^{(MI)}))^{1/2}, 0\})$ of (5.21), and to be 0, otherwise. Thus, we obtain an asymptotic $100(1-\alpha)\%$ confidence interval for φ as (Lui and Chang, 2010):

$$[\varphi_l^{(MI)}, \ \varphi_u^{(MI)}],$$
(5.23)

where

$$\varphi_l^{(MI)} = I(\hat{\varphi}^{(MI)}, \hat{Var}(\hat{\varphi}^{(MI)})) \max \{\hat{\varphi}^{(MI)} - Z_{\alpha/2}(\hat{Var}(\hat{\varphi}^{(MI)}))^{1/2}, 0\}$$
$$+ (1 - I(\hat{\varphi}^{(MI)}, \hat{Var}(\hat{\varphi}^{(MI)}))) \exp(-Z_{\alpha/2}(\hat{Var}(\log(\hat{\varphi}^{(MI)})))^{1/2}),$$

and

$$\varphi_u^{(MI)} = I(\hat{\varphi}^{(MI)}, \hat{Var}(\hat{\varphi}^{(MI)}))(\hat{\varphi}^{(MI)} + Z_{\alpha/2}(\hat{Var}(\hat{\varphi}^{(MI)}))^{1/2})$$
$$+ (1 - I(\hat{\varphi}^{(MI)}, \hat{Var}(\hat{\varphi}^{(MI)}))) \exp(Z_{\alpha/2}(\hat{Var}(\log(\hat{\varphi}^{(MI)})))^{1/2}).$$

We arbitrarily recommend setting the constant K to be 2.5 in application of the interval estimator (5.23).

Example 5.4   Consider the RED studying the effect of flu vaccine on the flu-rated hospitalization rate in Table 5.1. When employing estimators $\hat{\varphi}^{(MI)}$ (5.11), we obtain the point estimate for the OR of flu-related hospitalization rate between the vaccinated and nonvaccinated groups to be 0.856 (Lui and Chang, 2010). When employing interval estimators (5.21)–(5.23), we obtain the 95 % confidence intervals for the OR as [0.000, 6.491], [0.001, 618.329], and [0.000, 6.491], respectively. Because all these resulting 95 % confidence intervals cover 1, there is no significant evidence to support that taking flu vaccine can reduce the risk of flu-related hospitalization. This example also illustrates the situation in which use of the interval estimator (5.22) with the logarithmic transformation can cause a substantial loss of precision. Note that since the flu-related hospitalization rate among compliers in the control group is low (≈ 0.037) here, it is really not surprising to see that the point estimates $\hat{\gamma}^{(MI)} = 0.861$ for the PR (obtained in Example 5.3) and $\hat{\varphi}^{(MI)} = 0.856$ for the OR obtained here are similar to one another. Note also that because the sampling distribution for $\hat{\varphi}^{(MI)}$ is generally larger than $\hat{\gamma}^{(MI)}$, we can see that the length of the interval estimate for the OR is longer, as shown here, than that for the PR.

5.5   Sample size determination

It is essentially important that we can incorporate both noncompliance and subsequent missing outcomes into sample size calculation in a RED in which there are many patients not complying with their assigned treatment and/or dropping out from the trial, especially when the RED has a long duration. As noted previously, the estimated sample size obtained as dividing the resulting sample size calculated with assuming that patients all have known outcomes by the probability of nonmissing outcomes can be inaccurate (Lui and Chang, 2008a). In this section, we focus our attention on sample size calculation for testing superiority, noninferiority, and equivalence on the basis of the test procedures proposed in Sections 5.1–5.3 for a RCT with noncompliance and subsequent missing outcomes.

Define $k = n_0/n_1$ as the ratio of sample allocation between the standard and experimental treatments. Given a fixed ratio of sample allocation k, we concentrate our attentions on estimating the minimum required number of patients n_1 from the experimental treatment. The corresponding estimates of the minimum required number of patients from the standard treatment and the total minimum required number of patients for the entire trial are then given by $n_0 = kn_1$ and $n_T = (k + 1)n_1$, respectively.

5.5.1   Sample size calculation for testing superiority

Consider using procedure (5.4) to test the null hypothesis $H_0 : \Delta = 0$ versus $H_a : \Delta = \Delta_0 \neq 0$, where Δ_0 is a specified magnitude of clinical significance determined by clinicians. Note that $E_{rS}^{(g)}$'s can all be uniquely determined by the following parameters: the subpopulation proportions π_{+C}, and π_{+A} (and hence $\pi_{+N} = 1 - (\pi_{+C} + \pi_{+A})$), the conditional probabilities of a positive response in various subpopulations $\pi_{1|C}^{(0)}$, $\pi_{1|A}$, and $\pi_{1|N}$; the probability of nonmissing outcomes $\eta_C^{(g)}(g = 1, 0)$, η_N, and η_A; and the PD Δ. Thus, given a fixed ratio $k(= n_0/n_1)$, we can express $Var(\hat{\Delta}^{(MI)})$ (5.3) as a function of π_{+C}, π_{+A}, $\pi_{1|C}^{(0)}$, $\pi_{1|A}$, $\pi_{1|N}$, $\eta_C^{(1)}$, $\eta_C^{(0)}$, η_N, η_A, Δ, and k,

$$V_{PD}^{(MI)}(\pi_{+C}, \pi_{+A}, \pi_{1|C}^{(0)}, \pi_{1|A}, \pi_{1|N}, \eta_C^{(1)}, \eta_C^{(0)}, \eta_N, \eta_A, \Delta, k)/n_1. \quad (5.24)$$

For brevity in notations, we denote $V_{PD}^{(MI)}(\pi_{+C}, \pi_{+A}, \pi_{1|C}^{(0)}, \pi_{1|A}, \pi_{1|N}, \eta_C^{(1)}, \eta_C^{(0)}, \eta_N, \eta_A, \Delta, k)$ by $V_{PD}^{(MI)}$. Based on the test procedure (5.4) and

$V_{PD}^{(MI)}$ defined in (5.24), we can show that an estimate of the minimum required number of patients n_1 from the experimental treatment for a desired power $1 - \beta$ of detecting a given nonzero difference Δ_0 of clinical interest at the α-level is given by (Lui and Chang, 2008a):

$$n_1 = Ceil\{[Z_{\alpha/2}\sqrt{V_{PD}^{(MI)}} + Z_\beta\sqrt{V_{PD}^{(MI)}}/(1 - \Delta_0^2)]^2/[\tanh^{-1}(\Delta_0)]^2\},$$

$$(5.25)$$

where $Ceil\{x\}$ is the smallest integer $\geq x$. To allow readers appreciate the effect due to various sources on the estimate of the minimum required sample size n_1 (5.25), we summarize the resulting estimate n_1 in Table 5.2 for a desired power 80 % of detecting a given Δ_0 of clinical significance in testing $H_0 : \Delta = 0$ at the 5 % level in situations in which the sub-population proportions: $(\pi_{+C}, \pi_{+A}, \pi_{+N}) = (0.95, 0.03, 0.02)$, $(0.80, 0.15, 0.05)$, $(0.60, 0.25, 0.15)$; the conditional probabilities of a positive response: $\pi_{1|C}^{(0)} = 0.3$, $\pi_{1|A} = 0.50$, and $\pi_{1|N} = 0.25$; $\Delta_0 = 0.05, 0.10, 0.20$; the ratio of sample size allocation $k = 0.50, 1, 2, 4, 8$; and the vector of probabilities of nonmissing outcome $(\eta_C^{(1)}, \eta_C^{(0)}, \eta_N, \eta_A) = $ I, II, III, where I $= (1.0, 1.0, 1.0, 1.0)$, II $= (0.95, 0.85, 0.90, 0.80)$ and III $= (0.85, 0.75, 0.80, 0.70)$. For example, when $(\eta_C^{(1)}, \eta_C^{(0)}, \eta_N, \eta_A) = $ II, $(\pi_{+C}, \pi_{+A}, \pi_{+N}) = (0.95, 0.03, 0.02)$, $\Delta_0 = 0.10$, and $k (= n_0/n_1) = 2$, we need to take 327 patients from the experimental treatment for a desired power of 80 % at the 5 % level. This translates the estimate of the total number of patients needed for the entire RCT is 981 $(= 327 + 327 \times 2)$.

As shown in Table 5.2, we note that given all the other parameters fixed, the estimate of the minimum required sample size n_1 increases as either the proportion of compliers π_{+C} or the probability of nonmissing outcomes decreases (i.e. $(\eta_C^{(1)}, \eta_C^{(0)}, \eta_N, \eta_A)$ changing from pattern I to III). For example, when $(\eta_C^{(1)}, \eta_C^{(0)}, \eta_N, \eta_A) = $ II, $\Delta_0 = 0.10$, and $k (= n_0/n_1) = 1$, the estimate of the minimum required number of patients n_1 increases from 434 patients to 611 when $(\pi_{+C}, \pi_{+A}, \pi_{+N})$ changes from $(0.95, 0.03, 0.02)$ to $(0.80, 0.15, 0.05)$; the relative magnitude of this increase is as large as approximately 41 % $(\approx (611-434)/434)$. Therefore, if we wished to reduce the number of patients needed for a RCT, we should maximize the proportion

Table 5.2 The estimates of the minimum required number of patients n_1 (5.25) from the experimental treatment for the desired power of 80% of detecting superiority in testing $H_0 : \Delta = 0$ at 5% level in the situations in which the conditional probabilities of positive response: $\pi_{1|C}^{(0)} = 0.3$, $\pi_{1|A} = 0.50$, and $\pi_{1|N} = 0.25$, $\Delta_0 = 0.05, 0.10, 0.20$; the subpopulation proportions: $(\pi_{+C}, \pi_{+A}, \pi_{+N}) = (0.95, 0.03, 0.02)$, $(0.80, 0.15, 0.05), (0.60, 0.25, 0.15)$; the ratio of sample allocation $k = 0.50, 1, 2, 4, 8$; the vector of probabilities of nonmissing outcome $(\eta_C^{(1)}, \eta_C^{(0)}, \eta_N, \eta_A) = $ I, II, III where I $= (1.0, 1.0, 1.0, 1.0)$, II $= (0.95, 0.85, 0.90, 0.80)$ and III $= (0.85, 0.75, 0.80, 0.70)$.

				$(\eta_C^{(1)}, \eta_C^{(0)}, \eta_N, \eta_A) = $ I				
π_{+C}	π_{+A}	π_{+N}	Δ_0	$k = 0.5$	1	2	4	8
0.95	0.03	0.02	0.05	2265	1530	1162	978	886
			0.10	576	392	301	255	232
			0.20	146	100	77	66	60
0.80	0.15	0.05	0.05	3277	2208	1673	1406	1272
			0.10	826	560	428	361	328
			0.20	208	142	109	93	84
0.60	0.25	0.15	0.05	5894	3960	2993	2509	2268
			0.10	1473	995	756	637	577
			0.20	368	250	191	161	146

(Continued)

210   NONCOMPLIANCE AND SUBSEQUENT MISSING OUTCOMES

Table 5.2 (Continued)

π_{+C}	π_{+A}	π_{+N}	Δ_0	$k=0.5$	1	2	4	8
			$(\eta_C^{(1)}, \eta_C^{(0)}, \eta_N, \eta_A) = II$					
0.95	0.03	0.02	0.05	2554	1695	1265	1050	942
			0.10	649	434	327	273	246
			0.20	164	111	84	71	64
0.80	0.15	0.05	0.05	3629	2410	1800	1495	1343
			0.10	914	611	460	384	347
			0.20	230	155	117	98	89
0.60	0.25	0.15	0.05	6422	4268	3191	2653	2384
			0.10	1605	1073	807	673	607
			0.20	401	269	203	170	154
			$(\eta_C^{(1)}, \eta_C^{(0)}, \eta_N, \eta_A) = III$					
0.95	0.03	0.02	0.05	2880	1906	1420	1176	1055
			0.10	731	488	367	306	276
			0.20	185	125	94	79	72
0.80	0.15	0.05	0.05	4084	2707	2018	1674	1501
			0.10	1028	687	516	430	387
			0.20	259	174	131	110	99
0.60	0.25	0.15	0.05	7213	4787	3574	2968	2665
			0.10	1803	1203	903	753	678
			0.20	450	302	228	190	172

of compliers, but minimize the proportion of patients with subsequent missing outcomes.

Example 5.5   Consider the RED for studying the flu vaccine trial, in which the estimates for the parameters based on the data in Table 5.1 are: $\hat{\pi}_{+C} = 0.08$, $\hat{\pi}_{+A} = 0.14$, $\hat{\pi}_{1|C}^{(0)} = 0.04$, $\hat{\pi}_{1|A} = 0.10$, $\hat{\pi}_{1|N} = 0.09$, $\hat{\eta}_{C}^{(1)} = 1.00$, $\hat{\eta}_{C}^{(0)} = 0.91$, $\hat{\eta}_{N} = 0.52$, and $\hat{\eta}_{A} = 0.90$. Note that the estimate $\hat{\eta}_{C}^{(1)} (= (\hat{E}_{(2)CA}^{(1)} - \hat{E}_{(2)A}^{(0)})/\hat{\pi}_{+C})$ for the probability of nonmissing for compliers assigned to the intervention group of receiving reminders is actually larger than 1 based on the data in Table 5.1. Because the largest possible value for $\eta_{C}^{(1)}$ is 1, we arbitrarily set $\hat{\eta}_{C}^{(1)} = 1$. This occurrence of the resulting parameter estimates out of the parameter range can be due to either the sampling variation of our data or the invalidity of the assumed model. Suppose that we consider the situation in which parameters are given by the above estimates. Note that the flu-related hospitalization rate in the control group considered here is quite small (0.04). If we expect that patients receiving flu shots tend to have a lower risk of flu-rated hospitalization than those receiving no flu shots, then the absolute value of Δ can be no more than 0.04.

Say, we are interested in finding out what the estimate of the minimum required sample size n_1 (5.25) is for a desired power 80 % in detecting $\Delta = -0.02$ at 5 % level. When applying n_1 (5.25), we obtain 484 964, 362 337, 301 023, and 270 367 patients needed from the intervention group for $k = 1, 2, 4$, and 8, respectively. All these estimated sample sizes n_1 (5.25) are quite large partially due to the fact that both the proportion of compliers (π_{+C}) and the parameter Δ of interest considered here are relatively small. On the other hand, if one can increase the proportion of compliers to 0.30 (i.e. $\pi_{+C} = 0.30$, $\pi_{+A} = 0.14$) by developing a better and effective intervention program instead of using 'the computer-generated reminders', given all the other parameters fixed, the estimates of the minimum required sample size n_1 for the intervention group reduces to 29 020, 21 395, 17 583, and 15 677 patients for $k = 1, 2, 4$, and 8, respectively. One can easily see that the reduction in the required number of patients can be substantial as a result of an increase in the proportion of subpopulation compliers in the above case. This illustrates the importance of designing an effective intervention program in a RED.

5.5.2   Sample size calculation for testing noninferiority

The sample size formulae, which do not account for subsequent missing outcomes for testing noninferiority (discussed in Section 2.5.2), are not appropriate for use in a RED in which there can be many patients with subsequent missing outcomes. In this subsection, we incorporate both noncompliance and subsequent missing outcomes into sample size determination when testing noninferiority based on the PD, PR and OR.

5.5.2.1   Using the difference in proportions

Consider use of test statistic (5.5) for testing noninferiority based on the PD. Recall that the asymptotic variance $Var(\text{tanh}^{-1}(\hat{\Delta}^{(MI)}))$ can be approximated by

$$V_{PD}^{(MI)}/[n_1(1-\Delta^2)^2], \tag{5.26}$$

where $V_{PD}^{(MI)}$ is defined in (5.24). Thus, the estimate of the minimum required number of patients n_1 from the experimental treatment for a desired power $(1-\beta)$ of detecting noninferiority with a given specified value Δ_0 $(> -\varepsilon_l)$ at a nominal α-level is given by

$$n_1 = Ceil\{((Z_\alpha + Z_\beta)^2 V_{PD}^{(MI)}/[(1-\Delta_0^2)^2])/(\text{tanh}^{-1}(\varepsilon_l) + \text{tanh}^{-1}(\Delta_0))^2\}. \tag{5.27}$$

When there are no patients with missing outcomes (i.e. $(\eta_C^{(1)}, \eta_C^{(0)}, \eta_N, \eta_A) = (1.0, 1.0, 1.0, 1.0)$), the sample size formula (5.27) reduces to that (2.33) for no missing outcomes discussed in Chapter 2.

5.5.2.2   Using the ratio of proportions

Consider use of test statistic (5.9) for testing noninferiority based on the PR. For a given ratio of sample allocation $k = n_0/n_1$, we can re-express the asymptotic variance $Var(\log(\hat{\gamma}^{(MI)}))$ (5.8) as a function of π_{+C}, π_{+A}, $\pi_{1|C}^{(0)}$, $\pi_{1|A}$, $\pi_{1|N}$, $\eta_C^{(1)}$, $\eta_C^{(0)}$, η_N, η_A, γ, and k,

$$V_{LPR}^{(MI)}(\pi_{+C}, \pi_{+A}, \pi_{1|C}^{(0)}, \pi_{1|A}, \pi_{1|N}, \eta_C^{(1)}, \eta_C^{(0)}, \eta_N, \eta_A, \gamma, k)/n_1. \tag{5.28}$$

For simplicity, we denote $V_{LPR}^{(MI)}(\pi_{+C}, \pi_{+A}, \pi_{1|C}^{(0)}, \pi_{1|A}, \pi_{1|N}, \eta_C^{(1)}, \eta_C^{(0)},$ $\eta_N, \eta_A, \gamma, k)$ by $V_{LPR}^{(MI)}$. On the basis of the test statistic (5.9) and $V_{LPR}^{(MI)}$ defined in (5.28), the estimate of the minimum required number n_1 of patients for a desired power $(1-\beta)$ of detecting noninferiority with a given specified value $\gamma_0(> 1 - \gamma_l)$ at a nominal α-level is given by

$$n_1 = Ceil\{(Z_\alpha + Z_\beta)^2 V_{LPR}^{(MI)}/(\log(\gamma_0) - \log(1 - \gamma_l))^2\}. \qquad (5.29)$$

We can easily show that the sample size formula (5.29) includes the sample size formula (2.35) as a special case of no patients with subsequent missing outcomes.

5.5.2.3   Using the odds ratio of proportions

Consider use of test statistic (5.13) for testing noninferiority based on the OR. For a given ratio $k = n_0/n_1$ of sample allocation, we can re-express the asymptotic variance $Var(\log(\hat{\varphi}^{(MI)}))$ (5.12) as a function of $\pi_{+C}, \pi_{+A}, \pi_{1|C}^{(0)}, \pi_{1|A}, \pi_{1|N}, \eta_C^{(1)}, \eta_C^{(0)}, \eta_N, \eta_A, \varphi,$ and k,

$$V_{LOR}^{(MI)}(\pi_{+C}, \pi_{+A}, \pi_{1|C}^{(0)}, \pi_{1|A}, \pi_{1|N}, \eta_C^{(1)}, \eta_C^{(0)}, \eta_N, \eta_A, \varphi, k)/n_1. \qquad (5.30)$$

We abbreviate $V_{LOR}^{(MI)}(\pi_{+C}, \pi_{+A}, \pi_{1|C}^{(0)}, \pi_{1|A}, \pi_{1|N}, \eta_C^{(1)}, \eta_C^{(0)}, \eta_N, \eta_A, \varphi,$ $k)$ by $V_{LOR}^{(MI)}$. On the basis of the test statistic (5.13) and $V_{LOR}^{(MI)}$ defined in (5.30), the estimate of the minimum required number n_1 of patients for a desired power $(1-\beta)$ of detecting noninferiority with a given specified value $\varphi_0(> 1 - \varphi_l)$ at a nominal α-level is given by

$$n_1 = Ceil\{(Z_\alpha + Z_\beta)^2 V_{LOR}^{(MI)}/(\log(\varphi_0) - \log(1 - \varphi_l))^2\}. \qquad (5.31)$$

Note that the sample size formula (5.31) simplifies to the sample size formula (2.37) when there are no patients with subsequent missing outcomes.

5.5.3   Sample size calculation for testing equivalence

When deriving closed-form sample size formulae for detecting equivalence, as noted in Section 2.5.3, we need to make an additional approximation of the power function. If this power approximation is not good, the closed form sample size formulae presented in the following can lose accuracy. Therefore, the trial-and-error adjustment procedure as suggested in Chapter 2 should be employed if this occurs.

5.5.3.1   Using the difference in proportions

Recall that using the PD to measure the relative treatment effect in establishing equivalence. We want to demonstrate Δ to satisfy the inequality: $-\varepsilon_l < \Delta < \varepsilon_u$, where ε_l and ε_u (> 0) are the maximum clinically acceptable lower and upper margins determined by clinicians. Thus, the power function for testing $H_0 : \Delta \leq -\varepsilon_l$ or $\Delta \geq \varepsilon_u$ at the α-level based on the test procedure (5.14) for given a specified Δ_0 can be approximated by

$$\phi_{PD}(\Delta_0) = \Phi(\frac{\tanh^{-1}(\varepsilon_u) - \tanh^{-1}(\Delta_0)}{\sqrt{Var(\tanh^{-1}(\hat{\Delta}^{(MI)}))}} - Z_\alpha)$$
$$- \Phi(\frac{-\tanh^{-1}(\varepsilon_l) - \tanh^{-1}(\Delta_0)}{\sqrt{Var(\tanh^{-1}(\hat{\Delta}^{(MI)}))}} + Z_\alpha), \quad (5.32)$$

where $Var(\tanh^{-1}(\hat{\Delta}^{(MI)})) = V_{PD}^{(MI)}/[n_1(1 - \Delta_0^2)^2]$. When the number of patients assigned to both treatments is large and $-\varepsilon_l < \Delta_0 < 0$, we may further approximate the power function $\phi_{PD}(\Delta_0)$ (5.32) by

$$1 - \Phi(\frac{-\tanh^{-1}(\varepsilon_l) - \tanh^{-1}(\Delta_0)}{\sqrt{Var(\tanh^{-1}(\hat{\Delta}^{(MI)}))}} + Z_\alpha). \quad (5.33)$$

On the basis of the power function (5.33), we obtain an estimate of the minimum required number of patients n_1 from the experimental treatment for a desired power $(1-\beta)$ of detecting equivalence with a specified Δ_0 at a nominal α-level as

$$n_1 = Ceil\{((Z_\alpha + Z_\beta)^2 V_{PD}^{(MI)}/[(1 - \Delta_0^2)^2])/(\tanh^{-1}(\varepsilon_l) + \tanh^{-1}(\Delta_0))^2\}. \quad (5.34)$$

If the number of patients assigned to both treatments is large and $0 < \Delta_0 < \varepsilon_u$, we can approximate the power function $\phi_{PD}(\Delta_0)$ (5.32) by

$$\Phi(\frac{\tanh^{-1}(\varepsilon_u) - \tanh^{-1}(\Delta_0)}{\sqrt{Var(\tanh^{-1}(\hat{\Delta}^{(MI)}))}} - Z_\alpha). \quad (5.35)$$

On the basis of the power function (5.35), we obtain an estimate of the minimum required number of patients n_1 from the experimental treatment for a desired power $(1-\beta)$ of detecting equivalence with a specified Δ_0 at a nominal α-level as

$$n_1 = Ceil\{((Z_\alpha + Z_\beta)^2 V_{PD}^{(MI)}/[(1 - \Delta_0^2)^2])/(\tanh^{-1}(\varepsilon_u) - \tanh^{-1}(\Delta_0))^2\}. \tag{5.36}$$

When $\Delta_0 = 0$, the power function $\phi(\Delta_0)$ (5.32) becomes

$$\phi_{PD}(\Delta_0) = \Phi(\frac{\tanh^{-1}(\varepsilon_u)}{\sqrt{Var(\tanh^{-1}(\hat{\Delta}^{(MI)}))}} - Z_\alpha)$$
$$- \Phi(\frac{-\tanh^{-1}(\varepsilon_l)}{\sqrt{Var(\tanh^{-1}(\hat{\Delta}^{(MI)}))}} + Z_\alpha). \tag{5.37}$$

Based on (5.37) with assuming $\varepsilon_l = \varepsilon_u$, we obtain an estimate of the minimum required number of patients n_1 from the experimental treatment for a desired power $(1-\beta)$ of detecting equivalence with $\Delta_0 = 0$ at a nominal α-level as

$$n_1 = Ceil\{((Z_\alpha + Z_{\beta/2})^2 V_{PD}^{(MI)})/(\tanh^{-1}(\varepsilon_u))^2\}. \tag{5.38}$$

Note that using n_1 (5.34) (or n_1 (5.36)) will tend to underestimate the minimum required sample size if the approximation of the power function (5.32) by the power function (5.33) (or by the power function (5.35)) is not accurate. This is because the latter tends to be larger than the former by a nonnegligible magnitude when the estimate n_1 of the minimum required number of patients is not large. This can occur when the acceptable margins are chosen not to be small or when the chosen value $\Delta_0 (\neq 0)$ of interest is in the neighborhood of 0. Thus, in this case we may wish to use n_1 (5.34) (or n_1 (5.36)) as an initial estimate and apply the trial-and-error procedure to find the minimum positive integer n_1 such that the power function $\phi_{PD}(\Delta_0)$ (5.32) is larger than or equal to the desired power $1 - \beta$.

5.5.3.2 Using the ratio of proportions

When testing equivalence between two treatments based on using the PR, we want to reject the null hypothesis $H_0 : \gamma \leq 1 - \gamma_l$ or $\gamma \geq 1 + \gamma_u$

and claim that the two treatment are equivalent when the underlying PR γ_0 falls in $1 - \gamma_l < \gamma_0 < 1 + \gamma_u$. On the basis of the test procedure (5.15), we obtain the power function,

$$\phi_{PR}(\gamma_0) = \Phi(\frac{\log(1 + \gamma_u) - \log(\gamma_0)}{\sqrt{Var(\log(\hat{\gamma}^{(MI)}))}} - Z_\alpha)$$
$$-\Phi(\frac{\log(1 - \gamma_l) - \log(\gamma_0)}{\sqrt{Var(\log(\hat{\gamma}^{(MI)}))}} + Z_\alpha), \qquad (5.39)$$

where $1 - \gamma_l < \gamma_0 < 1 + \gamma_u$. If the resulting sample size n_1 is large, we may follow the same arguments as for deriving sample size formulae (5.34). (5.36), and (5.38), and obtain an estimates of the minimum required number n_1 of patients from the experimental treatment for a desired power $(1-\beta)$ of detecting equivalence with a given specified value γ_0 (where $1 - \gamma_l < \gamma_0 < 1 + \gamma_u$) at a nominal α-level as given by (Lui and Chang, 2008b)

$$n_1 = Ceil\{(Z_\alpha + Z_\beta)^2 V_{LPR}^{(MI)}/(\log(\gamma_0) - \log(1 - \gamma_l))^2\}$$
$$\text{for } 1 - \gamma_l < \gamma_0 < 1, \qquad (5.40)$$

$$n_1 = Ceil\{(Z_\alpha + Z_\beta)^2 V_{LPR}^{(MI)}/(\log(\gamma_0) - \log(1 + \gamma_u))^2\}$$
$$\text{for } 1 < \gamma_0 < 1 + \gamma_u, \qquad (5.41)$$

and

$$n_1 = Ceil\{(Z_\alpha + Z_{\beta/2})^2 V_{LPR}^{(MI)}/(\log(1 + \gamma_u))^2\}$$
$$\text{for } \gamma_0 = 1 \text{ and } \log(1 + \gamma_u) = -\log(1 - \gamma_l). \qquad (5.42)$$

When the acceptable margins γ_l and γ_u are chosen not to be small (say, $1 - \gamma_l = 0.50$ and $1 + \gamma_u = 2.0$) or when the chosen value $\gamma_0(\neq 1)$ is in the neighborhood of 1, using n_1 (5.40) (or (5.41)) tends to underestimate the minimum required sample size. As suggested before, we may wish to use n_1 (5.40) (or (5.41)) as an initial estimate and employ the trial-and-error procedure to find the minimum positive integer such that the power function $\phi_{PR}(\gamma_0)$ (5.39) is larger than or equal to the desired power $1 - \beta$.

To illustrate the use of closed-form sample size formulae n_1 (5.40)–(5.42), we set $\gamma_l = 0.20$ and $\gamma_u = 0.25$ (so that $\log(1 + \gamma_u) = -\log(1 - \gamma_l)$). We assume that the underlying conditional probabilities of a positive response in different subpopulations for the standard treatment are: $\pi_{1|C}^{(0)} = 0.30$, $\pi_{1|A} = 0.50$, and $\pi_{1|N} = 0.25$. We assume further that the conditional probability of a positive response among compliers for the experimental treatment is $\pi_{1|C}^{(1)} = \gamma \pi_{1|C}^{(0)}$, where $1 - \gamma_l < \gamma < 1 + \gamma_u$. We consider the situations in which the ratio of probabilities of a positive response between compliers in two treatments $\gamma_0 = 0.90, 1.0, 1.1$; the subpopulation proportions $(\pi_{+C}, \pi_{+A}, \pi_{+N}) = (0.95, 0.03, 0.02), (0.80, 0.15, 0.05), (0.60, 0.25, 0.15)$; the ratio of sample allocation between two treatments $k = 0.5, 1, 2, 4, 8$; and the vector of probabilities of nonmissing outcome $(\eta_C^{(1)}, \eta_C^{(0)}, \eta_A, \eta_N) = $ I, II, III, where I $= (1.0, 1.0, 1.0, 1.0)$, II $= (0.95, 0.85, 0.90, 0.80)$ and III $= (0.85, 0.75, 0.80, 0.70)$.

We summarize in Table 5.3 the minimum required number n_1 of patients needed from the experimental treatment for the desired power of 80 % to detect equivalence when $\gamma_0 = 0.90, 1.0, 1.1$ at 0.05-level in the situations determined by combinations of the above parameter values. For example, when $(\eta_C^{(1)}, \eta_C^{(0)}, \eta_A, \eta_N) = $ II, $(\pi_{+C}, \pi_{+A}, \pi_{+N}) = (0.95, 0.03, 0.02)$, $\gamma_0 = 1$, and $k (= n_0/n_1) = 2$, we need to have 735 $(= n_1)$ patients assigned to the experimental treatment for 80 % power at 5 % level (Table 5.3). This translates the estimate of the minimum total number of patients needed for the entire RCT is 2205 $(= 735 + 735 \times 2)$. Finally, given all the other parameters fixed, we see that the estimate of the minimum required sample size n_1 seems to increase as either the subpopulation proportion of compliers π_{+C} or the probability of non-missing outcomes decreases. For example, when $(\eta_C^{(1)}, \eta_C^{(0)}, \eta_A, \eta_N) = $ II, $\gamma_0 = 1$, and $k (= n_0/n_1) = 1$, the estimate of the minimum required number of patients n_1 for the experimental treatment increases from 997 patients to 1437 patients when $(\pi_{+C}, \pi_{+A}, \pi_{+N})$ changes from II $= (0.95, 0.03, 0.02)$ to III $= (0.80, 0.15, 0.05)$; the relative magnitude of this increase in n_1 is as large as 44 % $(= (1437\text{-}997)/997)$.

5.5.3.3   Using the odds ratio of proportions

When using the OR $(\varphi = (\pi_{1|C}^{(1)} \pi_{2|C}^{(0)})/(\pi_{2|C}^{(1)} \pi_{1|C}^{(0)}))$ to measure the relative treatment effect in testing equivalence, we wish to have a desired power of claiming that the two treatments are equivalent when the underlying φ falls in $1 - \varphi_l < \varphi < 1 + \varphi_u$. On the basis of the test procedure (5.16),

Table 5.3 The estimates of the minimum required number of patients n_1 (5.40)–(5.42) from the experimental treatment for the desired power 80% of detecting equivalence with the maximum acceptable levels $\gamma_l = 0.20$ and $\gamma_u = 0.25$ at the 5% level in the situations in which the conditional probabilities of a positive response: $\pi_{1|C}^{(1)} = \pi_{1|C}^{(0)}\gamma$, $\pi_{1|A} = 0.50$, and $\pi_{1|N} = 0.25$, where $\pi_{1|C}^{(0)} = 0.3$, $\gamma_0 = 0.9, 1.0, 1.1$; the subpopulation proportions: $(\pi_{+C}, \pi_{+A}, \pi_{+N}) = (0.95, 0.03, 0.02), (0.80, 0.15, 0.05), (0.60, 0.25, 0.15)$; the ratio of sample size allocation $k = 0.5, 1, 2, 4, 8$; the vector of probabilities of nonmissing outcome $(\eta_C^{(1)}, \eta_C^{(0)}, \eta_N, \eta_A) = I$, II, III, where I = (1.0, 1.0, 1.0, 1.0), II = (0.95, 0.85, 0.90, 0.80) and III = (0.85, 0.75, 0.80, 0.70).#

| | | | | $(\eta_C^{(1)}, \eta_C^{(0)}, \eta_N, \eta_A) = I$ | | | | |
π_{+C}	π_{+A}	π_{+N}	γ_0	$k = 0.5$	1	2	4	8
0.95	0.03	0.02	0.90	3706	2529	1940	1646	1499
			1.00	1348	899	674	562	506
			1.10	2818	1839	1349	1104	982
0.80	0.15	0.05	0.90	5601	3803	2904	2455	2230
			1.00	1974	1316	987	823	741
			1.10	4029	2639	1943	1596	1422
0.60	0.25	0.15	0.90	10382	7013	5329	4487	4066
			1.00	3588	2392	1794	1495	1346
			1.10	7209	4743	3509	2893	2584

$(\eta_C^{(1)}, \eta_C^{(0)}, \eta_N, \eta_A) = \text{II}$

0.95	0.03	0.02	0.90	4166	2793	2107	1764	1592
			1.00	1521	997	735	604	538
			1.10	3194	2049	1476	1190	1047
0.80	0.15	0.05	0.90	6163	4127	3110	2601	2346
			1.00	2186	1437	1062	875	781
			1.10	4489	2897	2101	1703	1504
0.60	0.25	0.15	0.90	11228	7511	5652	4723	4258
			1.00	3908	2578	1913	1580	1414
			1.10	7901	5140	3759	3069	2724

$(\eta_C^{(1)}, \eta_C^{(0)}, \eta_N, \eta_A) = \text{III}$

0.95	0.03	0.02	0.90	4695	3141	2364	1976	1781
			1.00	1716	1122	825	677	602
			1.10	3604	2307	1658	1334	1172
0.80	0.15	0.05	0.90	6931	4634	3485	2911	2624
			1.00	2461	1614	1191	980	874
			1.10	5055	3256	2357	1907	1682
0.60	0.25	0.15	0.90	12609	8423	6330	5284	4761
			1.00	4390	2892	2143	1768	1581
			1.10	8881	5769	4213	3435	3046

we may obtain the power function as given by

$$\phi_{OR}(\varphi_0) = \Phi(\frac{\log(1+\varphi_u) - \log(\varphi_0)}{\sqrt{Var(\log(\hat{\varphi}^{(MI)}))}} - Z_\alpha)$$
$$-\Phi(\frac{\log(1-\varphi_l) - \log(\varphi_0)}{\sqrt{Var(\log(\hat{\varphi}^{(MI)}))}} + Z_\alpha), \qquad (5.43)$$

where $1 - \varphi_l < \varphi_0 < 1 + \varphi_u$. As for deriving sample size formulae (5.34), (5.36), and (5.38), we may obtain an estimate of the minimum required number n_1 of patients from the experimental treatment for a desired power $(1-\beta)$ of detecting equivalence with a given specified value $1 - \varphi_l < \varphi_0 < 1 + \varphi_u$ at a nominal α-level as

$$n_1 = Ceil\{(Z_\alpha + Z_\beta)^2 V_{LOR}^{(MI)} / (\log(\varphi_0) - \log(1 - \varphi_l))^2\}$$
$$\text{for } 1 - \varphi_l < \varphi_0 < 1, \qquad (5.44)$$

$$n_1 = Ceil\{(Z_\alpha + Z_\beta)^2 V_{LOR}^{(MI)} / (\log(\varphi_0) - \log(1 + \varphi_u))^2\}$$
$$\text{for } 1 < \varphi_0 < 1 + \varphi_u, \qquad (5.45)$$

and

$$n_1 = Ceil\{(Z_\alpha + Z_{\beta/2})^2 V_{LOR}^{(MI)} / (\log(1 + \varphi_u))^2\}$$
$$\text{for } \varphi_0 = 1 \quad \text{and} \quad \log(1 + \varphi_u) = -\log(1 - \varphi_l). \qquad (5.46)$$

Note that when the acceptable margins φ_l and φ_u are chosen not relatively small (say, $\varphi_l = 0.50$ and $\varphi_u = 1.0$), or when the chosen value $\varphi_0 (\neq 1)$ is in the neighborhood of 1, using n_1 (5.44) and (5.45) tends to underestimate the minimum required sample size n_1. In this case, we can use n_1 (5.44) (or (5.45)) as an initial estimate and then apply the trial-and-error procedure to search for the minimum positive integer n_1 such that the power function (5.43) $\phi_{OR}(\varphi_0) \geq 1 - \beta$.

To illustrate the use of closed-from sample size formulae n_1 (5.44)–(5.46) and compare the resulting estimate of the needed sample size based on the OR and PR, we set $\varphi_l = 0.20$ and $\varphi_u = 0.25$ (so that $\log(1 + \varphi_u) = -\log(1 - \varphi_l)$). We arbitrarily consider the situations in which the underlying conditional probabilities of a positive response in different subpopulations for the standard treatment are: $\pi_{1|C}^{(0)} = 0.30$, $\pi_{1|A} = 0.50$, and $\pi_{1|N} = 0.25$. We assume that the conditional probability of a positive response among compliers for the experimental treatment is $\pi_{1|C}^{(1)} = \varphi_0 \pi_{1|C}^{(0)}/(\varphi \pi_{1|C}^{(0)} + (1 - \pi_{1|C}^{(0)}))$, where $1 - \varphi_l < \varphi_0 < 1 + \varphi_u$. We consider the situations in which the OR of probabilities of a positive response between compliers in two treatments $\varphi_0 = 0.90, 1.0, 1.1$; the subpopulation proportions $(\pi_{+C}, \pi_{+A}, \pi_{+N}) = (0.95, 0.03, 0.02), (0.80, 0.15, 0.05), (0.60, 0.25, 0.15)$; the ratio of sample allocation between two treatments $k = 0.5, 1, 2, 4, 8$; and the vector of probabilities of nonmissing outcome $(\eta_C^{(1)}, \eta_C^{(0)}, \eta_A, \eta_N) = $ I, II, III, where I $ = (1.0, 1.0, 1.0, 1.0)$, II $ = (0.95, 0.85, 0.90, 0.80)$ and III $= (0.85, 0.75, 0.80, 0.70)$.

We summarize in Table 5.4 the estimate of the minimum required number n_1 of patients from the experimental treatment for the desired power of 80 % to detect equivalence when $\varphi_0 = 0.90, 1.0, 1.1$ at the 0.05-level. From Table 5.4, for example, when $(\eta_C^{(1)}, \eta_C^{(0)}, \eta_A, \eta_N) = $ II, $(\pi_{+C}, \pi_{+A}, \pi_{+N}) = (0.95, 0.03, 0.02)$, $\varphi_0 = 1$, and $k (= n_0/n_1) = 2$, we need $1499 (= n_1)$ patients assigned to the experimental treatment for 80 % power at 5 % level. This translates the total required number of patients for the entire RCT is $4497 (= 1499 + 1499 \times 2)$. Finally, given the other parameters fixed, we see that the estimate of the minimum required sample size n_1 increases as either the proportion of compliers π_{+C} or the probability of nonmissing outcomes decreases. When comparing the resulting minimum required sample sizes between Table 5.3 and Table 5.4, we can see that the estimate of the minimum required sample size for the desired power 80 % of detecting equivalence with a given OR, say, $\varphi_0 = 1$, is generally much larger than that of detecting equivalence with a given $\gamma_0 = 1$ under the same configurations. This may be because the sampling variation of $\log(\hat{\varphi}^{(MI)})$ tends to be larger than that of $\log(\hat{\gamma}^{(MI)})$ (see the length of the resulting interval estimates in Examples 5.3 and 5.4). This can also be due to the fact that when $\pi_{1|C}^{(0)} = 0.30$, the acceptance range on the PD scale corresponding to $0.80 < \varphi_0 < 1.25$ based on the OR in Table 5.4 is $-0.045 < \Delta_0 < 0.049$, that is narrower than $-0.06 < \Delta_0 < 0.075$, the acceptance range on the PD scale corresponding to $0.80 < \gamma_0 < 1.25$ based on the PR in Table 5.3.

5.6   An alternative missing at random (MAR) model

The compound exclusion restriction assumes that the probability of non-missing for always-takers and never-takers depends on the assigned

Table 5.4   The estimates of the minimum required number of patients n_1 (5.44)–(5.46) from the experimental treatment for the desired power 80 % of detecting equivalence with the maximum acceptable levels $\varphi_l = 0.20$ and $\varphi_u = 0.25$ at the 5 % level in the situations in which the conditional probabilities of a positive response: $\pi_{1|C}^{(1)} = \pi_{1|C}^{(0)}\varphi_0/(\pi_{1|C}^{(0)}\varphi_0 + (1 - \pi_{1|C}^{(0)}))$, $\pi_{1|A} = 0.50$, and $\pi_{1|N} = 0.25$, where $\pi_{1|C}^{(0)} = 0.3$, $\varphi_0 = 0.9, 1.0, 1.1$; the subpopulation proportions: $(\pi_{+C}, \pi_{+A}, \pi_{+N}) = (0.95, 0.03, 0.02), (0.80, 0.15, 0.05), (0.60, 0.25, 0.15)$; the ratio of sample size allocation $k = 0.5, 1, 2, 4, 8$; the vector of probabilities of nonmissing outcome $(\eta_C^{(1)}, \eta_C^{(0)}, \eta_N, \eta_A) = $ I, II, III, where I $= (1.0, 1.0, 1.0, 1.0)$, II $= (0.95, 0.85, 0.90, 0.80)$ and III $= (0.85, 0.75, 0.80, 0.70)$.

| | | | | $(\eta_C^{(1)}, \eta_C^{(0)}, \eta_N, \eta_A) = $ I | | | | |
π_{+C}	π_{+A}	π_{+N}	φ_0	$k = 0.5$	1	2	4	8
0.95	0.03	0.02	0.90	7263	4876	3682	3086	2787
			1.00	2750	1833	1375	1146	1031
			1.10	5957	3949	2945	2443	2192
0.80	0.15	0.05	0.90	10808	7245	5464	4574	4129
			1.00	4028	2686	2014	1679	1511
			1.10	8624	5723	4272	3547	3184
0.60	0.25	0.15	0.90	19850	13287	10005	8365	7544
			1.00	7322	4882	3661	3051	2746
			1.10	15547	10329	7720	6416	5764

$(\eta_C^{(1)}, \eta_C^{(0)}, \eta_N, \eta_A) = \text{II}$

$\eta_C^{(1)}$	$\eta_C^{(0)}$	η_N	η_A					
0.95	0.03	0.02	0.90	8187	5402	4009	3313	2964
			1.00	3104	2034	1499	1232	1098
			1.10	6734	4388	3214	2628	2334
0.80	0.15	0.05	0.90	11937	7891	5868	4856	4351
			1.00	4462	2932	2168	1785	1594
			1.10	9572	6260	4605	3777	3363
0.60	0.25	0.15	0.90	21553	14279	10642	8824	7915
			1.00	7975	5260	3903	3224	2885
			1.10	16974	11155	8245	6790	6063

$(\eta_C^{(1)}, \eta_C^{(0)}, \eta_N, \eta_A) = \text{III}$

$\eta_C^{(1)}$	$\eta_C^{(0)}$	η_N	η_A					
0.95	0.03	0.02	0.90	9232	6078	4500	3712	3318
			1.00	3501	2289	1683	1380	1229
			1.10	7596	4938	3610	2945	2613
0.80	0.15	0.05	0.90	13431	8863	6579	5437	4866
			1.00	5021	3294	2431	1999	1783
			1.10	10775	7034	5164	4229	3761
0.60	0.25	0.15	0.90	24211	16019	11923	9875	8851
			1.00	8959	5902	4373	3608	3226
			1.10	19073	12516	9238	7599	6780

treatment g only through the treatment actually received d (i.e. $\eta_A^{(1)} = \eta_A^{(0)} = \eta_A$ and $\eta_N^{(1)} = \eta_N^{(0)} = \eta_N$). However, this assumption is not really testable. In certain situations, the nonmissing outcome for always-takers (or never-takers) can actually depend on the treatment assignment and the treatment receipt. For example, an always-taker (or a never-taker) assigned to the placebo may be more likely to withdraw from a trial than he/she does when the patient is assigned to a treatment especially under a nonblind RCT. Therefore, the probability of nonmissing outcomes $\eta_d^{(g)}$ may actually depend on both the assigned treatment g ($= 1$ for experimental, $g = 0$ for standard) and the received treatment d ($= 1$ for experimental, $g = 0$ for standard) instead of the underlying potential treatment receipt status S. For convenience in the following discussion, we define $\pi_{rCA}^{(1)} = \pi_{rC}^{(1)} + \pi_{rA}$ and $\pi_{rCN}^{(0)} = \pi_{rC}^{(0)} + \pi_{rN}$ for $r = 1, 2$. Under the assumed MAR model, we may summarize the latent probability structure of the observed data for patients assigned to the experimental ($g = 1$) treatment by use of the following table (Lui, 2008a; Lui and Cumberland, 2008; Mealli, Imbens and Ferro $et~al.$, 2004):

Assigned experimental treatment ($g = 1$)

		Treatment received		
		Experimental (CA)	Standard (N)	Total
Outcome	Positive	$\eta_1^{(1)}\pi_{1CA}^{(1)}$	$\eta_0^{(1)}\pi_{1N}$	$\eta_1^{(1)}\pi_{1CA}^{(1)} + \eta_0^{(1)}\pi_{1N}$
	Negative	$\eta_1^{(1)}\pi_{2CA}^{(1)}$	$\eta_0^{(1)}\pi_{2N}$	$\eta_1^{(1)}\pi_{2CA}^{(1)} + \eta_0^{(1)}\pi_{2N}$
	Unknown	$(1 - \eta_1^{(1)})\pi_{+CA}^{(1)}$	$(1 - \eta_0^{(1)})\pi_{+N}$	$(1 - \eta_1^{(1)})\pi_{+CA}^{(1)}$ $+ (1 - \eta_0^{(1)})\pi_{+N}$
	Total	$\pi_{+CA}^{(1)}$ $(= \pi_{+C} + \pi_{+A})$	π_{+N}	1.0

For convenience, we let $F_{rS}^{(1)}$ denote the cell probability of row r ($= 1, 2, 3$) and column S ($= CA, N$) in the above table. For example, the parameter $F_{1CA}^{(1)} = \eta_1^{(1)}\pi_{1CA}^{(1)}$ denotes the cell probability that a randomly selected patient assigned to the experimental treatment has a known positive response and receives the assigned (experimental) treatment. As another example, the parameter $F_{3CA}^{(1)} = (1 - \eta_1^{(1)})\pi_{+CA}^{(1)}$ denotes the cell probability that a randomly selected patient assigned to the experimental treatment has the missing outcome and complies with his/her assigned (experimental) treatment. Thus, we have $F_{+CA}^{(1)} = \pi_{+CA}^{(1)} = \pi_{+C} + \pi_{+A}$ and $F_{+N}^{(1)} = \pi_{+N}$. Also, we have $F_{r+}^{(1)} = \eta_1^{(1)}\pi_{rCA}^{(1)} + \eta_0^{(1)}\pi_{rN}$ for $r = 1$, 2, and $F_{3+}^{(1)} = (1 - \eta_1^{(1)})\pi_{+CA}^{(1)} + (1 - \eta_0^{(1)})\pi_{+N}$. Similarly, we may summarize the latent probability structure of the observed data for patients assigned to the standard treatment $(g = 0)$ under the assumed MAR model by use of the following table:

Assigned standard treatment $(g = 0)$

		Treatment received		
		Standard (CN)	Experimental (A)	Total
Outcome	Positive	$\eta_0^{(0)}\pi_{1CN}^{(0)}$	$\eta_1^{(0)}\pi_{1A}$	$\eta_0^{(0)}\pi_{1CN}^{(0)} + \eta_1^{(0)}\pi_{1A}$
	Negative	$\eta_0^{(0)}\pi_{2CN}^{(0)}$	$\eta_1^{(0)}\pi_{2A}$	$\eta_0^{(0)}\pi_{2CN}^{(0)} + \eta_1^{(0)}\pi_{2A}$
	Unknown	$(1 - \eta_0^{(0)})\pi_{+CN}^{(0)}$	$(1 - \eta_1^{(0)})\pi_{+A}$	$(1 - \eta_0^{(0)})\pi_{+CN}^{(0)}$ $+ (1 - \eta_1^{(0)})\pi_{+A}$
	Total	$\pi_{+CN}^{(0)}$ $(= \pi_{+C} + \pi_{+N})$	π_{+A}	1.0

Again, we let $F_{rS}^{(0)}$ denote the cell probability of row $r (= 1, 2, 3)$ and column $S (= CN, A)$ in the above table. Thus, we have $F_{rCN}^{(0)} = \eta_0^{(0)}\pi_{rCN}^{(0)}$, $F_{rA}^{(0)} = \eta_1^{(0)}\pi_{rA}(r = 1, 2)$, $F_{3CN}^{(0)} = (1 - \eta_0^{(0)})\pi_{+CN}^{(0)}$, and $F_{3A}^{(0)} = (1 - \eta_1^{(0)})\pi_{+A}$. Similarly, we have the marginal probabilities: $F_{+CN}^{(0)} = \pi_{+CN}^{(0)} = \pi_{+C} + \pi_{+N}$, $F_{+A}^{(0)} = \pi_{+A}$, $F_{r+}^{(0)} = \eta_0^{(0)}\pi_{rCN}^{(0)} + \eta_1^{(0)}\pi_{rA}$ for $r = 1$, 2, and $F_{3+}^{(0)} = (1 - \eta_0^{(0)})\pi_{+CN}^{(0)} + (1 - \eta_1^{(0)})\pi_{+A}$. Note that $\hat{\Delta}^{(MI)}$ (5.2) derived under the compound exclusion restriction model is no longer a consistent estimator of Δ under the assumed MAR model (Exercise 5.10).

Let $n_{rS}^{(g)}(r = 1, 2, 3, S = CA, N$ for $g = 1$, or $S = CN, A$ for $g = 0$) denote the number of patients falling in the cell with probability $F_{rS}^{(g)}$

among n_g subjects assigned to treatment g. The MLE for $F_{rS}^{(g)}$ is given by $\hat{F}_{rS}^{(g)} = n_{rS}^{(g)}/n_g$. Define $F_{(2)S}^{(g)} = (F_{1S}^{(g)} + F_{2S}^{(g)})$ and $\hat{F}_{(2)S}^{(g)} = (\hat{F}_{1S}^{(g)} + \hat{F}_{2S}^{(g)})$, where $g = 1, 0$, and $S = CA, N$ for $g = 1$, or $S = CN, A$ for $g = 0$. Note that the MAR model assumed here is a saturated model. Note also that because the probability of nonmissing outcomes $\eta_1^{(1)}$ for patients who received their assigned experimental treatment equals $F_{(2)CA}^{(1)}/F_{+CA}^{(1)}$, the MLE for $\eta_1^{(1)}$ is $\hat{\eta}_1^{(1)} = \hat{F}_{(2)CA}^{(1)}/\hat{F}_{+CA}^{(1)}$. Following similar arguments, we obtain the MLEs for the other parameters $\eta_d^{(g)}$ as given by $\hat{\eta}_0^{(1)} = \hat{F}_{(2)N}^{(1)}/\hat{F}_{+N}^{(1)}$, $\hat{\eta}_1^{(0)} = \hat{F}_{(2)A}^{(0)}/\hat{F}_{+A}^{(0)}$, and $\hat{\eta}_0^{(0)} = \hat{F}_{(2)CN}^{(0)}/\hat{F}_{+CN}^{(0)}$. Thus, the MLEs for $\pi_{rCA}^{(1)}$ and $\pi_{rN}^{(1)}(r = 1, 2)$ are $\hat{\pi}_{rCA}^{(1)} = \hat{F}_{rCA}^{(1)}/\hat{\eta}_1^{(1)}$ and $\hat{\pi}_{rN}^{(1)} = \hat{F}_{rN}^{(1)}/\hat{\eta}_0^{(1)}$, respectively. Also, the MLEs for $\pi_{rCN}^{(0)}$ and $\pi_{rA}^{(0)}(r = 1, 2)$ are given by $\hat{\pi}_{rCN}^{(0)} = \hat{F}_{rCN}^{(0)}/\hat{\eta}_0^{(0)}$ and $\hat{\pi}_{rA}^{(0)} = \hat{F}_{rA}^{(0)}/\hat{\eta}_1^{(0)}$, respectively.

5.6.1   Estimation of the proportion difference

In terms of parameters $\eta_d^{(g)}$ and $F_{rS}^{(g)}$, we can re-write Δ (2.1) as

$$\Delta = [(F_{1CA}^{(1)}/\eta_1^{(1)} + F_{1N}^{(1)}/\eta_0^{(1)}) - (F_{1CN}^{(0)}/\eta_0^{(0)} + F_{1A}^{(0)}/\eta_1^{(0)})]/(F_{+CA}^{(1)} - F_{+A}^{(0)}).$$
(5.47)

On the basis of the above resulting estimates, we obtain the MLE for Δ under the alternative MAR model assumed here as (Lui, 2008a),

$$\hat{\Delta}^{(AMI)} = [(\hat{F}_{1CA}^{(1)}/\hat{\eta}_1^{(1)} + \hat{F}_{1N}^{(1)}/\hat{\eta}_0^{(1)})$$
$$-(\hat{F}_{1CN}^{(0)}/\hat{\eta}_0^{(0)} + \hat{F}_{1A}^{(0)}/\hat{\eta}_1^{(0)})]/(\hat{F}_{+CA}^{(1)} - \hat{F}_{+A}^{(0)}). \quad (5.48)$$

Using the delta method (Agresti, 1990), we obtain an estimated asymptotic variance $\hat{Var}(\hat{\Delta}^{(AMI)})$ to be given by (Exercise 5.11):

$$\hat{Var}(\hat{\Delta}^{(AMI)}) = \{\hat{Var}(\hat{F}_{1CA}^{(1)}/\hat{\eta}_1^{(1)}) + \hat{Var}(\hat{F}_{1N}^{(1)}/\hat{\eta}_0^{(1)}) + \hat{Var}(\hat{F}_{1A}^{(0)}/\hat{\eta}_1^{(0)})$$
$$+ \hat{Var}(\hat{F}_{1CN}^{(0)}/\hat{\eta}_0^{(0)}) + 2\hat{Cov}(\hat{F}_{1CA}^{(1)}/\hat{\eta}_1^{(1)}, \hat{F}_{1N}^{(1)}/\hat{\eta}_0^{(1)}) + 2\hat{Cov}(\hat{F}_{1A}^{(0)}/\hat{\eta}_1^{(0)},$$
$$\hat{F}_{1CN}^{(0)}/\hat{\eta}_0^{(0)}) + (\hat{\Delta}^{(AMI)})^2 \hat{Var}(\hat{F}_{+CA}^{(1)} - \hat{F}_{+A}^{(0)}) - 2\hat{\Delta}^{(AMI)}\hat{Cov}(\hat{F}_{1CA}^{(1)}/\hat{\eta}_1^{(1)}$$
$$+ \hat{F}_{1N}^{(1)}/\hat{\eta}_0^{(1)}, \hat{F}_{+CA}^{(1)}) - 2\hat{\Delta}^{(AMI)}\hat{Cov}(\hat{F}_{1A}^{(0)}/\hat{\eta}_1^{(0)} + \hat{F}_{1CN}^{(0)}/\hat{\eta}_0^{(0)}, \hat{F}_{+A}^{(0)})\}/$$
$$(\hat{F}_{+CA}^{(1)} - \hat{F}_{+A}^{(0)})^2, \quad (5.49)$$

where

$$\hat{Var}(\hat{F}_{1CA}^{(1)}/\hat{\eta}_1^{(1)}) = [\hat{F}_{1CA}^{(1)}(1 - \hat{F}_{1CA}^{(1)}) + (\hat{\pi}_{1CA}^{(1)})^2\hat{\eta}_1^{(1)}(1/\hat{F}_{+CA}^{(1)} - \hat{\eta}_1^{(1)})$$
$$- 2\hat{\pi}_{1CA}^{(1)}(\hat{F}_{1CA}^{(1)})(1/\hat{F}_{+CA}^{(1)} - \hat{\eta}_1^{(1)}) + 3(\hat{F}_{1CA}^{(1)})^2(1 - \hat{F}_{+CA}^{(1)})/\hat{F}_{+CA}^{(1)}$$
$$- 2\hat{\pi}_{1CA}^{(1)}(\hat{F}_{1CA}^{(1)})\hat{\eta}_1^{(1)}(1 - \hat{F}_{+CA}^{(1)})/\hat{F}_{+CA}^{(1)}]/[n_1(\hat{\eta}_1^{(1)})^2],$$

$$\hat{Var}(\hat{F}_{1N}^{(1)}/\hat{\eta}_0^{(1)}) = [\hat{F}_{1N}^{(1)}(1 - \hat{F}_{1N}^{(1)}) + (\hat{\pi}_{1N}^{(1)})^2\hat{\eta}_0^{(1)}(1/\hat{F}_{+N}^{(1)} - \hat{\eta}_0^{(1)})$$
$$- 2\hat{\pi}_{1N}^{(1)}(\hat{F}_{1N}^{(1)})(1/\hat{F}_{+N}^{(1)} - \hat{\eta}_0^{(1)}) + 3(\hat{F}_{1N}^{(1)})^2(1 - \hat{F}_{+N}^{(1)})/\hat{F}_{+N}^{(1)}$$
$$- 2\hat{\pi}_{1N}^{(1)}(\hat{F}_{1N}^{(1)})\hat{\eta}_0^{(1)}(1 - \hat{F}_{+N}^{(1)})/\hat{F}_{+N}^{(1)}]/[n_1(\hat{\eta}_0^{(1)})^2],$$

$$\hat{Var}(\hat{F}_{1CN}^{(0)}/\hat{\eta}_0^{(0)}) = [\hat{F}_{1CN}^{(0)}(1 - \hat{F}_{1CN}^{(0)}) + (\hat{\pi}_{1CN}^{(0)})^2\hat{\eta}_0^{(0)}(1/\hat{F}_{+CN}^{(0)} - \hat{\eta}_0^{(0)})$$
$$- 2\hat{\pi}_{1CN}^{(0)}(\hat{F}_{1CN}^{(0)})(1/\hat{F}_{+CN}^{(0)} - \hat{\eta}_0^{(0)}) + 3(\hat{F}_{1CN}^{(0)})^2(1 - \hat{F}_{+CN}^{(0)})/\hat{F}_{+CN}^{(0)}$$
$$- 2\hat{\pi}_{1CN}^{(0)}(\hat{F}_{1CN}^{(0)})\hat{\eta}_0^{(0)}(1 - \hat{F}_{+CN}^{(0)})/\hat{F}_{+CN}^{(0)}]/[n_0(\hat{\eta}_0^{(0)})^2],$$

$$\hat{Var}(\hat{F}_{1A}^{(0)}/\hat{\eta}_1^{(0)}) = [\hat{F}_{1A}^{(0)}(1 - \hat{F}_{1A}^{(0)}) + (\hat{\pi}_{1A}^{(0)})^2\hat{\eta}_1^{(0)}(1/\hat{F}_{+A}^{(0)} - \hat{\eta}_1^{(0)})$$
$$- 2\hat{\pi}_{1A}^{(0)}(\hat{F}_{1A}^{(0)})(1/\hat{F}_{+A}^{(0)} - \hat{\eta}_1^{(0)}) + 3(\hat{F}_{1A}^{(0)})^2(1 - \hat{F}_{+A}^{(0)})/\hat{F}_{+A}^{(0)}$$
$$- 2\hat{\pi}_{1A}^{(0)}(\hat{F}_{1A}^{(0)})\hat{\eta}_1^{(0)}(1 - \hat{F}_{+A}^{(0)})/\hat{F}_{+A}^{(0)}]/[n_0(\hat{\eta}_1^{(0)})^2],$$

$$\hat{Cov}(\hat{F}_{1CA}^{(1)}/\hat{\eta}_1^{(1)}, \hat{F}_{1N}^{(1)}/\hat{\eta}_0^{(1)}) = -\hat{\pi}_{1CA}^{(1)}\hat{\pi}_{1N}^{(1)}/n_1,$$

$$\hat{Cov}(\hat{F}_{1A}^{(0)}/\hat{\eta}_1^{(0)}, \hat{F}_{1CN}^{(0)}/\hat{\eta}_0^{(0)}) = -\hat{\pi}_{1A}^{(0)}\hat{\pi}_{1CN}^{(0)}/n_0,$$

$$\hat{Var}(\hat{F}_{+CA}^{(1)} - \hat{F}_{+A}^{(0)}) = \hat{F}_{+CA}^{(1)}(1 - \hat{F}_{+CA}^{(1)})/n_1 + \hat{F}_{+A}^{(0)}(1 - \hat{F}_{+A}^{(0)})/n_0,$$

$$\hat{Cov}(\hat{F}_{1CA}^{(1)}/\hat{\eta}_1^{(1)} + \hat{F}_{1N}^{(1)}/\hat{\eta}_0^{(1)}, \hat{F}_{+CA}^{(1)}) = (\hat{\pi}_{1CA}^{(1)} - \hat{\pi}_{1+}^{(1)}\hat{F}_{+CA}^{(1)})/n_1,$$

and

$$\hat{Cov}(\hat{F}_{1A}^{(0)}/\hat{\eta}_1^{(0)} + \hat{F}_{1CN}^{(0)}/\hat{\eta}_0^{(0)}, \hat{F}_{+A}^{(0)}) = (\hat{\pi}_{1A}^{(0)} - \hat{\pi}_{1+}^{(0)}\hat{F}_{+A}^{(0)})/n_0.$$

Note that when $\eta_d^{(g)} = 1$ for all g and d (and hence $\hat{\eta}_d^{(g)} = 1$), both $\hat{\Delta}^{(AMI)}$ (5.48) and $\hat{Var}(\hat{\Delta}^{(AMI)})$ (5.49) reduce to those (2.5) and (2.6) (Exercise 5.12) for the case of nonmissing outcomes, respectively. On the basis of (5.48) and (5.49), we can do testing superiority, noninferiority, and equivalence, as well as interval estimation when using the PD to measure the relative treatment effect. For brevity, we discuss only interval estimation in the following.

When employing Wald's statistic based on the MLE, we may obtain an asymptotic $100(1 - \alpha)\%$ confidence interval for Δ as

$$[\max\{\hat{\Delta}^{(AMI)} - Z_{\alpha/2}(\hat{Var}(\hat{\Delta}^{(AMI)}))^{1/2}, -1\},$$
$$\min\{\hat{\Delta}^{(AMI)} + Z_{\alpha/2}(\hat{Var}(\hat{\Delta}^{(AMI)}))^{1/2}, 1\}], \qquad (5.50)$$

where $\hat{\Delta}^{(AMI)}$ and $\hat{Var}(\hat{\Delta}^{(AMI)})$ are given (5.48) and (5.49), respectively.

When considering use of $\tanh^{-1}(x)(= \frac{1}{2}\log((1 + x)/(1 - x)))$ transformation on $\hat{\Delta}^{(AMI)}$, we obtain an asymptotic $100\ (1 - \alpha)$ percent confidence interval for Δ as

$$[\tanh(\tanh^{-1}(\hat{\Delta}^{(AMI)}) - Z_{\alpha/2}\sqrt{\hat{Var}(\tanh^{-1}(\hat{\Delta}^{(AMI)}))},$$
$$\tanh(\tanh^{-1}(\hat{\Delta}^{(AMI)}) + Z_{\alpha/2}\sqrt{\hat{Var}(\tanh^{-1}(\hat{\Delta}^{(AMI)}))})] \qquad (5.51)$$

where $\hat{Var}(\tanh^{-1}(\hat{\Delta}^{(AMI)})) = \hat{Var}(\hat{\Delta}^{(AMI)})/(1 - (\hat{\Delta}^{(AMI)})^2)^2$.

Lui (2008a) assumed a structural constant risk additive model (see Section 2.6.1) and discussed interval estimation of the PD under the MAR model. Using Monte Carlo simulations, Lui (2008a) evaluated three asymptotic interval estimators, including interval estimators (5.50) and (5.51). Lui (2008a) found that both interval estimators (5.50) and (5.51) could perform well with respect to the coverage probability in a variety of situations. Lui noted that the interval estimator (5.51) was preferable to the interval estimator (5.50), because the former was generally more precise than the latter. Lui also noted that the estimated average length of both interval estimators increased as either the probability of noncompliance or the probabilities of missing outcomes increased. Thus, it would be essentially important to increase the probability of compliance or nonmissing outcomes if one wished to increase the precision. Furthermore, as noted in Exercise 5.10, the estimator $\hat{\Delta}^{(MI)}$ (5.2) derived under the compound exclusion restriction assumption can be robust under the alternative MAR model assumed here when the subpopulation proportion of compliers π_{+C} is large (≈ 1).

Example 5.6   Consider the data regarding the frequencies of patients with flu-related hospitalization according to the receipt of reminders and the status of flu shots in Table 5.1. Given these data, the MLE $\hat{\Delta}^{(AMI)}$ (5.48) is 0.018. When employing interval estimators (5.50), and (5.51), we obtain the 95 % confidence intervals for Δ to be $[-0.335, 0.371]$ and $[-0.323, 0.355]$, respectively. Because these resulting interval estimates cover 0, there is no significant evidence that flu vaccination can affect the risk of flu-related hospitalization. This nonsignificant finding is the same as that obtained previously under the compound exclusion restriction model. Note that while obtaining a negative estimate $\hat{\Delta}^{(MI)}(= -0.005)$ under the compound exclusion restriction model, we obtain a positive estimate $\hat{\Delta}^{(AMI)}(= 0.018)$ under the MAR model. Because both of these estimates are quite close to 0, we may argue that these different signs can simply occur by chance alone. On the other hand, since the resulting estimate $\hat{\Delta}^{(AMI)}$ with a positive sign seems to be against our general belief that the vaccine tends to be protective. Thus, the compound exclusion restriction model may be preferable to the MAR model for the data in Table 5.1.

5.6.2   Estimation of the proportion ratio

Under the MAR model, we can re-express the PR γ (2.8) in terms of parameters $\eta_d^{(g)}$ and $F_{rS}^{(g)}$ as

$$\gamma = (F_{1CA}^{(1)}/\eta_1^{(1)} - F_{1A}^{(0)}/\eta_1^{(0)})/(F_{1CN}^{(0)}/\eta_0^{(0)} - F_{1N}^{(1)}/\eta_0^{(1)}). \qquad (5.51)$$

When substituting the MLEs $\hat{F}_{rS}^{(g)}$ and $\hat{\eta}_d^{(g)}$ for $F_{rS}^{(g)}$ and $\eta_d^{(g)}$ in (5.51), respectively, we obtain the MLE for γ as (Lui and Cumberland, 2008)

$$\hat{\gamma}^{(AMI)} = (\hat{F}_{1CA}^{(1)}/\hat{\eta}_1^{(1)} - \hat{F}_{1A}^{(0)}/\hat{\eta}_1^{(0)})/(\hat{F}_{1CN}^{(0)}/\hat{\eta}_0^{(0)} - \hat{F}_{1N}^{(1)}/\hat{\eta}_0^{(1)}) \qquad (5.52)$$

Using the delta method again, we obtain an asymptotic variance $\hat{V}ar(\log(\hat{\gamma}^{(AMI)}))$ for the point estimator $\hat{\gamma}^{(AMI)}$ (5.52) using the logarithmic transformation as (Exercise 5.13):

$$\begin{aligned}
\hat{V}ar(\log(\hat{\gamma}^{(AMI)})) = &\{\hat{V}ar(\hat{F}_{1CA}^{(1)}/\hat{\eta}_1^{(1)}) + \hat{V}ar(\hat{F}_{1A}^{(0)}/\hat{\eta}_1^{(0)}) \\
&+ (\hat{\gamma}^{(AMI)})^2[\hat{V}ar(\hat{F}_{1CN}^{(0)}/\hat{\eta}_0^{(0)}) + \hat{V}ar(\hat{F}_{1N}^{(1)}/\hat{\eta}_0^{(1)})] \\
&+ 2\hat{\gamma}^{(AMI)}[\hat{C}ov(\hat{F}_{1CA}^{(1)}/\hat{\eta}_1^{(1)}, \hat{F}_{1N}^{(1)}/\hat{\eta}_0^{(1)}) + \hat{C}ov(\hat{F}_{1A}^{(0)}/\hat{\eta}_1^{(0)}, \hat{F}_{1CN}^{(0)}/\hat{\eta}_0^{(0)})]\}/ \\
&(\hat{F}_{1CA}^{(1)}/\hat{\eta}_1^{(1)} - \hat{F}_{1A}^{(0)}/\hat{\eta}_1^{(0)})^2. \qquad (5.53)
\end{aligned}$$

Note that when $\eta_d^{(g)} = 1$ for all g and d (and hence $\hat{\eta}_d^{(g)} = 1$), both $\hat{\gamma}^{(AMI)}$ (5.52) and $\hat{V}ar(\log(\hat{\gamma}^{(AMI)}))$ (5.53) simplify to (2.9) and (2.10) for the case of nonmissing outcomes. Note also that under the assumption of MCAR (i.e. $\eta_1^{(1)} = \eta_0^{(1)} = \eta_1^{(0)} = \eta_0^{(0)}$), one can easily show that γ equals $(F_{1CA}^{(1)} - F_{1A}^{(0)})/(F_{1CN}^{(0)} - F_{1N}^{(1)})$. Thus, the estimator $\hat{\gamma}^{(AMI)}$ (5.52) reduces to the same form as estimator (2.9) with $\hat{\pi}_{1S}^{(g)}$ replaced by $\hat{F}_{1S}^{(g)}$, where $S = CA$, N for $g = 1$, or $S = CN$, A for $g = 0$. Using the same arguments as for deriving interval estimators (5.18)–(5.20), we can derive the corresponding asymptotic $100(1-\alpha)\%$ confidence interval for γ based on $\hat{\gamma}^{(AMI)}$ (5.52) and $\hat{Var}(\log(\hat{\gamma}^{(AMI)}))$ (5.53) as well.

5.6.3 Estimation of the odds ratio

Under the MAR model, we can re-express φ (2.12) in terms of parameters $\eta_d^{(g)}$ and $F_{rS}^{(g)}$, as

$$\varphi = [(F_{1CA}^{(1)}/\eta_1^{(1)} - F_{1A}^{(0)}/\eta_1^{(0)})(F_{2CN}^{(0)}/\eta_0^{(0)} - F_{2N}^{(1)}/\eta_0^{(1)})]/$$
$$[(F_{2CA}^{(1)}/\eta_1^{(1)} - F_{2A}^{(0)}/\eta_1^{(0)})(F_{1CN}^{(0)}/\eta_0^{(0)} - F_{1N}^{(1)}/\eta_0^{(1)})]. \quad (5.54)$$

When substituting the MLEs $\hat{F}_{rS}^{(g)}$ and $\hat{\eta}_d^{(g)}$ for $F_{rS}^{(g)}$ and $\eta_d^{(g)}$ in (5.54), respectively, we obtain the MLE for φ under the alternative MAR model as

$$\hat{\varphi}^{(AMI)} = [(\hat{F}_{1CA}^{(1)}/\hat{\eta}_1^{(1)} - \hat{F}_{1A}^{(0)}/\hat{\eta}_1^{(0)})(\hat{F}_{2CN}^{(0)}/\hat{\eta}_0^{(0)} - \hat{F}_{2N}^{(1)}/\hat{\eta}_0^{(1)})]/$$
$$[(\hat{F}_{2CA}^{(1)}/\hat{\eta}_1^{(1)} - \hat{F}_{2A}^{(0)}/\hat{\eta}_1^{(0)})(\hat{F}_{1CN}^{(0)}/\hat{\eta}_0^{(0)} - \hat{F}_{1N}^{(1)}/\hat{\eta}_0^{(1)})]. \quad (5.55)$$

Using the delta method again, we obtain an asymptotic variance $\hat{Var}(\log(\hat{\varphi}^{(AMI)}))$ for the point estimator $\hat{\varphi}^{(AMI)}$ (5.55) with the logarithmic transformation as (Exercise 5.14):

$$\hat{Var}(\log(\hat{\varphi}^{(AMI)})) = \{\hat{Var}(\hat{F}_{1CA}^{(1)}/\hat{\eta}_1^{(1)}) + \hat{Var}(\hat{F}_{1A}^{(0)}/\hat{\eta}_1^{(0)})\}/(\hat{F}_{1CA}^{(1)}/\hat{\eta}_1^{(1)} - \hat{F}_{1A}^{(0)}/\hat{\eta}_1^{(0)})^2$$
$$+ \{\hat{Var}(\hat{F}_{2CN}^{(0)}/\hat{\eta}_0^{(0)}) + \hat{Var}(\hat{F}_{2N}^{(1)}/\hat{\eta}_0^{(1)})\}/(\hat{F}_{2CN}^{(0)}/\hat{\eta}_0^{(0)} - \hat{F}_{2N}^{(1)}/\hat{\eta}_0^{(1)})^2$$
$$+ \{\hat{Var}(\hat{F}_{2CA}^{(1)}/\hat{\eta}_1^{(1)}) + \hat{Var}(\hat{F}_{2A}^{(0)}/\hat{\eta}_1^{(0)})\}/(\hat{F}_{2CA}^{(1)}/\hat{\eta}_1^{(1)} - \hat{F}_{2A}^{(0)}/\hat{\eta}_1^{(0)})^2$$
$$+ \{\hat{Var}(\hat{F}_{1CN}^{(0)}/\hat{\eta}_0^{(0)}) + \hat{Var}(\hat{F}_{1N}^{(1)}/\hat{\eta}_0^{(1)})\}/(\hat{F}_{1CN}^{(0)}/\hat{\eta}_0^{(0)} - \hat{F}_{1N}^{(1)}/\hat{\eta}_0^{(1)})^2$$
$$- 2\{\hat{COV}(\hat{F}_{1CA}^{(1)}/\hat{\eta}_1^{(1)}, \hat{F}_{2N}^{(1)}/\hat{\eta}_0^{(1)}) + \hat{COV}(\hat{F}_{2CN}^{(0)}/\hat{\eta}_0^{(0)}, \hat{F}_{1A}^{(0)}/\hat{\eta}_1^{(0)})\}/$$
$$[(\hat{F}_{1CA}^{(1)}/\hat{\eta}_1^{(1)} - \hat{F}_{1A}^{(0)}/\hat{\eta}_1^{(0)})(\hat{F}_{2CN}^{(0)}/\hat{\eta}_0^{(0)} - \hat{F}_{2N}^{(1)}/\hat{\eta}_0^{(1)})]$$
$$- 2\{\hat{COV}(\hat{F}_{1CA}^{(1)}/\hat{\eta}_1^{(1)}, \hat{F}_{2CA}^{(1)}/\hat{\eta}_1^{(1)}) + \hat{COV}(\hat{F}_{2A}^{(0)}/\hat{\eta}_1^{(0)}, \hat{F}_{1A}^{(0)}/\hat{\eta}_1^{(0)})\}/$$
$$[(\hat{F}_{1CA}^{(1)}/\hat{\eta}_1^{(1)} - F_{1A}^{(0)}/\hat{\eta}_1^{(0)})(\hat{F}_{2CA}^{(1)}/\hat{\eta}_1^{(1)} - \hat{F}_{2A}^{(0)}/\hat{\eta}_1^{(0)})]$$
$$+ 2\{\hat{COV}(\hat{F}_{1CA}^{(1)}/\hat{\eta}_1^{(1)}, \hat{F}_{1N}^{(1)}/\hat{\eta}_0^{(0)}) + \hat{COV}(\hat{F}_{1A}^{(0)}/\hat{\eta}_1^{(0)}, \hat{F}_{1CN}^{(0)}/\hat{\eta}_0^{(0)})\}/$$
$$[(\hat{F}_{1CA}^{(1)}/\hat{\eta}_1^{(1)} - \hat{F}_{1A}^{(0)}/\hat{\eta}_1^{(0)})(\hat{F}_{1CN}^{(0)}/\hat{\eta}_0^{(0)} - \hat{F}_{1N}^{(1)}/\hat{\eta}_0^{(1)})]$$

$$+ 2\{C\hat{O}V(\hat{F}_{2CN}^{(0)}/\hat{\eta}_0^{(0)}, \hat{F}_{2A}^{(0)}/\hat{\eta}_1^{(0)}) + C\hat{O}V(\hat{F}_{2N}^{(1)}/\hat{\eta}_0^{(1)}, \hat{F}_{2CA}^{(1)}/\hat{\eta}_1^{(1)})\}/$$
$$[(\hat{F}_{2CN}^{(0)}/\hat{\eta}_0^{(0)} - \hat{F}_{2N}^{(1)}/\hat{\eta}_0^{(1)})(\hat{F}_{2CA}^{(1)}/\hat{\eta}_1^{(1)} - \hat{F}_{2A}^{(0)}/\hat{\eta}_1^{(0)})]$$
$$- 2\{C\hat{O}V(\hat{F}_{1CN}^{(0)}/\hat{\eta}_0^{(0)}, \hat{F}_{2CN}^{(0)}/\hat{\eta}_0^{(0)}) + C\hat{O}V(\hat{F}_{1N}^{(1)}/\hat{\eta}_0^{(1)}, \hat{F}_{2N}^{(1)}/\hat{\eta}_0^{(1)})\}/$$
$$[(\hat{F}_{2CN}^{(0)}/\hat{\eta}_0^{(0)} - \hat{F}_{2N}^{(1)}/\hat{\eta}_0^{(1)})(\hat{F}_{1CN}^{(0)}/\hat{\eta}_0^{(0)} - \hat{F}_{1N}^{(1)}/\hat{\eta}_0^{(1)})]$$
$$- 2\{C\hat{O}V(\hat{F}_{2CA}^{(1)}/\hat{\eta}_1^{(1)}, \hat{F}_{1N}^{(1)}/\hat{\eta}_0^{(1)}) + C\hat{O}V(\hat{F}_{2A}^{(0)}/\hat{\eta}_1^{(0)}, \hat{F}_{1CN}^{(0)}/\hat{\eta}_0^{(0)})\}/$$
$$[(\hat{F}_{2CA}^{(1)}/\hat{\eta}_1^{(1)} - \hat{F}_{2A}^{(0)}/\hat{\eta}_1^{(0)})(\hat{F}_{1CN}^{(0)}/\hat{\eta}_0^{(0)} - \hat{F}_{1N}^{(1)}/\hat{\eta}_0^{(1)})], \tag{5.56}$$

where

$$\hat{Var}(\hat{F}_{rCA}^{(1)}/\hat{\eta}_1^{(1)}) = [\hat{F}_{rCA}^{(1)}(1 - \hat{F}_{rCA}^{(1)}) + (\hat{\pi}_{rCA}^{(1)})^2\hat{\eta}_1^{(1)}(1/\hat{F}_{+CA}^{(1)} - \hat{\eta}_1^{(1)})$$
$$- 2\hat{\pi}_{rCA}^{(1)}(\hat{F}_{rCA}^{(1)})(1/\hat{F}_{+CA}^{(1)} - \hat{\eta}_1^{(1)}) + 3(\hat{F}_{rCA}^{(1)})^2(1 - \hat{F}_{+CA}^{(1)})/\hat{F}_{+CA}^{(1)}$$
$$- 2\hat{\pi}_{rCA}^{(1)}(\hat{F}_{rCA}^{(1)})\hat{\eta}_1^{(1)}(1 - \hat{F}_{+CA}^{(1)})/\hat{F}_{+CA}^{(1)}]/[n_1(\hat{\eta}_1^{(1)})^2],$$

$$\hat{Var}(\hat{F}_{rN}^{(1)}/\hat{\eta}_0^{(1)}) = [\hat{F}_{rN}^{(1)}(1 - \hat{F}_{rN}^{(1)}) + (\hat{\pi}_{rN}^{(1)})^2\hat{\eta}_0^{(1)}(1/\hat{F}_{+N}^{(1)} - \hat{\eta}_0^{(1)})$$
$$- 2\hat{\pi}_{rN}^{(1)}(\hat{F}_{rN}^{(1)})(1/\hat{F}_{+N}^{(1)} - \hat{\eta}_0^{(1)}) + 3(\hat{F}_{rN}^{(1)})^2(1 - \hat{F}_{+N}^{(1)})/\hat{F}_{+N}^{(1)}$$
$$- 2\hat{\pi}_{rN}^{(1)}(\hat{F}_{rN}^{(1)})\hat{\eta}_0^{(1)}(1 - \hat{F}_{+N}^{(1)})/\hat{F}_{+N}^{(1)}]/[n_1(\hat{\eta}_0^{(1)})^2],$$

$$\hat{Var}(\hat{F}_{rCN}^{(0)}/\hat{\eta}_0^{(0)}) = [\hat{F}_{rCN}^{(0)}(1 - \hat{F}_{rCN}^{(0)}) + (\hat{\pi}_{rCN}^{(0)})^2\hat{\eta}_0^{(0)}(1/\hat{F}_{+CN}^{(0)} - \hat{\eta}_0^{(0)})$$
$$- 2\hat{\pi}_{rCN}^{(0)}(\hat{F}_{rCN}^{(0)})(1/\hat{F}_{+CN}^{(0)} - \hat{\eta}_0^{(0)}) + 3(\hat{F}_{rCN}^{(0)})^2(1 - \hat{F}_{|CN}^{(0)})/\hat{F}_{+CN}^{(0)}$$
$$- 2\hat{\pi}_{rCN}^{(0)}(\hat{F}_{rCN}^{(0)})\hat{\eta}_0^{(0)}(1 - \hat{F}_{+CN}^{(0)})/\hat{F}_{+CN}^{(0)}]/[n_0(\hat{\eta}_0^{(0)})^2],$$

$$\hat{Var}(\hat{F}_{rA}^{(0)}/\hat{\eta}_1^{(0)}) = [\hat{F}_{rA}^{(0)}(1 - \hat{F}_{rA}^{(0)}) + (\hat{\pi}_{rA}^{(0)})^2\hat{\eta}_1^{(0)}(1/\hat{F}_{+A}^{(0)} - \hat{\eta}_1^{(0)})$$
$$- 2\hat{\pi}_{rA}^{(0)}(\hat{F}_{rA}^{(0)})(1/\hat{F}_{+A}^{(0)} - \hat{\eta}_1^{(0)}) + 3(\hat{F}_{rA}^{(0)})^2(1 - \hat{F}_{+A}^{(0)})/\hat{F}_{+A}^{(0)}$$
$$- 2\hat{\pi}_{rA}^{(0)}(\hat{F}_{rA}^{(0)})\hat{\eta}_1^{(0)}(1 - \hat{F}_{+A}^{(0)})/\hat{F}_{+A}^{(0)}]/[n_0(\hat{\eta}_1^{(0)})^2], \quad \text{for } r = 1, 2$$

$$C\hat{O}V(\hat{F}_{rCA}^{(1)}/\hat{\eta}_1^{(1)}, \hat{F}_{r'N}^{(1)}/\hat{\eta}_0^{(1)}) = -\hat{\pi}_{rCA}^{(1)}\hat{\pi}_{r'N}^{(1)}/n_1,$$

$$C\hat{O}V(\hat{F}_{rCN}^{(0)}/\hat{\eta}_0^{(0)}, \hat{F}_{r'A}^{(0)}/\hat{\eta}_1^{(0)}) = -\hat{\pi}_{rCN}^{(0)}\hat{\pi}_{r'A}^{(0)}/n_0, \text{ for } r = 1, 2 \text{ and } r' = 1, 2.$$

$$C\hat{O}V(\hat{F}_{1CA}^{(1)}/\hat{\eta}_1^{(1)}, \hat{F}_{2CA}^{(1)}/\hat{\eta}_1^{(1)}) = \hat{\pi}_{1CA}^{(1)}(1 - \hat{F}_{+CA}^{(1)})/n_1 - \hat{Var}(\hat{F}_{1CA}^{(1)}/\hat{\eta}_1^{(1)})$$

$$C\hat{O}V(\hat{F}_{1N}^{(1)}/\hat{\eta}_0^{(1)}, \hat{F}_{2N}^{(1)}/\hat{\eta}_0^{(1)}) = \hat{\pi}_{1N}^{(1)}(1 - \hat{F}_{+N}^{(1)})/n_1 - \hat{Var}(\hat{F}_{1N}^{(1)}/\hat{\eta}_0^{(1)})$$

$$C\hat{O}V(\hat{F}_{1CN}^{(0)}/\hat{\eta}_0^{(0)}, \hat{F}_{2CN}^{(0)}/\hat{\eta}_0^{(0)}) = \hat{\pi}_{1CN}^{(0)}(1 - \hat{F}_{+CN}^{(0)})/n_0 - \hat{Var}(\hat{F}_{1CN}^{(0)}/\hat{\eta}_0^{(0)})$$

$$C\hat{O}V(\hat{F}_{1A}^{(0)}/\hat{\eta}_1^{(0)}, \hat{F}_{2A}^{(0)}/\hat{\eta}_1^{(0)}) = \hat{\pi}_{1A}^{(0)}(1 - \hat{F}_{+A}^{(0)})/n_0 - \hat{Var}(\hat{F}_{1A}^{(0)}/\hat{\eta}_1^{(0)})$$

Note that when $\eta_d^{(g)} = 1$ for all g and d (and hence $\hat{\eta}_d^{(g)} = 1$), both $\hat{\varphi}^{(AMI)}$ (5.55) and $\hat{Var}(\log(\hat{\varphi}^{(AMI)}))$ (5.56) simplify to (2.13) and (2.14), respectively, for the case of nonmissing outcomes. Note also that under the MCAR, we can easily show that $\hat{\varphi}^{(AMI)}$ (5.55) reduces to the same form as $\hat{\varphi}$ (2.13) with $\hat{\pi}_{1S}^{(g)}$ replaced by $\hat{F}_{1S}^{(g)}$, where $S = CA, N$ for $g = 1$, or $S = CN, A$ for $g = 0$. Using the same idea as for deriving interval estimators (5.21)–(5.23), we can derive the corresponding asymptotic $100(1-\alpha)\%$ confidence interval for φ based on $\hat{\varphi}^{(AMI)}$ (5.55) and $\hat{Var}(\log(\hat{\varphi}^{(AMI)}))$ (5.56).

When comparing a new, enhanced, teaching treatment with a standard treatment of only receiving mailed information on the practice of breast self-examination (BSE), Mealli, Imbens and Ferro et al. (2004) contended that the exclusion restriction assumption on nonmissing outcomes for never-takers (as stated in the compound exclusion restriction assumption) appeared questionable. Mealli, Imbens and Ferro et al. (2004) claimed that never-takers who were assigned to the new treatment and explicitly refused to comply with their assigned treatment might plausibly induce them to refuse to respond and have missing outcome. Thus, Mealli, Imbens and Ferro et al. (2004) suggested that the exclusion restriction assumption for nonmissing outcomes should be applied to compliers rather than never-takers. Following Mealli, Imbens and Ferro et al. (2004), we present the latent probability structure by replacing the exclusion restriction assumption on nonmissing outcomes for never-takers in the compound exclusion restriction assumption by the exclusion restriction assumption on nonmissing outcomes for compliers in Exercise 5.15. Using the same ideas and arguments as those presented here, we can extend the results presented here to do hypothesis testing and estimation under the model proposed by Mealli, Imbens and Ferro et al. (2004) as well.

Finally, when collecting data using a multi-center design or combining the results from a few trials in meta-analysis, we may need to control the center or trial effects by forming strata determined by centers or trials. Following similar ideas as those suggested in Chapter 3, we can apply all the estimators and their asymptotic variances as presented here to do stratified analysis when there are many patients not complying with their assigned treatment and/or having subsequent missing outcomes.

Exercises

5.1 Show that under the compound exclusion restriction assumption and latent ignorability, we can completely and uniquely determine all the cell probability of observed data for both assigned treatments g (g = 1, 0) based on the set $\{\pi_{+C}, \pi_{+A}, \pi_{1|C}^{(0)},$ $\Delta, \pi_{1|A}, \pi_{1|N}, \eta_C^{(1)}, \eta_C^{(0)}, \eta_A, \eta_N\}$ containing 10 parameters.

5.2 Show that the parameter $E_{1+}^{(1)}/E_{(2)+}^{(1)} - E_{1+}^{(0)}/E_{(2)+}^{(0)}$ based on patients with known outcomes in the ITT analysis is generally not equal to 0 under $H_0 : \Delta = 0$. Thus, we can no longer apply the ITT analysis to test $H_0 : \Delta = 0$ as what is done (in Chapter 2) for a noncompliance RCT with no missing data. Can you provide the conditions such that $E_{1+}^{(1)}/E_{(2)+}^{(1)} - E_{1+}^{(0)}/E_{(2)+}^{(0)} = 0$ if and only if $\Delta = 0$ (Answers: $\eta_C^{(1)} = \eta_C^{(0)}$ or $\pi_{1|C} = (\eta_N\pi_{1N} + \eta_A\pi_{1A})/(\eta_N\pi_{+N} + \eta_A\pi_{+A})$, where $\pi_{1|C}$ denotes the common value of $\pi_{1|C}^{(1)} = \pi_{1|C}^{(0)}$ under $H_0 : \Delta = 0$.)

5.3 When there are no patients with missing outcomes (i.e. $\eta_C^{(1)} = \eta_C^{(0)} = \eta_N = \eta_A = 1$), show that the MLE $\hat{\Delta}^{(MI)}$ (5.2) is identical to $\hat{\Delta}$ (2.5).

5.4 Using the delta method, show that the asymptotic variance $Var(\hat{\Delta}^{(MI)})$ (Lui and Chang, 2008a) for the MLE $\hat{\Delta}^{(MI)}$ (5.2) is given by (5.3).

5.5 Show that an asymptotic variance $Var(\log(\hat{\gamma}^{(MI)}))$ for $\hat{\gamma}^{(MI)}$ (5.7) is given by (5.8).

5.6 Show that an asymptotic variance $Var(\log(\hat{\varphi}^{(MI)}))$ of $\hat{\varphi}^{(MI)}$ (5.11) is given by (5.12).

5.7 For simplicity, we often assume MCAR and analyze data conditional upon patients with known outcomes. Thus, we may employ the following estimator of the OR,

$$\hat{OR}_{MCAR}^{(MI)} = [(\hat{E}_{1CA}^{(1)}/\hat{E}_{(2)+}^{(1)} - \hat{E}_{1A}^{(0)}/\hat{E}_{(2)+}^{(0)})(\hat{E}_{2CN}^{(0)}/\hat{E}_{(2)+}^{(0)} - \hat{E}_{2N}^{(1)}/\hat{E}_{(2)+}^{(1)})]/$$
$$[(\hat{E}_{2CA}^{(1)}/\hat{E}_{(2)+}^{(1)} - \hat{E}_{2A}^{(0)}/\hat{E}_{(2)+}^{(0)})(\hat{E}_{1CN}^{(0)}/\hat{E}_{(2)+}^{(0)} - \hat{E}_{1N}^{(1)}/\hat{E}_{(2)+}^{(1)})]$$

where $E_{(2)+}^{(g)} = E_{1+}^{(g)} + E_{2+}^{(g)} = \eta_C^{(g)}\pi_{+C} + \eta_N\pi_{+N} + \eta_A\pi_{+A}$ for $g = 1, 0$. Show that when $\eta_C^{(1)} = \eta_C^{(0)}(= \eta_C)$, $\hat{OR}_{MCAR}^{(MI)}$ can be still a consistent estimator of the OR even when the probability of nonmissing η_J may vary between subpopulations ($J = C$, A, and N).

5.8 Consider the data in Table 5.1, what is the 95% confidence interval for Δ when we employ interval estimator $[\hat{\Delta}^{(MI)} - Z_{\alpha/2} \sqrt{\hat{Var}(\hat{\Delta}^{(MI)})}, \hat{\Delta}^{(MI)} + Z_{\alpha/2}\sqrt{\hat{Var}(\hat{\Delta}^{(MI)})}]$ without using $\tanh^{-1}(x)$ transformation? (Answer: $[-0.229, 0.219]$)

5.9 Discuss how can we check whether missing occurs completely at random? Is there evidence that we can claim that missing in Table 5.1 does not occur completely at random at the 5 %?

5.10 Show that $\hat{\Delta}^{(MI)}$ (5.2) is a consistent estimator of the parameter $(\eta_1^{(1)}\pi_{1C}^{(1)} + (\eta_1^{(1)} - \eta_1^{(0)})\pi_{1A})/(\eta_1^{(1)}\pi_{+C} + (\eta_1^{(1)} - \eta_1^{(0)})\pi_{+A}) - (\eta_0^{(0)}\pi_{1C}^{(0)} + (\eta_0^{(0)} - \eta_0^{(1)})\pi_{1N})/(\eta_0^{(0)}\pi_{+C} + (\eta_0^{(0)} - \eta_0^{(1)})\pi_{+N})$, which is no longer the same as $\Delta(= \pi_{1|C}^{(1)} - \pi_{1|C}^{(0)})$ under the alternative MAR model defined in Section 5.6. (Comments: If π_{+C} is large (or equivalently, both π_{+A} and π_{+N} are ≈ 0) or both $|\eta_d^{(1)} - \eta_d^{(0)}|$ for $d = 1, 0$ are ≈ 0, this parameter can be easily seen approximately equal to $\Delta(= \pi_{1|C}^{(1)} - \pi_{1|C}^{(0)})$. In other words, when the subpopulation proportion of compliers π_{+C} is high (≈ 1), $\hat{\Delta}^{(MI)}$ may still perform well under the alternative MAR model.)

5.11 Show that an estimated asymptotic variance $\hat{Var}(\hat{\Delta}^{(AMI)})$ for $\hat{\Delta}^{(AMI)}$ (5.48) under the alternative MAR model is given by (5.49).

5.12 Show that when $\eta_d^{(g)} = 1$ for all g and d (and hence $\hat{\eta}_d^{(g)} = 1$), both $\hat{\Delta}^{(AMI)}$ (5.48) and $\hat{Var}(\hat{\Delta}^{(AMI)})$ (5.49) reduce to those (2.5) and (2.6), respectively, for the case of nonmissing outcomes.

5.13 Show that an asymptotic variance $\hat{Var}(\log(\hat{\gamma}^{(AMI)}))$ for the point estimator $\hat{\gamma}^{(AMI)}$ (5.52) is given by (5.53) (Lui and Cumberland, 2008).

5.14 Show that an asymptotic variance $\hat{Var}(\log(\hat{\varphi}^{(AMI)}))$ for the point estimator $\hat{\varphi}^{(AMI)}$ (5.55) with the logarithmic transformation is given by (5.56).

5.15 Following Mealli, Imbens and Ferro *et al.* (2004), we may assume that the exclusion restriction assumption on the patient response holds for always-takers and never-takers, but the exclusion restriction assumption on a nonmissing outcome holds for always-takers and compliers (instead of never-takers). In other words, we may summarize the latent probability structure for the observed data of patients assigned to the experimental ($g = 1$) treatment by use of the following table.

Assigned experimental treatment ($g = 1$)

Treatment received	Experimental	Control	
	Compliers and always-takers (CA)	Never-takers (N)	Total
Outcome Positive	$\eta_C \pi_{1C}^{(1)} + \eta_A \pi_{1A}$	$\eta_N^{(1)} \pi_{1N}$	$\eta_C \pi_{1C}^{(1)} + \eta_A \pi_{1A} + \eta_N^{(1)} \pi_{1N}$
Negative	$\eta_C \pi_{2C}^{(1)} + \eta_A \pi_{2A}$	$\eta_N^{(1)} \pi_{2N}$	$\eta_C \pi_{2C}^{(1)} + \eta_A \pi_{2A} + \eta_N^{(1)} \pi_{2N}$
Unknown	$(1 - \eta_C)\pi_{+C} + (1 - \eta_A)\pi_{+A}$	$(1 - \eta_N^{(1)})\pi_{+N}$	$(1 - \eta_C)\pi_{+C} + (1 - \eta_A)\pi_{+A} + (1 - \eta_N^{(1)})\pi_{+N}$
Total	$\pi_{+C} + \pi_{+A}$	π_{+N}	1.0

Similarly, we may summarize the latent probability structure for the observed data of patients assigned to the standard treatment by use of the following table.

Assigned standard treatment ($g = 0$)

Treatment received	Control	Experimental	
	Compliers and never-takers (CN)	Always-takers (A)	Total
Outcome Positive	$\eta_C \pi_{1C}^{(0)} + \eta_N^{(0)} \pi_{1N}$	$\eta_A \pi_{1A}$	$\eta_C \pi_{1C}^{(0)} + \eta_N^{(0)} \pi_{1N} + \eta_A \pi_{1A}$
Negative	$\eta_C \pi_{2C}^{(0)} + \eta_N^{(0)} \pi_{2N}$	$\eta_A \pi_{2A}$	$\eta_C \pi_{2C}^{(0)} + \eta_N^{(0)} \pi_{2N} + \eta_A \pi_{2A}$

Treatment received	Control	Experimental	
	Compliers and never-takers (CN)	Always-takers (A)	Total
Unknown	$(1 - \eta_C)\pi_{+C}$ $+ (1 - \eta_N^{(0)})\pi_{+N}$	$(1 - \eta_A)\pi_{+A}$	$(1 - \eta_C)\pi_{+C}$ $+ (1 - \eta_N^{(0)})\pi_{+N}$ $+ (1 - \eta_A)\pi_{+A}$
Total	$\pi_{+C} + \pi_{+N}$	π_{+A}	1.0

For convenience we let $G_{rS}^{(g)}(r = 1, 2, 3,$ and $S = CA, N$ for $g = 1$, or $S = CN, A$ for $g = 0$) denote the corresponding cell probability for row r and column S in the assigned treatment g. Suppose that we randomly assign n_g patients to receive the experimental $(g = 1)$ and standard $(g = 0)$ treatments, respectively. Let $n_{rS}^{(g)}(r = 1, 2, 3,$ and $S = CA, N$ for $g = 1$ or $S = CN, A$ for $g = 0$) denote the number of patients falling in the cell with the probability $G_{rS}^{(g)}$ in the assigned treatment g. The MLE of $G_{rS}^{(g)}$ is then $\hat{G}_{rS}^{(g)} = n_{rS}^{(g)}/n_g$ due to the fact that the assumed model is a saturated model. Under the above model assumptions, derive the MLE for $\Delta = \pi_{1|C}^{(1)} - \pi_{1|C}^{(0)}$ (2.1), $\gamma = \pi_{1|C}^{(1)}/\pi_{1|C}^{(0)}$ (2.8) and $\varphi = \pi_{1|C}^{(1)}\pi_{2|C}^{(0)}/(\pi_{2|C}^{(1)}\pi_{1|C}^{(0)})$ (2.12) in terms of $\hat{G}_{rS}^{(g)}$. (Hint: Note that $\hat{\pi}_{+N} = \hat{G}_{+N}^{(1)}$ and $\hat{\pi}_{+A} = \hat{G}_{+A}^{(0)}$. Thus, we have $\hat{\pi}_{+C} = 1 - \hat{G}_{+N}^{(1)} - \hat{G}_{+A}^{(0)}$. Furthermore, we can easily obtain the MLEs for the corresponding parameters: $\hat{\eta}_C = (\hat{G}_{(2)CA}^{(1)} - \hat{G}_{(2)A}^{(0)})/\hat{\pi}_{+C}$, $\hat{\eta}_A = \hat{G}_{(2)A}^{(0)}/\hat{G}_{+A}^{(0)}$, $\hat{\eta}_N^{(1)} = \hat{G}_{(2)N}^{(1)}/\hat{G}_{+N}^{(1)}$, and $\hat{\eta}_N^{(0)} = [\hat{G}_{(2)CN}^{(0)} - \hat{G}_{(2)CA}^{(1)} + \hat{G}_{(2)A}^{(0)}]/\hat{G}_{+N}^{(1)}$. Thus, we obtain the MLE $\hat{\pi}_{1C}^{(1)} = (\hat{G}_{1CA}^{(1)} - \hat{G}_{1A}^{(0)})/\hat{\eta}_C$. Also, since $\hat{\pi}_{1N} = (\hat{G}_{1N}^{(1)})/\hat{\eta}_N^{(1)} = (\hat{G}_{1N}^{(1)}\hat{G}_{+N}^{(1)})/\hat{G}_{(2)N}^{(1)}$, we have the MLE $\hat{\pi}_{1C}^{(0)} = (\hat{G}_{1CN}^{(0)} - \hat{\eta}_N^{(0)}\hat{\pi}_{1N})/\hat{\eta}_C$. This leads us to obtain the MLE for Δ to be $\hat{\Delta}^{(MMI)} = [(\hat{G}_{1CA}^{(1)} - \hat{G}_{1A}^{(0)}) - (\hat{G}_{1CN}^{(0)} - \hat{\eta}_N^{(0)}\hat{\pi}_{1N})]/(\hat{G}_{(2)CA}^{(1)} - \hat{G}_{(2)A}^{(0)})$. We also obtain the MLE for the PR as $\hat{\gamma}^{(MMI)} = \hat{\pi}_{1C}^{(1)}/\hat{\pi}_{1C}^{(0)} = (\hat{G}_{1CA}^{(1)} - \hat{G}_{1A}^{(0)})/(\hat{G}_{1CN}^{(0)} - \hat{\eta}_N^{(0)}\hat{\pi}_{1N})$, where $\hat{\eta}_N^{(0)}\hat{\pi}_{1N} = [\hat{G}_{(2)CN}^{(0)} - \hat{G}_{(2)CA}^{(1)} + \hat{G}_{(2)A}^{(0)}]\hat{G}_{1N}^{(1)}/\hat{G}_{(2)N}^{(1)}$. Similarly, the MLE for the OR is $\hat{\varphi}^{(MMI)} = \hat{\pi}_{1C}^{(1)}(\hat{\pi}_{+C} - \hat{\pi}_{1C}^{(0)})/[(\hat{\pi}_{+C} - \hat{\pi}_{1C}^{(1)})\hat{\pi}_{1C}^{(0)}]$.)

5.16 Show that the estimator $\hat{\Delta}^{(MI)}$ (5.2) is not a consistent estimator of Δ under the model assumed in Exercise 5.15. Show that $\hat{\Delta}^{(MI)}$ can be still a consistent estimator if $\eta_N^{(1)} \approx \eta_N^{(0)}$ or $\pi_{+N} \approx 0$. Thus, when the proportion of compliers is high (i.e. $\pi_{+C} \approx 1$), $\hat{\Delta}^{(MI)}$ can be still an approximately consistent estimator for Δ. Based on Exercises 5.10 and 5.16, we may infer that if the proportion of noncompliers is minimal (or equivalently, $\pi_{+C} \approx 1$), the estimator $\hat{\Delta}^{(MI)}$ can be robust. Thus, one of the best strategies to deal with the effects resulting from noncompliance and subsequent missing outcomes is to minimize the proportion of noncompliers in trials.

5.17 On the basis of data in Table 5.1, what is the MLE for Δ (2.1) under the model assumed in Exercise 5.15? What is the MLE for γ (2.8) and the MLE for φ (2.12) under the model assumed in Exercise 5.15?

Appendix

Note that all sample size calculation formulae presented are derived on the basis of large sample theory. Thus, if the estimate of the minimum required sample size should not be large so as to assure the assumed normal approximation of the test statistic for a given configuration to be valid, the sample size calculation procedure presented here can be inaccurate.

The following is the SAS program for producing the estimate of the minimum required sample size for a desired power of 80 % in detecting superiority at the ($\alpha =$) 5 % level in Table 5.2. Readers may modify this program to accommodate the situations of their interest.

```
data step1;
*** This program is for calculation of the required sample size;
*** for testing superiority based on risk difference in randomized
    clinical;
*** trials with noncompliance and missing values in Table 5.2;
  array sam(m) samx1-samx5;
  array pow(m) epow1-epow5;
  array fail(m) efail1-efail5;
  za=1.96;
  zb=0.842;  ** for power of 80 percent;
  do pattern= 1, 2,3;
    put pattern 1-10;
  do marprob=1 to 3;
  if marprob eq 1 then do;
  pc=0.95; pa=0.03; pn=0.02;  ** proportion of populations in different;
                    end;     ** categories;
  if marprob eq 2 then do;
  pc=0.80; pa=0.15; pn=0.05;
  end;
  if marprob eq 3 then do;
  pc=0.60; pa=0.25; pn=0.15;
  end;
  rconc=0.30; rcona=0.50; rconn=0.25; ** conditional probability of a
                          positive response;
  desired=0.80;  ** desired power;
  do dd=0.05,0.10,0.20; ** true difference of interest between two
                          treatments;
  do numk=0.5,1,2,4,8;  ** ratio of sample allocation;
  if numk=0.5 then m=1;
  if numk=1 then m=2;
  if numk=2 then m=3;
  if numk=4 then m=4;
  if numk=8 then m=5;
  if pattern eq 1 then do;
```

```
nomissc1=1.0;
nomissc0=1.0;
nomissa=1.0;
nomissn=1.0;
end;
if pattern eq 2 then do;
nomissc1=0.95;
nomissc0=0.85;
nomissa=0.90;
nomissn=0.80;
end;
if pattern eq 3 then do;
nomissc1=0.85;
nomissc0=0.75;
nomissa=0.80;
nomissn=0.70;
end;
 xp1=pc*(rconc+dd)*nomissc1;
 xp2=pa*rcona*nomissa;
 xp3=pn*rconn*nomissn;
 xp4=pc*(1-(rconc+dd))*nomissc1;
 xp5=pa*(1-rcona)*nomissa;
 xp6=pn*(1-rconn)*nomissn;
 xp7=pc*(1-nomissc1);
 xp8=pa*(1-nomissa);
 xp9=pn*(1-nomissn);
 xpe1=xp1+xp2;
 xpe2=xp3;
 xpe3=xp4+xp5;
 xpe4=xp6;
 xpe5=xp7+xp8;
 xpe6=xp9;
 yp1=pc*rconc*nomissc0;
 yp2=pa*rcona*nomissa;
 yp3=pn*rconn*nomissn;
 yp4=pc*(1-rconc)*nomissc0;
 yp5=pa*(1-rcona)*nomissa;
 yp6=pn*(1-rconn)*nomissn;
 yp7=pc*(1-nomissc0);
 yp8=pa*(1-nomissa);
 yp9=pn*(1-nomissn);
 ype1=yp1+yp3;
 ype2=yp2;
 ype3=yp4+yp6;
 ype4=yp5;
 ype5=yp7+yp9;
 ype6=yp8;
 v1=(xpe1*(1-xpe1)+ype2*(1-ype2)/numk+
 (rconc+dd)**2*((xpe1+xpe3)*(1-(xpe1+xpe3))+
 (ype2+ype4)*(1-(ype2+ype4))/numk)-
  2*(rconc+dd)*(xpe1-xpe1*(xpe1+xpe3)+(ype2-ype2*(ype2+ype4))/numk))/
```

```
   ((xpe1+xpe3)-(ype2+ype4))**2;
v2=(xpe2*(1-xpe2)+ype1*(1-ype1)/numk+
   rconc**2*((xpe2+xpe4)*(1-(xpe2+xpe4))+
   (ype1+ype3)*(1-(ype1+ype3))/numk)-
  2*rconc*(xpe2-xpe2*(xpe2+xpe4)+(ype1-ype1*(ype1+ype3))/numk))/
   ((ype1+ype3)-(xpe2+xpe4))**2;
c12=(xpe1*xpe2+ype1*ype2/numk-
      rconc*(xpe1*(xpe2+xpe4)+ype2*(ype1+ype3)/numk)-
      (rconc+dd)*((xpe1+xpe3)*xpe2+(ype2+ype4)*ype1/numk)+
    rconc*(rconc+dd)*((xpe1+xpe3)*(xpe2+xpe4)+(ype1+ype3)*(ype2+ype4)/
    numk))/
   (((xpe1+xpe3)-(ype2+ype4))*((ype1+ype3)-(xpe2+xpe4)));
var0=v1+v2-2*c12;
var1=var0/(1-dd**2)**2;
td=0.5*log((1+dd)/(1-dd));
n1=ceil((za*sqrt(var0)+zb*sqrt(var1))**2/td**2);
sam=n1;
if m eq 5 then do;
put pc 1-5 2 pa 6-10 2 pn 11-15 2  dd 16-20 2
samx1 26-32 samx2 36-42 samx3 46-52 samx4 56-62 samx5 66-72;
 end;  ** end of do if m eq 4;
 end;  ** end of do numk;
 end;  ** end of do rr;
 end;  ** end of do marprob;
 end;  ** do pattern;
```

The following is the SAS program for producing the estimate of the minimum required sample size for a desired power of 80 % in detecting equivalence based on the proportion ratio at the ($\alpha =$) 5 % level in Table 5.3. Note that when the acceptable margins are chosen to be not relatively small (say, $\gamma_l = 0.50$ and $\gamma_u = 1.0$), we should treat the resulting estimate obtained from this program as an initial estimate and apply trial-and error procedure to find the minimum required sample size as described in the context.

```
data step1;
* This program is for calculation of the minimum required sample size;
* for assessing equivalence based on proportion ratio under a RCT;
* with noncompliance and missing outcomes in Table 5.3;
  array sam(m) samx1-samx5;
  za=1.645; ** the upper 5 percentile of the standard normal distribution;
  zb1=0.842;
  zb2=1.282;
do rconc=0.30;  ** conditional prob of positive response among compliers;
  rcona=0.50;   ** conditional prob of positive response for always-
                   takers is;
  rconn=0.25;   ** conditional prob of positive response for never-takers;
  put rconc 1-10 3;
```

```
do pattern= 1, 2,3;
   put pattern 10-30;
do marprob=1 to 3;
if marprob eq 1 then do;
pc=0.95; pa=0.03; pn=0.02;   ** proportion of subpopulations in
                                   different;
                  end;      ** compliance categories;
if marprob eq 2 then do;
pc=0.80; pa=0.15; pn=0.05;
                  end;
if marprob eq 3 then do;
pc=0.60; pa=0.25; pn=0.15;
                  end;
deltal=0.20;    ** maximum acceptance lower level for equivalence;
deltau=0.25;    ** maximum acceptance uper  level for equivalence;
do rr=0.90,1,1.1;  *true ratio of prop of response between two
                  treatments;
do numk=0.5,1,2,4,8; *ratio of sample allocation between two
                  treatments;
if numk=0.5 then m=1;
if numk=1 then m=2;
if numk=2 then m=3;
if numk=4 then m=4;
if numk=8 then m=5;
if pattern eq 1 then do;  ** prob of nonmissing outcomes;
nomissc1=1.0;  **for complier assigned to expermental  treatment;
nomissc0=1.0;  **for complier assigned to standard treatment;;
nomissa=1.0;   **for always takers;
nomissn=1.0;   **for never takers;
end;
if pattern eq 2 then do;
nomissc1=0.95;
nomissc0=0.85;
nomissa=0.90;
nomissn=0.80;
end;
if pattern eq 3 then do;
nomissc1=0.85;
nomissc0=0.75;
nomissa=0.80;
nomissn=0.70;
end;
 xp1=pc*rconc*rr*nomissc1;
 xp2=pa*rcona*nomissa;
 xp3=pn*rconn*nomissn;
 xp4=pc*(1-rconc*rr)*nomissc1;
 xp5=pa*(1-rcona)*nomissa;
 xp6=pn*(1-rconn)*nomissn;
 xp7=pc*(1-nomissc1);
 xp8=pa*(1-nomissa);
 xp9=pn*(1-nomissn);
```

```
    xpe1=xp1+xp2;
    xpe2=xp3;
    xpe3=xp4+xp5;
    xpe4=xp6;
    xpe5=xp7+xp8;
    xpe6=xp9;
    yp1=pc*rconc*nomissc0;
    yp2=pa*rcona*nomissa;
    yp3=pn*rconn*nomissn;
    yp4=pc*(1-rconc)*nomissc0;
    yp5=pa*(1-rcona)*nomissa;
    yp6=pn*(1-rconn)*nomissn;
    yp7=pc*(1-nomissc0);
    yp8=pa*(1-nomissa);
    yp9=pn*(1-nomissn);
    ype1=yp1+yp3;
    ype2=yp2;
    ype3=yp4+yp6;
    ype4=yp5;
    ype5=yp7+yp9;
    ype6=yp8;
    v1=((xpe2+xpe4)*(1-(xpe2+xpe4))+
       (ype1+ype3)*(1-(ype1+ype3))/numk)/((ype1+ype3)-(xpe2+xpe4))**2;
    v2=(xpe1*(1-xpe1)+
       ype2*(1-ype2)/numk)/(xpe1-ype2)**2;
    v3=((xpe1+xpe3)*(1-(xpe1+xpe3))+
       (ype2+ype4)*(1-(ype2+ype4))/numk)/((ype2+ype4)-(xpe1+xpe3))**2;
    v4=(xpe2*(1-xpe2)+
       ype1*(1-ype1)/numk)/(xpe2-ype1)**2;
    c12=(ype2*(ype1+ype3)/numk+xpe1*(xpe2+xpe4))/
        ((ype1+ype3-(xpe2+xpe4))*(xpe1-ype2));
    c13=((ype2+ype4)*(ype1+ype3)/numk+(xpe1+xpe3)*(xpe2+xpe4))/
        ((ype1+ype3-(xpe2+xpe4))*(xpe1+xpe3-(ype2+ype4)));
    c14=((ype1-ype1*(ype1+ype3))/numk+(xpe2-xpe2*(xpe2+xpe4)))/
        ((ype1+ype3-(xpe2+xpe4))*(ype1-xpe2));
    c23=((ype2-ype2*(ype2+ype4))/numk+(xpe1-xpe1*(xpe1+xpe3)))/
        ((xpe1-ype2)*(xpe1+xpe3-(ype2+ype4)));
    c24=(ype1*ype2/numk+xpe1*xpe2)/
        ((xpe1-ype2)*(ype1-xpe2));
    c34=((ype2+ype4)*ype1/numk+(xpe1+xpe3)*xpe2)/
        ((xpe1+xpe3-(ype2+ype4))*(ype1-xpe2));
    var=v1+v2+v3+v4+2*c12-2*c13-2*c14-2*c23-2*c24+2*c34;
    if  round(rr,0.00000001) lt 1.0 then n1=(za+zb1)**2*var/(log(rr)-log
(1-deltal))**2;
    if  round(rr,0.00000001) eq 1.0 then n1=(za+zb2)**2*var/(log(1+
deltau)**2);
    if  round(rr,0.00000001) gt 1.0 then n1=(za+zb1)**2*var/(log(rr)-log
(1+deltau))**2;
    sam=ceil(n1);
  if m eq 5 then do;
  put pc 1-5 2 pa 6-10 2 pn 11-15 2  rr 16-20 2
```

```
   samx1 26-32 samx2 36-42 samx3 46-52 samx4 56-62 samx5 66-72;
   end;   ** end of do if m eq 5;
   end;   ** end of do numk;
   end; ** end of do rr;
   end;   ** end of do marprob;
   end;   ** do pattern;
   end;   ** end of do rconc;
```

The following is the SAS program for producing the estimate of the minimum required sample size for a desired power of 80 % in detecting equivalence based on the odds ratio at the ($\alpha =$) 5 % level in Table 5.4. Note that when the acceptable margins are chosen to be not relatively small (say, $\varphi_l = 0.50$ and $\varphi_u = 1.0$), we should treat the resulting estimate obtained from this program as an initial estimate and apply trial and error procedure to find the minimum required sample size as described in the context.

```
data step1;
* This program is for calculation of the minimum required sample size;
* for assessing equivalence based on odds ratio under a RCT;
* with noncompliance and missing outcomes in Table 5.4;
  array sam(m) samx1-samx5;
za=1.645; **the upper 5 percentile of the standard normal distribution;
  zb1=0.842;
  zb2=1.282;
 do rconc=0.30; **conditional prob of positive response among compliers;
    rcona=0.50; **conditional prob of positive response for always-takers;
    rconn=0.25; **conditional prob of positive response for never-takers;
    put rconc 1-10 3;
  do pattern= 1, 2,3;
    put pattern 10-30;
  do marprob=1 to 3;
   if marprob eq 1 then do;
    pc=0.95;
    pa=0.03;
    pn=0.02;    ** proportion of subpopulations in different;
       end;     ** categories;
   if marprob eq 2 then do;
    pc=0.80; pa=0.15; pn=0.05;
       end;
   if marprob eq 3 then do;
    pc=0.60; pa=0.25; pn=0.15;
       end;
   delta1=0.20;   ** maximum acceptance lower level for equivalence;
   deltau=0.25;   ** maximum acceptance upper level for equivalence;
   do or=0.90,1,1.1;   *true odds ratio of prop of response between two
treatments;
```

```
   do numk=0.5,1,2,4,8; *ratio of sample allocation between two
treatments;
   if numk=0.5 then m=1;
   if numk=1 then m=2;
   if numk=2 then m=3;
   if numk=4 then m=4;
   if numk=8 then m=5;
   if pattern eq 1 then do;  ** prob of nonmissing outcomes;
   nomissc1=1.0;  **for complier assigned to experimental  treatment;
   nomissc0=1.0;  **for complier assigned to standard treatment;;
   nomissa=1.0;    **for always takers;
   nomissn=1.0;    **for never takers;
   end;
   if pattern eq 2 then do;
   nomissc1=0.95;
   nomissc0=0.85;
   nomissa=0.90;
   nomissn=0.80;
   end;
   if pattern eq 3 then do;
   nomissc1=0.85;
   nomissc0=0.75;
   nomissa=0.80;
   nomissn=0.70;
   end;
    rconce=(rconc*or)/(rconc*or+(1-rconc));
    xp1=pc*rconce*nomissc1;
    xp2=pa*rcona*nomissa;
    xp3=pn*rconn*nomissn;
    xp4=pc*(1-rconce)*nomissc1;
    xp5=pa*(1-rcona)*nomissa;
    xp6=pn*(1-rconn)*nomissn;
    xp7=pc*(1-nomissc1);
    xp8=pa*(1-nomissa);
    xp9=pn*(1-nomissn);
    xpe1=xp1+xp2;
    xpe2=xp3;
    xpe3=xp4+xp5;
    xpe4=xp6;
    xpe5=xp7+xp8;
    xpe6=xp9;
    yp1=pc*rconc*nomissc0;
    yp2=pa*rcona*nomissa;
    yp3=pn*rconn*nomissn;
    yp4=pc*(1-rconc)*nomissc0;
    yp5=pa*(1-rcona)*nomissa;
    yp6=pn*(1-rconn)*nomissn;
    yp7=pc*(1-nomissc0);
    yp8=pa*(1-nomissa);
    yp9=pn*(1-nomissn);
    ype1=yp1+yp3;
```

```
ype2=yp2;
ype3=yp4+yp6;
ype4=yp5;
ype5=yp7+yp9;
ype6=yp8;
v1=(xpe1*(1-xpe1)+ype2*(1-ype2)/numk)/(xpe1-ype2)**2;
v2=(xpe4*(1-xpe4)+
   ype3*(1-ype3)/numk)/(ype3-xpe4)**2;
v3=(xpe3*(1-xpe3)+
   ype4*(1-ype4)/numk)/(xpe3-ype4)**2;
v4=(xpe2*(1-xpe2)+
   ype1*(1-ype1)/numk)/(ype1-xpe2)**2;
c12=(ype2*ype3/numk+xpe1*xpe4)/
   ((ype3-xpe4)*(xpe1-ype2));
c13=(ype2*ype4/numk+xpe1*xpe3)/
   ((xpe1-ype2)*(xpe3-ype4));
c14=(xpe1*xpe2+ype1*ype2/numk)/
   ((xpe1-ype2)*(ype1-xpe2));
c23=(xpe3*xpe4+ype4*ype3/numk)/
   ((xpe3-ype4)*(ype3-xpe4));
c24=(ype1*ype3/numk+xpe2*xpe4)/
   ((ype1-xpe2)*(ype3-xpe4));
c34=(ype1*ype4/numk+xpe3*xpe2)/
   ((xpe3-ype4)*(ype1-xpe2));
var=v1+v2+v3+v4+2*c12+2*c13-2*c14-2*c23+2*c24+2*c34;
if  round(or,0.00000001) lt 1.0 then n1=(za+zb1)**2*var/(log(or)-
log(1-deltal))**2;
if  round(or,0.00000001) eq 1.0 then n1=(za+zb2)**2*var/(log(1+deltau)
**2);
if  round(or,0.00000001) gt 1.0 then n1=(za+zb1)**2*var/(log(or)-
log(1+deltau))**2;
 sam=ceil(n1);
if m eq 5 then do;
put pc 1-5 2 pa 6-10 2 pn 11-15 2  or 16-20 2
 samx1 26-32 samx2 36-42 samx3 46-52 samx4 56-62 samx5 66-72;
end;  ** end of do if m eq 5;
end;  ** end of do numk;
end;  ** end of do rr;
end;  ** end of do marprob;
end;  ** do pattern;
end;  ** end of do rconc;
```

6

Randomized clinical trials with noncompliance in repeated binary measurements

Because of the nature of administering certain medical treatments, we may encounter a randomized clinical trial (RCT), in which one applies a treatment repeatedly to a patient at several courses of therapies and takes a binary measurement from the patient after the application of the treatment at each course. The RCT with repeated binary measurements per patient as focused here can also arise when studied patients are rare or relatively expensive to obtain in a RCT, and the patient response of interest can recurrently occur. For example, consider the treatment for acute myeloid leukaemia (AML) (Ohno, Miyawaki and Hatake et al., 1997). Three courses of consolidation chemotherapies with different drug combinations were planned after one or two courses of remission induction chemotherapy. For reduction of febrile neutropenia events among AML patients, a prophylactic use of macrophage colony stimulating factor (M-CSF) was compared to placebo at three courses of intensive and different combinations of chemotherapies (Matsuyama, 2002; Sato, 2001; Ohno, Miyawaki and Hatake et al., 1997) and whether an occurrence of a febrile neutropenia event on a patient in each of these courses was recorded.

Binary Data Analysis of Randomized Clinical Trials with Noncompliance, First Edition. Kung-Jong Lui.
© 2011 John Wiley & Sons, Ltd. Published 2011 by John Wiley & Sons, Ltd.

Table 6.1 summarizes the observed proportions of patients with febrile neutropenia events for the intention-to-treat (ITT) analysis at each course of chemotherapies in the M-CSF trial. We can see that use of M-CSF consistently reduces the febrile neutropenia risk at all courses of therapies. As noted in Chapter 2, however, use of the ITT analysis tends to underestimate the relative treatment effect when there are patients not complying with their assigned treatment under certain commonly assumed conditions. Thus, the development of test procedures and consistent estimators accounting for noncompliance in repeated binary data under such a RCT should be of use and interest in practice. Note that it is inappropriate to employ stratified analysis with strata formed by different therapeutic courses here. This is because patient responses taken from the same group of patients between different courses are likely to be correlated and hence the methods presented in Chapter 3 are inapplicable to the situations considered in this chapter.

Table 6.1 The observed proportions of patients with febrile neutropenia incidence at each course of chemotherapies in the M-CSF trial.

Course $J =$	M-CSF	Placebo	Risk Difference
1	0.644	0.758	−0.115
2	0.598	0.697	−0.099
3	0.280	0.432	−0.152

Following Matsuyama (2002) and Sato (2001), we assume structural risk models for the potential outcomes of each patient when he/she receives the experimental treatment or placebo in repeated binary measurements. Under the commonly assumed assumptions for a RCT with noncompliance, including the stable unit treatment value assumption (SUTVA) (Rubin, 1978), the monotonicity assumption (Angrist, Imbens and Rubin, 1996; Brunner and Neumann, 1985; Zhou and Li, 2006), the exclusion restriction assumption for the patient responses (Angrist, Imbens and Rubin, 1996; Frangakis and Rubin, 1999) and the strong exclusion restriction assumption for the treatment-receipt among always-takers and never-takers defined here, we focus our attention on the situations in which a binary measurement is taken after the application of a treatment at each of multiple courses in the presence of noncompliance. In Section 6.1, we present procedures for testing superiority using the ITT analysis in a RCT with noncompliance. When using the proportion difference (PD) and proportion ratio (PR) to measure the relative treatment effect, we develop procedures accounting for noncompliance in testing noninferiority and equivalence in repeated binary data in Section 6.2 and Section 6.3, respectively. We further discuss interval estimation of the PD and PR under the assumed structural risk models in Section 6.4. Finally, we address sample size determination for testing superiority, noninferiority, and equivalence based on the proposed test procedures in Section 6.5. Note that the structural risk models for binary data proposed by Sato (2001) and Matsuyama (2002) are actually related to the general class of structural mean model (SMM) proposed and discussed elsewhere (Robins, 1994; Clarke and Windmeijer, 2010; Bellamy, Lin and Ten Have, 2007).

Suppose that we randomly assign n_g patients to an experimental treatment ($g = 1$) and a standard treatment (or placebo) ($g = 0$), respectively. For patient i ($= 1, 2, \ldots, n_g$) assigned to treatment g at course j ($= 1, 2, \ldots, J$), the patient would receive the assigned treatment if he/she accepted, or would receive the other, otherwise. We focus our discussion on the situation in which each patient receives exactly one of the two treatments under comparison at each course. To estimate the treatment efficacy, we make the SUTVA and the exclusion restriction assumption (Sato, 2001; Angrist, Imbens and Rubin, 1996; Matsuyama, 2002). The former is to assume that there is no interference between patients, while the latter is to assume that the response is not affected by the treatment assigned, but rather by the treatment actually received. Let $Y_{ij}^{(g)}$ denote the random variable of response for patient i assigned to treatment g at course j, and $Y_{ij}^{(g)} = 1$ if the patient has a positive response, and $= 0$, otherwise. Similarly, let $Z_{ij}^{(g)}$ denote the random variable of treatment receipt right before taking the response $Y_{ij}^{(g)}$ for the corresponding patient, and $Z_{ij}^{(g)} = 1$ if patient i assigned to treatment g at course j actually receives the experimental treatment, and $= 0$, otherwise. For each patient at the initial course ($j = 1$), we define the vector $(d(1), d(0))$ as his/her potential treatment-received status: $d(g) = 1$ if the patient assigned to treatment g actually receives the experimental treatment, and $d(g) = 0$ otherwise. Thus, we can divide our sampling population into four subpopulations on the basis of the potential treatment-received status at the initial course. These include compliers (C) ($d(1) = 1$ and $d(0) = 0$), never-takers (N) ($d(1) = d(0) = 0$), always-takers (A) ($d(1) = d(0) = 1$), and defiers (D) ($d(1) = 0$ and $d(0) = 1$). We assume monotonicity ($d(1) \geq d(0)$) or no defiers here. Note that, by definition, if $i \in A$ (always-takers), then $Z_{i1}^{(g)} = 1$ at course $j = 1$ regardless of his/her assigned treatment g ($g = 1, 0$). Similarly, if $i \in N$ (never-takers), then $Z_{i1}^{(g)} = 0$ despite of his/her assigned treatment g. Also, if $i \in C$ (compliers), then we have, by definition, $Z_{i1}^{(1)} = 1$ and $Z_{i1}^{(0)} = 0$. Because the effect due to an experimental treatment relative to the standard treatment (placebo) on a patient response may vary between subpopulations, we assume the following structural risk additive model for the underlying probability of a positive response on patient i ($i = 1, 2, \ldots, n_g$) assigned to treatment g ($g = 1, 0$) at course j ($j = 1, 2, \ldots, J$) (Lui, 2007c):

$$
\begin{aligned}
P(Y_{ij}^{(g)} = 1 | p_{ij}^{(g)}, z_{ij}^{(g)}) &= p_{ij}^{(g)} + \Delta_C z_{ij}^{(g)} \quad \text{if patient } i \in C, \\
&= p_{ij}^{(g)} + \Delta_A z_{ij}^{(g)} \quad \text{if patient } i \in A, \\
&= p_{ij}^{(g)} + \Delta_N z_{ij}^{(g)} \quad \text{if patient } i \in N, \quad (6.1)
\end{aligned}
$$

where $p_{ij}^{(g)}$ denotes the underlying basic probability of a positive response when patient i assigned to treatment g is assumed to receive the standard treatment (or placebo) at course j; Δ_S represents the excess effect due to the experimental treatment on the patient response from subpopulation S ($S = C, A, N$) over the standard treatment (or placebo). In other words, patient i assigned to treatment g from subpopulation S would have the probability $p_{ij}^{(g)} + \Delta_S$ of a positive response at course j if he/she took the experimental treatment, or the probability $p_{ij}^{(g)}$ of a positive response if he/she took the standard treatment (or placebo). Note that for each patient only one of the potential outcomes corresponding to these two probabilities can be observed in practice. This is often called the counterfactual approach. The parameter Δ_C defined in model (6.1) actually represents the complier average causal effect (CACE) and is the parameter of our focus here.

Note also that model (6.1) includes the constant risk additive model considered elsewhere (Sato, 2000, 2001; Matsuyama, 2002; Matsui, 2005; Lui, 2007g) as a special case when $\Delta_C = \Delta_A = \Delta_N$ (Lui, 2007c). As assumed elsewhere (Sato, 2001; Matsuyama, 2002), we assume that there is no carry over treatment effect in the following discussion as well. Because patients are randomly assigned to one of two treatments, the expected number of positive responses over J courses for a randomly selected patient i from the assigned experimental treatment and that for a randomly selected patient i' from the assigned standard treatment (or placebo) are expected to equal each other if patients are all assumed to receive the standard treatment (or placebo); that is, $E(p_{i+}^{(1)}) = E(p_{i'+}^{(0)})$, where $p_{i+}^{(g)} = \sum_j p_{ij}^{(g)}$. Define $Y_{i+}^{(g)} = \sum_j Y_{ij}^{(g)}$ and $Z_{i+}^{(g)} = \sum_j Z_{ij}^{(g)}$, which represent over J courses ($i = 1, 2, \ldots, n_g$) in the assigned treatment g ($g = 1, 0$) the number of times for patient i having a positive response and the number of times for patient i receiving the experimental treatment, respectively.

Note that whether a patient continues taking the same treatment as that at the previous course or switches to receive the other treatment can depend on the previous outcome. Thus, the expected number of times for receiving the experimental treatment for an always-taker $E(Z_{i+}^{(g)}|A)$ may not necessarily equal J. Similarly, the expected number of times for receiving the experimental treatment for a never-taker $E(Z_{i+}^{(g)}|N)$ may also not equal 0. However, we may reasonably assume that both $E(Z_{i+}^{(1)}|A) = E(Z_{i'+}^{(0)}|A)$ and $E(Z_{i+}^{(1)}|N) = E(Z_{i'+}^{(0)}|N)$ hold for given two randomly selected patients i and i' from the assigned experimental ($g = 1$) and standard ($g = 0$) treatments, respectively. This is because patients, who are always-takers (or never-takers), are randomly assigned to either of the two treatments in a RCT, come from the same sub-population, and begin with taking the same experimental (or standard) treatment at the initial course despite what treatment they are assigned to. Thus, we may reasonably assume that the random variable $Z_{ij}^{(g)}$ of treatment receipt for patients who are always-takers (or never-takers) follows the same stochastic process between the two assigned treatments, especially in a double-blind trial. We may call this the strong exclusion restriction assumption of treatment-receipt for always-takers and never-takers.

Note that both $Y_{i+}^{(g)}$ and $Z_{i+}^{(g)}$ can take one of the possible values: $0, 1, 2, \ldots, J$. Let $n_{rc}^{(g)}$ denote the number of patients with $(Y_{i+}^{(g)} = r, Z_{i+}^{(g)} = c)$, where $r = 0, 1, 2, \ldots, J$ and $c = 0, 1, 2, \ldots, J$, among n_g patients assigned to treatment g. Then the random numbers $\{n_{rc}^{(g)} | r = 0, 1, 2, \ldots, J$ and $c = 0, 1, 2, \ldots, J\}$ follow the multinomial distribution with parameters n_g and $\underline{\pi}'_g = (\pi_{00}^{(g)}, \pi_{01}^{(g)}, \ldots, \pi_{0J}^{(g)}, \pi_{10}^{(g)}, \pi_{11}^{(g)}, \ldots, \pi_{1J}^{(g)}, \ldots, \pi_{J0}^{(g)}, \pi_{J1}^{(g)}, \ldots, \pi_{JJ}^{(g)})$, where $\pi_{rc}^{(g)}$ denotes the cell probability that a randomly selected patient from the assigned treatment g has $(Y_{i+}^{(g)} = r, Z_{i+}^{(g)} = c)$. A commonly used unbiased consistent estimator for $\pi_{rc}^{(g)}$ is simply $\hat{\pi}_{rc}^{(g)} = n_{rc}^{(g)}/n_g$. Therefore, we can estimate the marginal probabilities $P(Y_{i+}^{(g)} = r) = \pi_{r+}^{(g)}$ and $P(Z_{i+}^{(g)} = c) = \pi_{+c}^{(g)}$ by $\hat{\pi}_{r+}^{(g)} = \sum_c n_{rc}^{(g)}/n_g$ and $\hat{\pi}_{+c}^{(g)} = \sum_r n_{rc}^{(g)}/n_g$, respectively.

Define $\overline{\overline{Y}}_{++}^{(g)} = \sum_i Y_{i+}^{(g)}/(n_g J) = \sum_r (r/J)\hat{\pi}_{r+}^{(g)}$, the proportion of a positive response over J repeated binary measurements among n_g patients assigned to treatment g ($g = 1, 0$). Furthermore, define $\overline{\overline{Z}}_{++}^{(g)} = \sum_i Z_{i+}^{(g)}/(n_g J) = \sum_c (c/J)\hat{\pi}_{+c}^{(g)}$ ($g = 1, 0$), the proportion of times for receiving the experimental treatment over J repeated binary measurements among n_g patients assigned to treatment g. Note that the PD estimator $\hat{\delta}^{(RE)} = \overline{\overline{Y}}_{++}^{(1)} - \overline{\overline{Y}}_{++}^{(0)}$ for the ITT analysis estimates, as noted in the previous chapters, the programmatic effectiveness rather than treatment efficacy. Based on the above model assumptions, we can show that (Exercise 6.1)

$$E(\hat{\delta}^{(RE)}) = \Delta_C E(\overline{\overline{Z}}_{++}^{(1)} - \overline{\overline{Z}}_{++}^{(0)})$$
$$= \Delta_C \left(\sum_c (c/J)\pi_{+c}^{(1)} - \sum_c (c/J)\pi_{+c}^{(0)} \right), \qquad (6.2)$$

where the multiplicative factor (MF) $(\sum_c (c/J)\pi_{+c}^{(1)} - \sum_c (c/J)\pi_{+c}^{(0)})$ represents the difference in the expected proportion of times for receiving the experimental treatment per patient between the assigned experimental treatment and the assigned standard treatment (or placebo). For the case of a single measurement per patient (i.e. $J = 1$), this MF simply represents the subpopulation proportion of compliers under the monotonicity assumption. When every patient complies his/her assigned treatment at all courses, the MF reaches its maximum value of 1, and thereby the ITT estimator $\hat{\delta}^{(RE)}$ is an unbiased estimator of Δ_C in this particular case. Note that the MF should be positive in most practically encountered cases. Note also that the above MF is often specific to a given RCT and can vary between trials. Thus, the programmatic effectiveness in the ITT analysis tends to, as noted in Chapter 2, vary between trials even for a given fixed treatment efficacy Δ_C. Note also that because the absolute value of MF always falls in the range $0 \leq MF \leq 1$, using $|\overline{\overline{Y}}_{++}^{(1)} - \overline{\overline{Y}}_{++}^{(0)}|$ is likely to attenuate the absolute treatment effect $|\Delta_C|$ in the presence of noncompliance under the above assumed conditions. Furthermore, we can easily show that an estimated variance for $\overline{\overline{Y}}_{++}^{(g)}$ (for $g = 1, 0$) is given by (Exercise 6.2):

$$\hat{Var}(\overline{\overline{Y}}_{++}^{(g)}) = [\sum_r (r/J)^2 \hat{\pi}_{r+}^{(g)} - (\sum_r (r/J)\hat{\pi}_{r+}^{(g)})^2]/n_g. \tag{6.3}$$

In the following discussion, when there is no confusion, we denote Δ_C by Δ for simplicity in notation. Note that the above results can be extended to a structural risk model accounting a possible variation of the experimental treatment effect between patients and repeated measurements under additional assumptions (Exercise 6.3).

6.1   Testing superiority

When comparing an experimental treatment with a standard treatment, we often want to test the superiority of the former to the latter with respect to the treatment efficacy. For ethical and safety reasons, however, we consider doing a two-sided test instead of a one-side test here (Fleiss, 1981). In other words, we want to test the null hypothesis $H_0 : \Delta = 0$ versus $H_a : \Delta \neq 0$. From Equation (6.2), we can see that the expectation $E(\hat{\delta}^{(RE)}) = E(\overline{\overline{Y}}_{++}^{(1)} - \overline{\overline{Y}}_{++}^{(0)}) = 0$ if and only if $\Delta = 0$ (unless the MF equals 0). Thus, we may consider applying the following test statistic based on $\hat{\delta}^{(RE)}$ ($= \overline{\overline{Y}}_{++}^{(1)} - \overline{\overline{Y}}_{++}^{(0)}$) for the ITT analysis to test $H_0 : \Delta = 0$:

$$Z = \hat{\delta}^{(RE)} / \sqrt{\hat{Var}(\hat{\delta}^{(RE)} | H_0)}, \tag{6.4}$$

where $\hat{Var}(\hat{\delta}^{(RE)}|H_0) = [\sum_r (r/J)^2 \hat{\bar{\pi}}_{r+}^{(p)} - (\sum_r (r/J)\hat{\bar{\pi}}_{r+}^{(p)})^2](1/n_1 + 1/n_0)$
and where $\hat{\bar{\pi}}_{r+}^{(p)} = (n_1\hat{\pi}_{r+}^{(1)} + n_0\hat{\pi}_{r+}^{(0)})/(n_1 + n_0)$ for $r = 0, 1, 2, \ldots, J$. If
the test statistic (6.4), $Z > Z_{\alpha/2}$ or $Z < -Z_{\alpha/2}$, we will reject $H_0 : \Delta = 0$
at the α-level. Furthermore, we will claim that the experimental treatment
is superior to the standard treatment if the test statistic (6.4), $Z > Z_{\alpha/2}$.
As noted in the previous chapters, we may also consider use of the
$\tanh^{-1}(x)$ transformation when employing the test statistic (6.4). Since
the asymptotic variance $\hat{Var}(\tanh^{-1}(\hat{\delta}^{(RE)}|H_0)) = \hat{Var}(\hat{\delta}^{(RE)}|H_0)$ under H_0,
this leads us to obtain the following statistic for testing $H_0 : \Delta = 0$:

$$Z = \tanh^{-1}(\hat{\delta}^{(RE)})/\sqrt{\hat{Var}(\hat{\delta}^{(RE)}|H_0)}. \tag{6.5}$$

We reject $H_0 : \Delta = 0$ at the α-level if the statistic (6.5), $Z > Z_{\alpha/2}$ or
$Z < -Z_{\alpha/2}$, and claim that the experimental treatment is superior to the
standard treatment if $Z > Z_{\alpha/2}$ holds. Note that when $J = 1$, test statistics (6.4) and (6.5) reduce to test statistics (2.3) and (2.4), respectively
(Exercise 6.4).

When the MF is greater than 0, we can easily see from Equation (6.2)
that

$$\Delta = (E(\overline{\overline{Y}}_{++}^{(1)}) - E(\overline{\overline{Y}}_{++}^{(0)}))/(E(\overline{\overline{Z}}_{++}^{(1)}) - E(\overline{\overline{Z}}_{++}^{(0)}))$$
$$= (\sum_r r\pi_{r+}^{(1)} - \sum_r r\pi_{r+}^{(0)})/(\sum_c c\pi_{+c}^{(1)} - \sum_c c\pi_{+c}^{(0)}). \tag{6.6}$$

Thus, we can substitute $\hat{\pi}_{r+}^{(g)}$ for $\pi_{r+}^{(g)}$, and $\hat{\pi}_{+c}^{(g)}$ for $\pi_{+c}^{(g)}$ in Equation (6.6),
and obtain a consistent estimator for Δ as

$$\hat{\Delta}^{(RE)} = (\sum_r r\hat{\pi}_{r+}^{(1)} - \sum_r r\hat{\pi}_{r+}^{(0)})/(\sum_c c\hat{\pi}_{+c}^{(1)} - \sum_c c\hat{\pi}_{+c}^{(0)}),$$
$$= (\overline{Y}_{++}^{(1)} - \overline{Y}_{++}^{(0)})/(\overline{Z}_{++}^{(1)} - \overline{Z}_{++}^{(0)}), \tag{6.7}$$

where $\overline{Y}_{++}^{(g)} = \sum_i Y_{i+}^{(g)}/n_g$ and $\overline{Z}_{++}^{(g)} = \sum_i Z_{i+}^{(g)}/n_g$, which denote the
average number of having positive responses per patient and the aver-
age time of receiving the experimental treatment per patient among n_g
subjects assigned to treatment g $(= 1, 0)$, respectively.

Sjölander (2008) noted that the constant risk model (i.e. $\Delta_C = \Delta_A = \Delta_N$) considered elsewhere (Sato, 2001; Matsuyama, 2002) implicitly
assumes that there are no latent covariate effects on the received treat-
ments and patient outcomes. Sjölander (2008) noted further that this

assumption is likely too strong to hold in most practically encountered situations. By contrast, we do allow the effect due to some latent covariates on the received treatments and patient outcomes through the status of the latent subpopulation under model (1). However, the estimator $\hat{\Delta}^{(RE)}$ (6.7) obtained here is actually identical to the estimator derived under a constant risk additive model proposed by Sato (2001) and Matsuyama (2002) based on a randomization-based approach. In other words, the estimator proposed by Sato (2001) and Matsuyama (2002) can be still valid for use under the risk additive model (1) assumed here. Note also that $\hat{\Delta}^{(RE)}$ (6.7) is an extension of the instrumental variable estimator (Angrist, Imbens and Rubin, 1996) to accommodate repeated binary measurements (Sato, 2001). When there is only a single measurement per patient (i.e. $J = 1$), the estimator $\hat{\Delta}^{(RE)}$ (6.7) reduces to $\hat{\Delta}$ (2.5) under the monotonicity assumption (see Section 2.6.3).

Example 6.1   Consider the data taken from a randomized multi-center double-blind trial in which we study the effect of taking M-CSF ($g = 1$) versus placebo ($g = 0$) on febrile neutropenia incidence for AML patients over three courses of intensive chemotherapies (Sato, 2001; Matsuyama, 2002; Ohno, Miyawaki and Hatake et al., 1997). There were 178 eligible patients who participated in the beginning of the trial. However, 7 patients were lost to follow-up at the end of the first course and 15 patients were lost to follow-up at the end of the second course. For illustration purpose only, we assume that missing completely at random (MCAR) and consider the data consisting of only the 156 patients with complete information over three courses. There were only two patients assigned to M-CSF treatment who did not comply with their assigned treatment at the third course, while every patients assigned to the placebo complied with their assigned treatment. We summarize the observed frequencies $n_{rs}^{(g)}$ patients with ($Y_{i+}^{(g)} = r$, $Z_{i+}^{(g)} = c$) in Table 6.2. Based on these data, we obtain the ITT estimate $\hat{\delta}^{(RE)}$ of the PD for febrile neutropenia incidence among AML patients between taking the M-CSF and placebo in the ITT analysis to be -0.111. By contrast, the estimate $\hat{\Delta}^{(RE)}$ (6.7) for the PD in compliers is -0.112. These two estimates are similar to each other due to the fact that compliance to the assigned treatment in this trial is quite high. When employing statistics (6.4) and (6.5) for testing superiority, we have found p-values to be 0.022 and 0.017, which of both suggest significant evidence that using M-CSF can reduce febrile neutropenia incidence among AML patients at the 5 % level.

6.2 Testing noninferiority

Since the establishment of superiority for an experimental treatment versus a standard treatment is much more difficult than that for an experimental treatment versus a placebo, we may often consider testing noninferiority of the experimental treatment to the standard treatment with respect to the treatment efficacy when it is unethical to have a placebo control. This is true especially when the former is less expensive and is easier to administer than the latter. In the following section, we discuss testing noninferiority in repeated binary measurements under a RCT with noncompliance.

6.2.1   Using the difference in proportions

When using the PD of a positive response to measure the relative treatment effect in assessing noninferiority, we want to test $H_0 : \Delta \leq -\varepsilon_l$ versus $H_a : \Delta > -\varepsilon_l$, where ε_l is the maximum clinically acceptable margin that the experimental treatment can be regarded as noninferior to the standard treatment when $\Delta > -\varepsilon_l$ holds. Note that the noninferiority of an experimental treatment to a standard treatment with respect to the programmatic effectiveness does not necessarily imply the noninferiority of the former to the latter with respect to the treatment efficacy (Exercise 2.7). Thus, we consider directly using the test statistic $\hat{\Delta}^{(RE)}$ (6.7) instead of $\hat{\delta}^{(RE)}(= \overline{\overline{Y}}_{++}^{(1)} - \overline{\overline{Y}}_{++}^{(0)})$ in testing noninferiority. Using the delta method (Agresti, 1990; Lui, 2004), we obtain the estimated asymptotic variance for $\hat{\Delta}^{(RE)}$ (6.7) as given by (Exercise 6.5):

$$
\begin{aligned}
\hat{Var}(\hat{\Delta}^{(RE)}) = \sum_g \Big\{ &\sum_r r^2 \hat{\pi}_{r+}^{(g)} - \Big(\sum_r r \hat{\pi}_{r+}^{(g)} \Big)^2 - 2\hat{\Delta}^{(RE)} \Big(\sum_r \sum_c rc \hat{\pi}_{rc}^{(g)} \\
&- \Big(\sum_r r\hat{\pi}_{r+}^{(g)} \Big) \Big(\sum_c c\hat{\pi}_{+c}^{(g)} \Big) \Big) + \hat{\Delta}^{(RE)^2} \Big(\sum_c c^2 \hat{\pi}_{+c}^{(g)} \\
&- \Big(\sum_c c\hat{\pi}_{+c}^{(g)} \Big)^2 \Big) \Big\} / [n_g (\sum_c c\hat{\pi}_{+c}^{(1)} - \sum_c c\hat{\pi}_{+c}^{(0)})^2].
\end{aligned} \tag{6.8}
$$

On the basis of the test statistic $\hat{\Delta}^{(RE)}$ (6.7) with the $\tanh^{-1}(x)$ transformation and the estimated variance $\hat{Var}(\hat{\Delta}^{(RE)})$ (6.8), we will reject $H_0 : \Delta \leq -\varepsilon_l$ at the α-level and claim that the experimental treatment is noninferior to the standard treatment if

$$Z = (\tanh^{-1}(\hat{\Delta}^{(RE)}) + \tanh^{-1}(\varepsilon_l))/\sqrt{\hat{Var}(\tanh^{-1}(\hat{\Delta}^{(RE)}))} > Z_\alpha, \quad (6.9)$$

where $\hat{Var}(\tanh^{-1}(\hat{\Delta}^{(RE)})) = \hat{Var}(\hat{\Delta}^{(RE)})/(1 - (\hat{\Delta}^{(RE)})^2)^2$. Note that the test statistic (6.9) reduces to statistic (2.7) for testing noninferiority when we take a single one measurement per patient under the monotonicity assumption (Exercise 6.6).

6.2.2   Using the ratio of proportions

When we may have the difficulty in determination of a pre-determined noninferior margin ε_l on the PD scale, we may consider use of the PR instead of the PD to measure the relative treatment efficacy in establishing noninferiority. This can occur when the underlying patient response rate for a standard treatment varies substantially between trials. Furthermore, when the experimental treatment effect relative to the standard treatment is believed to be multiplicative, it may also be logically appealing to use the PR (rather than the PD) to measure the treatment efficacy. Considering a possible variation of the relative effect of an experimental treatment to a standard treatment on the patient response between sub-populations, we assume the structural risk multiplicative model (Lui, 2007c) for the underlying probability of a positive response on patient i ($i = 1, 2, \ldots, n_g$) assigned to treatment g ($g = 1, 0$) at course j ($j = 1, 2, \ldots, J$) as given by:

$$P(Y_{ij}^{(g)} = 1 | p_{ij}^{(g)}, z_{ij}^{(g)}) = p_{ij}^{(g)} \gamma_C^{z_{ij}^{(g)}} \quad \text{if patient } i \in C,$$

$$= p_{ij}^{(g)} \gamma_A^{z_{ij}^{(g)}} \quad \text{if patient } i \in A,$$

$$= p_{ij}^{(g)} \gamma_N^{z_{ij}^{(g)}} \quad \text{if patient } i \in N, \quad (6.10)$$

where $p_{ij}^{(g)}$ denotes the underlying probability of a positive response when patient i assigned to treatment g is assumed to receive the standard treatment (or placebo) at course j; and γ_S (> 0) represents the experimental treatment effect relative to the standard treatment (or placebo) effect on the positive response of a patient from subpopulation S for $S = C, A, N$. Therefore, patient i assigned to treatment g from population S would have the probability $p_{ij}^{(g)} \gamma_S$ of a positive response at course j if he/she received the experimental treatment (i.e. $z_{ij}^{(g)} = 1$), or the probability $p_{ij}^{(g)}$ of a positive response if he/she received the standard treatment or placebo (i.e. $z_{ij}^{(g)} = 0$). We define $X_{i+}^{(g)} = \sum_j Y_{ij}^{(g)} Z_{ij}^{(g)}$ and $X_{i+}^{(g)^*} = \sum_j Y_{ij}^{(g)} (1 - Z_{ij}^{(g)})$, representing the number of positive responses over J repeated binary measurements on patient i assigned to treatment g when he/she takes the experimental treatment and that when he/she takes the standard treatment, respectively.

Note that because the total number $\sum_j Y_{ij}^{(g)}$ ($= X_{i+}^{(g)} + X_{i+}^{(g)^*}$) of positive responses for a patient despite what treatment he/she actually receives cannot exceed the maximum possible number of responses over J therapeutic courses, the case of $(X_{i+}^{(g)} = r, X_{i+}^{(g)^*} = c)$ with $r + c > J$ has the structure probability equal to 0. Let $f_{rc}^{(g)}$ denote the number of patients among n_g patients assigned to treatment g with the bivariate vector $(X_{i+}^{(g)} = r, X_{i+}^{(g)^*} = c)$, where $r = 0, 1, 2, \ldots, J$, and $c = 0, 1, 2, \ldots, J - r$. We may assume that the random numbers $\{f_{rc}^{(g)} | r = 0, 1, 2, \ldots, J, c = 0, 1, 2, \ldots, J - r\}$ follow the multinomial distribution with parameters n_g and $\{E_{rc}^{(g)} | r = 0, 1, 2, \ldots, J, c = 0, 1, 2, \ldots, J - r\}$, where $E_{rc}^{(g)}$ denotes the cell probability that a randomly selected patient i from the assigned treatment g has the bivariate vector $(X_{i+}^{(g)} = r, X_{i+}^{(g)^*} = c)$. A commonly used unbiased consistent estimator for $E_{rc}^{(g)}$ is simply $\hat{E}_{rc}^{(g)} = f_{rc}^{(g)} / n_g$ and thereby, we can estimate the marginal probabilities: $P(X_{i+}^{(g)} = r) = E_{r+}^{(g)}$ and $P(X_{i+}^{(g)^*} = c) = E_{+c}^{(g)}$ by $\hat{E}_{r+}^{(g)} = \sum_c f_{rc}^{(g)} / n_g$ and $\hat{E}_{+c}^{(g)} = \sum_r f_{rc}^{(g)} / n_g$, respectively. We here assume that there is no carry over treatment effects as well. The parameter γ_C for compliers is of our interest and is denoted by γ for simplicity. Under the model assumption (6.10) and the strong exclusion restriction assumption for the treatment-receipt for always-takers and never-takers as described previously, we can show that (Exercise 6.7):

$$\gamma = [E(X_{i+}^{(1)}) - E(X_{i'+}^{(0)})] / [E(X_{i'+}^{(0)^*}) - E(X_{i+}^{(1)^*})]$$

$$= \left(\sum_r r E_{r+}^{(1)} - \sum_r r E_{r+}^{(0)}\right) / \left(\sum_c c E_{+c}^{(0)} - \sum_c c E_{+c}^{(1)}\right) \quad (6.11)$$

when $E(X_{i'+}^{(0)*}) - E(X_{i+}^{(1)*}) = \sum_c cE_{+c}^{(0)} - \sum_c cE_{+c}^{(1)} > 0$. By substituting $\hat{E}_{r+}^{(g)}$ for $E_{r+}^{(g)}$ and $\hat{E}_{+c}^{(g)}$ for $E_{+c}^{(g)}$ in (6.11), we obtain the consistent estimator for γ as given by

$$\hat{\gamma}^{(RE)} = (\sum_r r\hat{E}_{r+}^{(1)} - \sum_r r\hat{E}_{r+}^{(0)})/(\sum_c c\hat{E}_{+c}^{(0)} - \sum_c c\hat{E}_{+c}^{(1)}). \qquad (6.12)$$

Note that the estimator $\hat{\gamma}^{(RE)}$ (6.12) is identical to the estimator for γ derived under a constant risk multiplicative model discussed elsewhere (Sato, 2000, 2001; Matsuyama, 2002; Matsui, 2005; Lui, 2007b). Note further that $\hat{\gamma}^{(RE)}$ reduces to $\hat{\gamma}$ (2.9) for the PR when we take a single one measurement per patient under the monotonicity assumption. When applying the delta method, we can show that the estimated asymptotic variance for $\hat{\gamma}^{(RE)}$ (6.12) is given by (Exercise 6.8):

$$\hat{Var}(\hat{\gamma}^{(RE)}) = \sum_g \{\sum_r r^2 \hat{E}_{r+}^{(g)} - (\sum_r r\hat{E}_{r+}^{(g)})^2 + 2\hat{\gamma}^{(RE)}(\sum_r \sum_c rc\hat{E}_{rc}^{(g)}$$
$$- (\sum_r r\hat{E}_{r+}^{(g)})(\sum_c c\hat{E}_{+c}^{(g)})) + \hat{\gamma}^{(RE)^2}(\sum_c c^2 \hat{E}_{+c}^{(g)}$$
$$- (\sum_c c\hat{E}_{+c}^{(g)})^2)\}/[n_g(\sum_c c\hat{E}_{+c}^{(0)} - \sum_c c\hat{E}_{+c}^{(1)})^2]. \qquad (6.13)$$

For assessing noninferiority, we want to test $H_0 : \gamma \leq 1 - \gamma_l$ versus $H_a : \gamma > 1 - \gamma_l$, where γ_l is the maximum clinically acceptable margin such that the experimental treatment can be regarded as noninferior to the standard treatment. On the basis of the statistic $\hat{\gamma}^{(RE)}$ (6.12) and the estimated variance $\hat{Var}(\hat{\gamma}^{(RE)})$ (6.13), we may consider the following test statistic with the logarithmic transformation,

$$Z = (\log(\hat{\gamma}^{(RE)}) - \log(1 - \gamma_l))/\sqrt{\hat{Var}(\log(\hat{\gamma}^{(RE)}))}, \qquad (6.14)$$

where $\hat{Var}(\log(\hat{\gamma}^{(RE)})) = \hat{Var}(\hat{\gamma}^{(RE)})/\hat{\gamma}^{(RE)^2}$. We reject $H_0 : \gamma \leq 1 - \gamma_l$ and claim that the experimental treatment is noninferior to the standard treatment at the α-level when the test statistic (6.14), $Z > Z_\alpha$. Note that when $J = 1$, the test statistic (6.14) reduces to the test statistic (2.11) for a single measurement per patient (Exercise 6.9).

6.3   Testing equivalence

When a generic drug is developed, we may sometimes wish to test equivalence rather than noninferiority with respect to the therapeutic efficacy due to the concern of toxicity (Dunnett and Gent, 1977; Westlake, 1974 and 1979). For brevity, we only outline the test procedures for assessing equivalence under a RCT with noncompliance in repeated binary measurements in the following.

6.3.1   Using the difference in proportions

When using the PD of a positive response to measure the relative treatment effect in establishing equivalence, we want to test $H_0 : \Delta \leq -\varepsilon_l$ or $\Delta \geq \varepsilon_u$ versus $H_a : -\varepsilon_l < \Delta < \varepsilon_u$, where ε_l and ε_u (> 0) are the maximum clinically acceptable lower and upper margins that an experimental treatment can be regarded as equivalent to a standard treatment and are pre-determined by clinicians. Using the Intersection-Union test (Casella and Berger, 1990), we will reject the null hypothesis $H_0 : \Delta \leq -\varepsilon_l$ or $\Delta \geq \varepsilon_u$ at the α-level and claim that the two treatments are equivalent if the test statistic $\tanh^{-1}(\hat{\Delta}^{(RE)})$ simultaneously satisfies the following two inequalities:

$$(\tanh^{-1}(\Delta^{(RE)}) + \tanh^{-1}(\varepsilon_l))/\sqrt{\hat{Var}(\tanh^{-1}(\hat{\Delta}^{(RE)}))} > Z_\alpha$$

$$\text{and} \quad (\tanh^{-1}(\hat{\Delta}^{(RE)}) - \tanh^{-1}(\varepsilon_u))/\sqrt{\hat{Var}(\tanh^{-1}(\hat{\Delta}^{(RE)}))} < -Z_\alpha,$$

$$(6.15)$$

where $\hat{Var}(\tanh^{-1}(\hat{\Delta}^{(RE)})) = \hat{Var}(\hat{\Delta}^{(RE)})/(1 - (\hat{\Delta}^{(RE)})^2)^2$, $\hat{\Delta}^{(RE)}$ and $\hat{Var}(\hat{\Delta}^{(RE)})$ are given in (6.7) and (6.8), respectively.

6.3.2   Using the ratio of proportions

When considering use of the PR to measure the relative treatment effect in establishing equivalence, we want to test $H_0 : \gamma \leq 1 - \gamma_l$ or $\gamma \geq 1 + \gamma_u$ versus $H_a : 1 - \gamma_l < \gamma < 1 + \gamma_u$ where γ_l and γ_u (> 0) are the maximum clinically acceptable lower and upper margins that the experimental treatment can be regarded as equivalent to the standard treatment. We will reject $H_0 : \gamma \leq 1 - \gamma_l$ or $\gamma \geq 1 + \gamma_u$ at the α-level and claim that two treatments are equivalent if the test statistic $\log(\hat{\gamma}^{(RE)})$ simultaneously satisfies the following two inequalities:

$$(\log(\hat{\gamma}^{(RE)}) - \log(1 - \gamma_l))/\sqrt{\hat{Var}(\log(\hat{\gamma}^{(RE)}))} > Z_\alpha.$$

$$\text{and} \quad (\log(\hat{\gamma}^{(RE)}) - \log(1 + \gamma_u))/\sqrt{\hat{Var}(\log(\hat{\gamma}^{(RE)}))} < -Z_\alpha, \quad (6.16)$$

where $\hat{Var}(\log(\hat{\gamma}^{(RE)})) = \hat{Var}(\hat{\gamma}^{(RE)})/(\hat{\gamma}^{(RE)})^2$, $\hat{\gamma}^{(RE)}$ and $\hat{Var}(\hat{\gamma}^{(RE)})$ are given in (6.12) and (6.13), respectively.

6.4   Interval estimation

When reporting the efficacy of an experimental treatment, we often present an interval estimate of the index used to measure the treatment effect in a RCT. This is because the confidence level and the width of a good interval estimator can provide us with the useful information on both the accuracy and the precision of our inference. Furthermore, the range of a confidence interval may also give us the magnitude of the underlying treatment effect. We discuss interval estimation of the PD and PR under a RCT with noncompliance in repeated binary measurements in this section.

6.4.1   Estimation of the proportion difference

First, we consider interval estimation of the PD Δ $(= \Delta_C)$ under model (6.1). On the basis of $\hat{\Delta}^{(RE)}$ (6.7) and $\hat{Var}(\hat{\Delta}^{(RE)})$ (6.8), we may obtain an asymptotic $100 (1 - \alpha) \%$ confidence interval using Wald's statistic for Δ as

$$[\max\{\hat{\Delta}^{(RE)} - Z_{\alpha/2}(\hat{Var}(\hat{\Delta}^{(RE)}))^{1/2}, -1\}, \min\{\hat{\Delta}^{(RE)} + Z_{\alpha/2}(\hat{Var}(\hat{\Delta}^{(RE)}))^{1/2}, 1\}],$$

$$(6.17)$$

where $\max\{a, b\}$ and $\min\{a, b\}$ are the maximum and minimum of a and b, respectively.

Note that $\hat{\Delta}^{(RE)}$ (6.7) is a ratio of two random variables, and hence its sampling distribution can be skewed when n_g is not large. Attempting to improve the performance of the interval estimator (6.17), we may consider use of $\tanh^{-1}(x)$ transformation (Edwardes, 1995; Lui, 2002). This leads us to obtain an asymptotic $100\,(1-\alpha)\,\%$ confidence interval for Δ as

$$[\tanh(\tanh^{-1}(\hat{\Delta}^{(RE)}) - Z_{\alpha/2}\sqrt{\hat{Var}(\tanh^{-1}(\hat{\Delta}^{(RE)}))}),$$

$$\tanh(\tanh^{-1}(\hat{\Delta}^{(RE)}) + Z_{\alpha/2}\sqrt{\hat{Var}(\tanh^{-1}(\hat{\Delta}^{(RE)}))})], \qquad (6.18)$$

where $\hat{Var}(\tanh^{-1}(\hat{\Delta}^{(RE)})) = \hat{Var}(\hat{\Delta}^{(RE)})/(1 - (\hat{\Delta}^{(RE)})^2)^2$.

To avoid our inference based on a ratio of two random variables, we may also consider use of the idea behind Fieller's Theorem (Casella and Berger, 1990). Define $T_{PD}^{(RE)} = (\overline{Y}_{++}^{(1)} - \overline{Y}_{++}^{(0)}) - \Delta(\overline{Z}_{++}^{(1)} - \overline{Z}_{++}^{(0)})$, where $\overline{Y}_{++}^{(g)} = \sum_i Y_{i+}^{(g)}/n_g$ and $\overline{Z}_{++}^{(g)} = \sum_i Z_{i+}^{(g)}/n_g$. From Equation (6.2), we can easily see that the expectation $E(T_{PD}^{(RE)}) = 0$ under model (6.1) (Exercise 6.10). Furthermore, we obtain the variance $Var(T_{PD}^{(RE)})$ as (Exercise 6.11):

$$Var(T_{PD}^{(RE)}) = \sum_g [\sum_r r^2\pi_{r+}^{(g)} - (\sum_r r\pi_{r+}^{(g)})^2]/n_g + \Delta^2 \sum_g [\sum_c c^2\pi_{+c}^{(g)}$$

$$- (\sum_c c\pi_{+c}^{(g)})^2]/n_g - 2\Delta \sum_g [\sum_r \sum_c rc\pi_{rc}^{(g)}$$

$$- (\sum_r r\pi_{r+}^{(g)})(\sum_c c\pi_{+c}^{(g)})]/n_g. \qquad (6.19)$$

As both n_g are large, we have $P(\{(T_{PD}^{(RE)})^2/Var(T_{PD}^{(RE)})\} \le Z_{\alpha/2}^2) \approx 1 - \alpha$. This leads us to consider the following quadratic equation (Exercise 6.12):

$$A^{(RE)}\Delta^2 - 2B^{(RE)}\Delta + C^{(RE)} \le 0, \qquad (6.20)$$

where

$$A^{(RE)} = (\overline{Z}_{++}^{(1)} - \overline{Z}_{++}^{(0)})^2 - Z_{\alpha/2}^2 \sum_g [\sum_c c^2\hat{\pi}_{+c}^{(g)} - (\sum_c c\hat{\pi}_{+c}^{(g)})^2]/n_g,$$

$$B^{(RE)} = (\overline{Y}_{++}^{(1)} - \overline{Y}_{++}^{(0)})(\overline{Z}_{++}^{(1)} - \overline{Z}_{++}^{(0)}) - Z_{\alpha/2}^2 \sum_g [\sum_r \sum_c rc\hat{\pi}_{rc}^{(g)}$$

$$- (\sum_r r\hat{\pi}_{r+}^{(g)})(\sum_c c\hat{\pi}_{+c}^{(g)})]/n_g,$$

and

$$C^{(RE)} = (\overline{Y}_{++}^{(1)} - \overline{Y}_{++}^{(0)})^2 - Z_{\alpha/2}^2 \sum_g [\sum_r r^2\hat{\pi}_{r+}^{(g)} - (\sum_r r\hat{\pi}_{r+}^{(g)})^2]/n_g.$$

Thus, if $A^{(RE)} > 0$ and $(B^{(RE)})^2 - A^{(RE)}C^{(RE)} > 0$, an asymptotic 100 $(1 - \alpha)\%$ confidence interval for Δ would be given by

$$[\max\{(B^{(RE)} - \sqrt{(B^{(RE)})^2 - A^{(RE)}C^{(RE)}})/A^{(RE)}, -1\},$$
$$\min\{(B^{(RE)} + \sqrt{(B^{(RE)})^2 - A^{(RE)}C^{(RE)}})/A^{(RE)}, 1\}]. \qquad (6.21)$$

Lui (2007g) assumed a constant risk additive model and applied Monte Carlo simulation to compare the performance of interval estimators (6.17), (6.18), (6.21) with an interval estimator derived from the randomization-based approach proposed elsewhere (Matsuyama, 2002). Lui (2007g) noted that they all can perform well with respect to the coverage probability for given an adequate number of patients in a variety of situations. Lui (2007g) further noted that while the interval estimator derived from the randomization-based approach (Matsuyama, 2002) may cause a slight loss of precision, the interval estimator (6.18) with the $\tanh^{-1}(x)$ transformation is likely to be the most precise with respect to the estimated average length among interval estimators considered here. When the number of patients in both treatments is large, however, all interval estimators are essentially equivalent with respect to both the coverage probability and the average length.

Example 6.2   To illustrate the use of interval estimators (6.17), (6.18) and (6.21), we consider the data in Table 6.2 in a double-blind RCT studying the effect of M-CSF ($g = 1$) versus the placebo ($g = 0$) on reducing the febrile neutropenia incidence for AML patients (Sato, 2001; Ohno, Miyawaki and Hatake *et al.*, 1997). When employing interval estimators (6.17), (6.18) and (6.21), we obtain the 95 % confidence intervals for Δ as $[-0.206, -0.018]$, $[-0.205, -0.017]$, and $[-0.206, -0.018]$, respectively. These resulting interval estimates are all similar to one another. Because all the upper limits of these confidence intervals are below 0, there is significant evidence that taking M-CSF can reduce the risk of febrile neutropenia incidence among the AML patients at the 5 % level. This is consistent with the result found in Example 6.1.

Example 6.3   To illustrate the use of interval estimators (6.17), (6.18) and (6.21) in the presence of a nonnegligible percentage of noncompliance, we consider in Table 6.3 the simulated data regarding 'no febrile

Table 6.2   Observed frequency ($n_{rs}^{(g)}$) for patients with ($Y_{i+}^{(g)} = r$, $Z_{i+}^{(g)} = c$), where r and c denote the number of febrile neutropenia events and the number of times taking M-CSF over three courses of chemotherapies in the M-CSF trial.

	M-CSF group (g = 1)				
	c				
r	0	1	2	3	Total
0	0	0	0	11	11
1	0	0	1	26	27
2	0	0	1	24	25
3	0	0	0	12	12
Total	0	0	2	73	75

	Placebo group (g = 0)				
	c				
r	0	1	2	3	Total
0	5	0	0	0	5
1	22	0	0	0	22
2	35	0	0	0	35
3	19	0	0	0	19
Total	81	0	0	0	81

neutropenia incidence' as a positive response based on parameter estimates obtained from the double-blind RCT studying the effect of M-CSF on reducing the febrile neutropenia incidence among AML patients (Lui, 2007g). Based on these data (Table 6.3), we obtain $\hat{\delta}^{(RE)}(= \overline{\overline{Y}}_{++}^{(1)} - \overline{\overline{Y}}_{++}^{(0)}) = 0.036$ and $\hat{\Delta}^{(RE)} = 0.069$. This illustrates that as compared with $\hat{\Delta}^{(RE)}$, using $\hat{\delta}^{(RE)}$ for the ITT analysis tends to underestimate the treatment efficacy Δ. Furthermore, when using interval estimators (6.17), (6.18) and (6.21), we obtain the 95 % confidence for Δ intervals as [−0.088, 0.226], [−0.089, 0.223], and [−0.088, 0.230], respectively. Again, these

Table 6.3 Simulated data $(n_{rc}^{(g)})$ for patients with $(Y_{i+}^{(1)} = r, Z_{i+}^{(g)} = c)$, where r and c denote the number of no febrile neutropenia events and the number of times taking the M-CSF over three courses of chemotherapies in the M-CSF trial.

	M-CSF group (g = 1)				
	c				
r	0	1	2	3	Total
0	0	1	4	5	10
1	0	4	19	16	39
2	1	5	10	12	28
3	0	2	5	3	10
Total	1	12	38	36	87

	Placebo group (g = 0)				
	c				
r	0	1	2	3	Total
0	7	7	1	0	15
1	15	17	4	0	36
2	16	14	4	1	35
3	1	3	1	0	5
Total	39	41	10	1	91

interval estimates are similar to one another, but the interval estimate (6.18) with the $\tanh^{-1}(x)$ transformation has the shortest length among these three interval estimates. This is consistent with the finding that the interval estimator (6.18) is likely to be more precise than interval estimators (6.17) and (6.21) based on Monte Carlo simulations (Lui, 2007g).

Note that the two random variables $Y_{ij-1}^{(g)}$ and $Z_{ij}^{(g)}$ are likely dependent in practical situations. A patient at course j ($j \geq 2$) would more likely continue taking the same treatment as that he/she took previously if he/she had a positive response (i.e. $Y_{ij-1}^{(g)} = 1$) at course $j - 1$, and would more likely switch to receive the other treatment, otherwise. Thus, we may assume the following stochastic model for the random variable of the treatment receipt $Z_{ij}^{(g)}$ of patient $i \in S$ ($= C, A, N$) assigned to treatment g (Lui, 2007f) for $j \geq 2$:

$$
\begin{aligned}
P(Z_{ij}^{(g)} = 1 | \underline{Y}_{ij-1}^{(g)}, \underline{Z}_{ij-1}^{(g)}, S) = 1_{\{Z_{ij-1}^{(g)}=1\}} \{ P(Z_{ij-1}^{(g)} = 1 | \underline{Y}_{ij-2}^{(g)}, \underline{Z}_{ij-2}^{(g)}, S) \\
\times (1 - \rho_S) + \rho_S Y_{ij-1}^{(g)} \} + (1 - 1_{\{Z_{ij-1}^{(g)}=1\}}) \\
\times \{ P(Z_{ij-1}^{(g)} = 1 | \underline{Y}_{ij-2}^{(g)}, \underline{Z}_{ij-2}^{(g)}, S)(1 - \rho_S) + \rho_S(1 - Y_{ij-1}^{(g)}) \},
\end{aligned}
$$

(6.22)

where $1_{\{equality\}}$ is an indicator function, and $1_{\{equality\}} = 1$ when the equality in braces holds, and $= 0$, otherwise; $\underline{Y}_{ij-1}^{(g)} = (Y_{i1}^{(g)}, \ldots, Y_{ij-1}^{(g)})'$ and $\underline{Z}_{ij-1}^{(g)} = (Z_{i1}^{(g)}, \ldots, Z_{ij-1}^{(g)})'$; $0 \leq \rho_S \leq 1$ is a measure of dependence for patient's selection of a treatment on his/her previous outcome. Note that in model (6.23) we define $P(Z_{i1}^{(g)} = 1 | \underline{Y}_{i0}^{(g)}, \underline{Z}_{i0}^{(g)}, S) = P(Z_{i1}^{(g)} = 1 | S)$ as the probability of taking the experimental treatment for patient i assigned to treatment g at the initial course. Note that when $\rho_S = 0$, we have $P(Z_{ij}^{(g)} = 1 | S) = P(Z_{ij-1}^{(g)} = 1 | S) = \cdots = P(Z_{i1}^{(g)} = 1 | S)$ (Exercise 6.13). In other words, the probability that a patient complies with his/her assigned treatment at course j does not depend on his/her previous outcome at course j-1. Note that at the initial course ($j = 1$), by definition, we have $P(Z_{i1}^{(g)} = 1 | A) = 1$, $P(Z_{i1}^{(g)} = 1 | N) = 0$, $P(Z_{i1}^{(1)} = 1 | C) = 1$, and $P(Z_{i1}^{(0)} = 1 | C) = 0$. Therefore, the commonly assumed ideal situation, in which every patient complies with his/her assigned treatment, is simply a special case for $P(C) = 1$, $P(A) = P(N) = 0$, and $\rho_C = 0$. On the other hand, when $\rho_S = 1$, the compliance to an assigned treatment for a given patient is completely determined by his/her previous outcome based on the model (6.23). In this extreme case, a patient at course j would continue taking the same treatment as that he/she took at course $j - 1$ if he/she had a positive response, and would automatically switch to take the other treatment if he/she had a negative response. In practice, we may wish to assure the parameter ρ_C to be small to avoid the loss of precision (or efficiency) (Lui, 2007f). To provide readers with an insight into the relations between $\pi_{r+}^{(g)}$'s (or $\pi_{+c}^{(g)}$'s) and the parameter ρ_S in model (6.23), as well as the effect due to ρ_S and $P(S)$ on Δ (6.6), we study in detail the case for $J = 2$ in Exercise 6.14. As shown here, however, we can do hypothesis testing and interval estimation for the treatment efficacy measured by Δ based on statistics $(Y_{i+}^{(g)}, Z_{i+}^{(g)})$ without the need of modeling the dependence relation between $Y_{ij-1}^{(g)}$ and $Z_{ij}^{(g)}$, or estimating these nuisance parameters ρ_S and $P(S)$ for $S = C, A$, and N.

When patients are difficult to recruit into a RCT, we may employ a multi-center design to facilitate the collection of data (Fleiss, 1981). Because patients attending various centers may possess different characteristics, the underlying probability of a patient response for a standard treatment and the extent of noncompliance to an assigned treatment may vary between centers. Thus, we may consider employing stratified analysis as discussed in Chapter 3 with strata formed by centers to control the center effect. Also, if there are unbalanced pre-treatment covariates which can affect patient outcomes of interest and the extent of noncompliance in a RCT, we may also wish to apply stratified analysis with strata determined by a combination of these covariates to control their confounding effects on estimation as well. Sato (2001) proposed, for example, the Mantel-Haenszel (MH) type estimator for repeated binary measurements as given by

$$\hat{\Delta}_{MH}^{(RE)} = \sum_l w_l (\sum_r r\hat{\pi}_{r+|l}^{(1)} - \sum_r r\hat{\pi}_{r+|l}^{(0)}) / \sum_l w_l (\sum_c c\hat{\pi}_{+c|l}^{(1)} - \sum_c c\hat{\pi}_{+c|l}^{(0)}),$$

(6.23)

where $w_l = n_{1l}n_{0l}/(n_{1l} + n_{0l})$, n_{gl} is the sample size for the assigned treatment g ($= 1$ for experimental and $= 0$ for standard or placebo) in stratum l, $\hat{\pi}_{r+|l}^{(g)}$ and $\hat{\pi}_{+c|l}^{(g)}$ are simply calculated as $\hat{\pi}_{r+}^{(g)}$ and $\hat{\pi}_{+c}^{(g)}$ in (6.7) (for $g = 1, 0$) by using the data from stratum l. Note that when we take only a single one measurement per patient and when every patient complies with his/her assigned treatment, the above $\hat{\Delta}_{MH}^{(RE)}$ reduces to the commonly used MH estimator for the RD in sparse data (Greenland and Robins, 1985). Note also that we can derive the asymptotic variance for $\hat{\Delta}_{MH}^{(RE)}$ (6.22) by again using the delta method.

6.4.2 Estimation of the proportion ratio

Because the PR, just like the PD, can be easily appreciated by clinicians, the PR is a popular index to measure the treatment efficacy in a RCT. Recall that when the PR represents the ratio of probabilities of adverse events between an experimental treatment and a standard treatment (or placebo), we call the PR the relative risk or risk ratio (RR). When RR is less than 1, 1-RR is called the relative difference (Sheps, 1958 and 1959) or the relative risk reduction (Laupacis, Sackett and Roberts, 1988; Fleiss 1981; Lui, 2004). In this section, we consider interval estimation of the PR for repeated binary measurements with noncompliance in a RCT.

On the basis of $\hat{\gamma}^{(RE)}$ (6.12) and $\hat{Var}(\hat{\gamma}^{(RE)})$ (6.13), we may first consider the asymptotic $100 (1 - \alpha)\%$ confidence interval for γ using the logarithmic transformation as given by (Lui, 2007b)

$$[\hat{\gamma}^{(RE)} \exp(-Z_{\alpha/2}(\hat{Var}(\log(\hat{\gamma}^{(RE)})))^{1/2}),$$
$$\hat{\gamma}^{(RE)} \exp(Z_{\alpha/2}(\hat{Var}(\log(\hat{\gamma}^{(RE)})))^{1/2})], \qquad (6.24)$$

where $\hat{Var}(\log(\hat{\gamma}^{(RE)})) = \hat{Var}(\hat{\gamma}^{(RE)}) / (\hat{\gamma}^{(RE)})^2$.

To avoid our inference based on a ratio of two statistics, of which the sampling distribution is possibly skewed when the number of patients per treatment is not large, as for deriving interval estimator (6.20), we may also consider use of the idea behind Fieller's Theorem (Casella and Berger, 1990). We define $T_{PR}^{(RE)} = (\overline{X}_{++}^{(1)} - \overline{X}_{++}^{(0)}) - \gamma(\overline{X}_{++}^{(0)*} - \overline{X}_{++}^{(1)*})$, where $\overline{X}_{++}^{(g)} = \sum_i X_{i+}^{(g)}/n_g$ and $\overline{X}_{++}^{(g)*} = \sum_i X_{i+}^{(g)*}/n_g$. We can easily show that the expectation $E(T_{PR}^{(RE)}) = 0$. We can further show that the variance $Var(T_{PR}^{(RE)})$ is given by

$$Var(T_{PR}^{(RE)}) = \sum_g [\sum_r r^2 E_{r+}^{(g)} - (\sum_r r E_{r+}^{(g)})^2]/n_g$$
$$+ \gamma^2 \sum_g [\sum_c c^2 E_{+c}^{(g)} - (\sum_c c E_{+c}^{(g)})^2]/n_g$$
$$+ 2\gamma \sum_g [\sum_r \sum_c rc E_{rc}^{(g)} - (\sum_r r E_{r+}^{(g)})(\sum_c c E_{+c}^{(g)})]/n_g.$$
$$(6.25)$$

As both n_g are large, we have $P(\{(T_{PR}^{(RE)})^2/Var(T_{PR}^{(RE)})\} \leq Z_{\alpha/2}^2) \approx 1 - \alpha$. This leads us to consider the following quadratic equation in γ:

$$a^{(RE)}(\gamma)^2 - 2b^{(RE)}(\gamma) + c^{(RE)} \leq 0, \tag{6.26}$$

where

$$a^{(RE)} = (\overline{X}_{++}^{(0)*} - \overline{X}_{++}^{(1)*})^2 - Z_{\alpha/2}^2 \sum_g [\sum_c c^2 \hat{E}_{+c}^{(g)} - (\sum_c c\hat{E}_{+c}^{(g)})^2]/n_g,$$

$$b^{(RE)} = (\overline{X}_{++}^{(1)} - \overline{X}_{++}^{(0)})(\overline{X}_{++}^{(0)*} - \overline{X}_{++}^{(1)*}) + Z_{\alpha/2}^2 \sum_g [\sum_r \sum_c rc\hat{E}_{rc}^{(g)}$$

$$- (\sum_r r\hat{E}_{r+}^{(g)})(\sum_c c\hat{E}_{+c}^{(g)})]/n_g,$$

and

$$c^{(RE)} = (\overline{X}_{++}^{(1)} - \overline{X}_{++}^{(0)})^2 - Z_{\alpha/2}^2 \sum_g [\sum_r r^2 \hat{E}_{r+}^{(g)} - (\sum_r r\hat{E}_{r+}^{(g)})^2]/n_g.$$

Thus, we obtain an asymptotic $100(1 - \alpha)\%$ confidence interval for γ as

$$[\max\{(b^{(RE)} - \sqrt{b^{(RE)^2} - a^{(RE)}c^{(RE)}})/a^{(RE)}, 0\},$$

$$(b^{(RE)} + \sqrt{b^{(RE)^2} - a^{(RE)}c^{(RE)}})/a^{(RE)}]. \tag{6.27}$$

Finally, we discuss the randomization-based approach discussed elsewhere (Sato, 2001; Matsuyama, 2002). We consider the counterfactual population consisting of $u_i^{(g)} = x_{i+}^{(g)} + \gamma x_{i+}^{(g)*}$ for $i = 1, 2, \ldots, n_g$ and $g = 1, 0$. Note that $t_{PR}^{(RE)} = \sum_i u_i^{(1)}/n_1 - \sum_i u_i^{(0)}/n_0$, which can be regarded as a realization of $T_{PR}^{(RE)}$, of which the expectation is 0. We consider the sampling distribution of the statistic $t_{PR}^{(RE)}$ with respect to random combination (Cochran, 1977) and obtain the following randomization-based variance (Exercise 6.15):

$$V_{RB}(t_{PR}^{(RE)}) = [(n_1 + n_0)^2/[n_1 n_0(n_1 + n_0 - 1)]]\{[\sum_r r^2 \hat{\overline{E}}_{r+}^{(p)}$$

$$- (\sum_r r\hat{\overline{E}}_{r+}^{(p)})^2] + \gamma^2 [\sum_c c^2 \hat{\overline{E}}_{+c}^{(p)} - (\sum_c c\hat{\overline{E}}_{+c}^{(p)})^2]$$

$$+ 2\gamma [\sum_r \sum_c rc\hat{\overline{E}}_{rc}^{(p)} - (\sum_r r\hat{\overline{E}}_{r+}^{(p)})(\sum_c c\hat{\overline{E}}_{+c}^{(p)})]\},$$

$$\tag{6.28}$$

where $\hat{\bar{E}}_{rc}^{(p)} = (n_1 \hat{E}_{rc}^{(1)} + n_0 \hat{E}_{rc}^{(0)})/(n_1 + n_0)$, $\hat{\bar{E}}_{r+}^{(p)} = \sum_c \hat{\bar{E}}_{rc}^{(p)}$, and $\hat{\bar{E}}_{+c}^{(p)} = \sum_r \hat{\bar{E}}_{rc}^{(p)}$. As both n_g are large, we have $P(\{(t_{PR}^{(RE)})^2 / V_{RB}(t_{PR}^{(RE)})\} \leq Z_{\alpha/2}^2) \approx 1 - \alpha$. This leads us to consider the following quadratic equation:

$$a_{RB}^{(RE)} \gamma^2 - 2b_{RB}^{(RE)} \gamma + c_{RB}^{(RE)} \leq 0, \tag{6.29}$$

where

$$a_{RB}^{(RE)} = (\overline{X}_{++}^{(0)*} - \overline{X}_{++}^{(1)*})^2 - Z_{\alpha/2}^2 (n_1 + n_0)^2 /$$
$$[n_1 n_0 (n_1 + n_0 - 1)][\sum_c c^2 \hat{\bar{E}}_{+c}^{(p)} - (\sum_c c \hat{\bar{E}}_{+c}^{(p)})^2],$$

$$b_{RB}^{(RE)} = (\overline{X}_{++}^{(1)} - \overline{X}_{++}^{(0)})(\overline{X}_{++}^{(0)*} - \overline{X}_{++}^{(1)*}) + Z_{\alpha/2}^2 (n_1 + n_0)^2 /$$
$$[n_1 n_0 (n_1 + n_0 - 1)][\sum_r \sum_c rc \hat{\bar{E}}_{rc}^{(p)} - (\sum_r r \hat{\bar{E}}_{r+}^{(p)})(\sum_c c \hat{\bar{E}}_{+c}^{(p)})],$$

and

$$c_{RB}^{(RE)} = (\overline{X}_{++}^{(1)} - \overline{X}_{++}^{(0)})^2 - Z_{\alpha/2}^2 (n_1 + n_0)^2 /$$
$$[n_1 n_0 (n_1 + n_0 - 1)][\sum_r r^2 \hat{\bar{E}}_{r+}^{(p)} - (\sum_r r \hat{\bar{E}}_{r+}^{(p)})^2].$$

This leads us to obtain an asymptotic $100(1 - \alpha)\%$ confidence interval for γ as

$$[\max\{(b_{RB}^{(RE)} - \sqrt{(b_{RB}^{(RE)})^2 - a_{RB}^{(RE)} c_{RB}^{(RE)}})/a_{RB}^{(RE)}, 0\},$$
$$(b_{RB}^{(RE)} + \sqrt{(b_{RB}^{(RE)})^2 - a_{RB}^{(RE)} c_{RB}^{(RE)}})/a_{RB}^{(RE)}]. \tag{6.30}$$

Lui (2007b) assumed a constant multiplicative model and used Monte Carlo simulation to evaluate the performance of several interval estimators, including (6.24), (6.27) and (6.30) presented here. Lui found that all interval estimators (6.24), (6.27) and (6.30) can perform well with respect to the coverage probability when the number of patients is reasonably large. Lui (2007b) further found that the interval estimator (6.24) using the logarithmic transformation is generally more precise than interval estimators (6.27) and (6.30) with respect to the average length, and all interval estimators lose precision as the extent of noncompliance increases. Note that when there are repeated measurements and an adequate extent of compliance, the denominator $\sum_c c E_{+c}^{(0)} - \sum_c c E_{+c}^{(1)}$ of γ

(6.11) is likely to lie farther away from 0 as compared with the case of a single measurement per patient. Thus, the problem of using the logarithmic transformation in interval estimation of the PR can cause, as noted in Chapter 2, a substantial loss of precision for a single measurement per patient should be of less concern in data with repeated binary measurements.

To allow readers appreciate the relations between parameters $E_{r+}^{(g)}$'s (or $E_{+c}^{(g)}$'s) under the structural risk multiplicative model (6.10) and the other parameters γ_S, ρ_S and $P(S)$ in model (6.23), we discuss in details the case for $J = 2$ in Exercise 6.16. As noted before, we can do testing hypothesis and interval estimation for the PR γ ($= \gamma_C$) under the risk multiplicative model (6.10) based on test statistics $(X_{i+}^{(g)}, X_{i+}^{(g)*})$ without the need of modeling the dependence relation between $Y_{ij-1}^{(g)}$ and $Z_{ij}^{(g)}$.

When we use a multi-center trial design to collect data or when there are confounders in a RCT, we may employ stratified analysis to control the confounding effect due to these centers or confounders. As suggested elsewhere (Sato, 2001), we may consider the MH type estimator as given by

$$\hat{\gamma}_{MH}^{(RE)} = \sum_l w_l (\sum_r r\hat{E}_{r+|l}^{(1)} - \sum_r r\hat{E}_{r+|l}^{(0)}) / \sum_l w_l (\sum_c c\hat{E}_{+c|l}^{(0)} - \sum_c c\hat{E}_{+c|l}^{(1)}), \qquad (6.31)$$

where $w_l = n_{1l}n_{0l}/(n_{1l} + n_{0l})$, n_{gl} is the number of patients assigned to treatment g in stratum l and $\hat{E}_{r+|l}^{(g)} = \sum_c f_{rc|l}^{(g)}/n_{gl}$ and $\hat{E}_{+c|l}^{(g)} = \sum_r f_{rc|l}^{(g)}/n_{gl}$, $f_{rc|l}^{(g)}$ is the frequency of patients corresponding to the cell $(X_{i+|l}^{(g)} = r, X_{i+|l}^{(g)*} = c)$ among n_{gl} patients assigned to treatment g based on the data in stratum l, and where $X_{i+|l}^{(g)}$ and $X_{i+|l}^{(g)*}$ denote for patient i assigned to treatment g in stratum l the total number of positive responses when he/she receives the experimental treatment and the total number of positive responses when he/she receives the standard treatment (or placebo), respectively. When the number of course is ($j =$) 1 and every patient complies with his/her assigned treatment in each stratum, the above estimator $\hat{\gamma}_{MH}^{(RE)}$ (6.31) reduces to the commonly used MH estimator for PR in sparse data (Greenland and Robins, 1985; Lui, 2005). We may also apply the delta method to derive the asymptotic variance of

$\hat{\gamma}_{MH}^{(RE)}$ with the logarithmic transformation for doing hypothesis testing and interval estimation of γ based on $\hat{\gamma}_{MH}^{(RE)}$ (6.31) in a stratified RCT with repeated binary measurements.

Example 6.4   To illustrate the use of interval estimators (6.24), (6.27) and (6.30), we consider the data consisting of 156 patients with complete information over three courses as described in Example 6.1. We summarize in Table 6.4 the frequency $f_{rs}^{(g)}$ of patients with the bivariate

Table 6.4   Observed frequency $(n_{rs}^{(g)})$ for patients with $(X_{i+}^{(g)} = r, X_{i+}^{(g)^*} = c)$, where r and c denote the number of febrile neutropenia events when the patient took M-CSF and the number of febrile neutropenia events when the patient took placebo in the assigned treatment group g (= 1 for the M-CSF and = 0 for the placebo), respectively.

M-CSF group (g = 1)				
		c		
r	0	1	2	3	Total
0	11	0	0	0	11
1	27	0	0	–	27
2	25	0	–	–	25
3	12	–	–	–	12
Total	75	0	0	0	75

Placebo group (g = 0)				
		c		
r	0	1	2	3	Total
0	5	22	35	19	81
1	0	0	0	–	0
2	0	0	–	–	0
3	0	–	–	–	0
Total	5	22	35	19	81

– indicates the structure probability of 0

random vector $(X_{i+}^{(g)} = r, X_{i+}^{(g)^*} = c)$. Given these data, we obtain the estimate of the PR, $\hat{\gamma}^{(RE)} = 0.819$ (Lui, 2007b). The resulting 95 % confidence intervals for γ using (6.24), (6.27), and (6.30) are $[0.689, 0.973]$, $[0.685, 0.970]$, and $[0.686, 0.971]$, respectively. Since all these resulting upper limits are below 1, there is significant evidence that taking M-CSF reduces febrile neutropenia incidence at the 5 %.

6.5 Sample size determination

Whether a patient receives a treatment at a time point may depend on his/her previous response when repeated binary measurements are taken from a patient. Furthermore, the structure of this dependence is most probably unknown and is likely to be much more complicated than the assumed model (6.23) in reality. As noted previously, however, we can avoid modeling this dependence and the intraclass correlation between repeated measurements taken from the patient by considering the joint distribution of the marginal number of possessing positive responses and the marginal number of times taking the experimental treatment on each patient. Following this idea, we discuss sample size calculation for testing procedures discussed in Sections 6.1–6.3 in repeated binary measurements under a RCT with noncompliance.

Define $k = n_0/n_1$ as the ratio of sample allocation between the standard and experimental treatments. Given a fixed ratio k, we focus our attention on estimating the minimum required number of patients n_1 from the experimental treatment in the following. The corresponding estimates of the minimum required number of patients from the standard treatment and the total minimum required number of patients for the entire RCT are then given by $n_0 = kn_1$ and $n_T = (k + 1)n_1$, respectively.

6.5.1 Sample size calculation for testing superiority

Consider sample size determination in use of statistic (6.5) for the ITT analysis to test the superiority of an experimental treatment to a standard treatment (or placebo). Note that the variance of the test statistic $\hat{\delta}^{(RE)}$ for the ITT analysis can be re-expressed as

$$Var(\hat{\delta}^{(RE)}) = V_{ITTPD}^{(RE)}(\underline{\pi}_{r+}^{(1)}, \underline{\pi}_{r+}^{(0)}, k)/n_1, \tag{6.32}$$

where $\underline{\pi}_{r+}^{(g)} = (\pi_{0+}^{(g)}, \pi_{1+}^{(g)}, \pi_{2+}^{(g)}, \ldots, \pi_{J+}^{(g)})'$ for $g = 1, 0$, and

$$V_{ITTPD}^{(RE)}(\underline{\pi}_{r+}^{(1)}, \underline{\pi}_{r+}^{(0)}, k) = \{[\sum_r (r/J)^2 \pi_{r+}^{(1)} - (\sum_r (r/J)\pi_{r+}^{(1)})^2]$$
$$+ [\sum_r (r/J)^2 \pi_{r+}^{(0)} - (\sum_r (r/J)\pi_{r+}^{(0)})^2]/k\}.$$

Furthermore, the variance $Var(\hat{\delta}^{(RE)})$ (6.32) under $H_0 : \Delta = 0$ may reduce to

$$Var(\hat{\delta}^{(RE)}|H_0) = V_{ITTPD}^{(RE)}(\underline{\pi}_{r+}^{(1)}, \underline{\pi}_{r+}^{(0)}, k|H_0)/n_1, \qquad (6.33)$$

where $V_{ITTPD}^{(RE)}(\underline{\pi}_{r+}^{(1)}, \underline{\pi}_{r+}^{(0)}, k|H_0) = [\sum_r (r/J)^2 \overline{\pi}_{r+}^{(p)} - (\sum_r (r/J)\overline{\pi}_{r+}^{(p)})^2](1 + 1/k)$, and $\overline{\pi}_{r+}^{(p)} = (\pi_{r+}^{(1)} + k\pi_{r+}^{(0)})/(1 + k)$. On the basis of the test statistic (6.5) and (6.33), we obtain an estimate of the minimum required number of patients n_1 from the experimental treatment for a desired power $1 - \beta$ of detecting a given difference Δ_0 (> 0) at the α-level (two-sided test) as

$$n_1 = Ceil\{(Z_{\alpha/2}\sqrt{V_{ITTPD}^{(RE)}(\underline{\pi}_{r+}^{(1)}, \underline{\pi}_{r+}^{(0)}, k|H_0)} + Z_\beta\sqrt{V_{ITTPD}^{(RE)}(\underline{\pi}_{r+}^{(1)}, \underline{\pi}_{r+}^{(0)}, k)}/$$
$$[1 - (\Delta_0 MF)^2])^2/[\tanh^{-1}(\Delta_0 MF)]^2\}, \qquad (6.34)$$

where $Ceil\{x\}$ is the smallest integer $\geq$ x and $MF = (\sum_c (c/J)\pi_{+c}^{(1)} - \sum_c (c/J)\pi_{+c}^{(0)})$. We can easily show that the above sample size formula n_1 (6.34) reduces to the sample size formula (2.31) for testing superiority when there is only a single one measurement ($j = 1$) per patient under the monotonicity assumption (Exercise 6.17). When employing sample size calculation formula (6.34), we need to determine the individual value for $\pi_{r+}^{(g)}$'s, which are generally difficult to obtain in practice for $J \geq 2$. Recall that $V_{ITTPD}^{(RE)}(\underline{\pi}_{r+}^{(1)}, \underline{\pi}_{r+}^{(0)}, k)$ simply represents $n_1 Var(\hat{\delta}^{(RE)}) = n_1(Var(\overline{Y}_{++}^{(1)}) + Var(\overline{Y}_{++}^{(0)}))$. Given the data in a pilot study, say, we randomly take m_g patients from group g ($= 1, 0$). Thus, we can estimate $V_{ITTPD}^{(RE)}(\underline{\pi}_{r+}^{(1)}, \underline{\pi}_{r+}^{(0)}, k)$ by simply $[(S_{y_{i+}^{(1)}}^2) + (S_{y_{i+}^{(0)}}^2)/k]/J^2$, where $S_{y_{i+}^{(g)}}^2 = \sum_i (Y_{i+}^{(g)} - \overline{Y}_{++}^{(g)})^2/m_g$, the sample variance estimator of $Var(Y_{i+}^{(g)})$. Similarly, we can estimate $V_{ITTPD}^{(RE)}(\underline{\pi}_{r+}^{(1)}, \underline{\pi}_{r+}^{(0)}, k|H_0)$ by $\hat{V}_{ITTPD}^{(RE)}(\underline{\pi}_{r+}^{(1)}, \underline{\pi}_{r+}^{(0)}, k|H_0) = (1 + 1/k)[\sum_g \sum_i (Y_{i+}^{(g)})^2 - (\sum_g \sum_i Y_{i+}^{(g)})^2/(m_1 + m_0)]/[(m_1 + m_0)J^2]$. Furthermore, we may estimate the MF from a pilot study by

$(\sum_i Z_{i+}^{(1)}/m_1 - \sum_i Z_{i+}^{(0)}/m_0)/J$ instead of determining the individual value for $\pi_{+c}^{(g)}$'s separately in application of n_1 (6.34).

6.5.2   Sample size calculation for testing noninferiority

When assessing the noninferiority of an experimental treatment to a standard treatment, we may consider taking more than a single measurement per patient to reduce the expense or the number of patients needed for our trials. In this section, we discuss sample size determination based on procedures for testing noninferiority when using the PD and the PR to measure the treatment efficacy in repeated binary data for a RCT with noncompliance.

6.5.2.1   Using the difference in proportions

Consider use of the test procedure (6.9) to test noninferiority. For a given fixed ratio $k = n_0/n_1$ of sample allocation between the standard and experimental treatments, we can re-express $Var(\hat{\Delta}^{(RE)})$ as a function of $\underline{\pi}_1, \underline{\pi}_2, \Delta$ and k,

$$V_{PD}^{(RE)}(\underline{\pi}_1, \underline{\pi}_2, \Delta, k)/n_1, \qquad (6.35)$$

where $\underline{\pi}_g$ is the column vector consisting of $\pi_{rc}^{(g)}$'s, and

$$
\begin{aligned}
V_{PD}^{(RE)}(\underline{\pi}_1, \underline{\pi}_2, \Delta, k) = &\{[\sum_r r^2\pi_{r+}^{(1)} - (\sum_r r\pi_{r+}^{(1)})^2 \\
&- 2\Delta(\sum_r \sum_c rc\pi_{rc}^{(1)} - (\sum_r r\pi_{r+}^{(1)})(\sum_c c\pi_{+c}^{(1)})) + \Delta^2(\sum_c c^2\pi_{+c}^{(1)} \\
&- (\sum_c c\pi_{+c}^{(1)})^2] + [\sum_r r^2\pi_{r+}^{(0)} - (\sum_r r\pi_{r+}^{(0)})^2 - 2\Delta(\sum_r \sum_c rc\pi_{rc}^{(0)} \\
&- (\sum_r r\pi_{r+}^{(0)})(\sum_c c\pi_{+c}^{(0)})) + \Delta^2(\sum_c c^2\pi_{+c}^{(0)} - (\sum_c c\pi_{+c}^{(0)})^2)]/k\}/ \\
&(\sum_c c\pi_{+c}^{(1)} - \sum_c c\pi_{+c}^{(0)})^2.
\end{aligned}
$$

Thus, the asymptotic variance $Var(\tanh^{-1}(\hat{\Delta}^{(RE)}))$ for statistic $\tanh^{-1}(\hat{\Delta}^{(RE)})$ is simply equal to $V_{PD}^{(RE)}(\underline{\pi}_1, \underline{\pi}_2, \Delta, k)/[n_1(1 - \Delta^2)^2]$. Based on the test procedure (6.9) and (6.35), we obtain an estimate of the minimum required number of patients n_1 from the experimental treatment for a desired power $(1 - \beta)$ of detecting noninferiority with a given specified value Δ_0 $(> -\varepsilon_l)$ at a nominal α-level as

$$
\begin{aligned}
n_1 = Ceil\{((Z_\alpha + Z_\beta)^2 V_{PD}^{(RE)}(\underline{\pi}_1, \underline{\pi}_2, \Delta_0, k)/[(1 - \Delta_0^2)^2]) / \\
(\tanh^{-1}(\varepsilon_l) + \tanh^{-1}(\Delta_0))^2\},
\end{aligned}
\tag{6.36}
$$

where $Ceil\{x\}$ is the smallest integer $\geq x$. Note that when there is a single measurement per patient (i.e. $J = 1$), the sample size formula n_1 (6.36) reduces to n_1 (2.33) under the monotonicity assumption. Note also that in application of n_1 (6.36), we need to determine the value for $V_{PD}^{(RE)}(\underline{\pi}_1, \underline{\pi}_2, \Delta_0, k)$, which is a function of $\pi_{rc}^{(g)}$'s. In practice, we may have the difficulty in assigning these individual cell probabilities in use of (6.36). However, we can determine the approximate value for $V_{PD}^{(RE)}(\underline{\pi}_1, \underline{\pi}_2, \Delta_0, k)$ from data in a pilot study via the following formula:

$$
\{[S_{y_{i+}^{(1)}}^2 - 2\Delta_0 S_{y_{i+}^{(1)}, z_{i+}^{(1)}} + (\Delta_0)^2 S_{z_{i+}^{(1)}}^2] + [S_{y_{i+}^{(0)}}^2 - 2\Delta_0 S_{y_{i+}^{(0)}, z_{i+}^{(0)}} + (\Delta_0)^2 S_{z_{i+}^{(0)}}^2]/k\}/
$$
$$
(\overline{Z}_{++}^{(1)} - \overline{Z}_{++}^{(0)})^2,
\tag{6.37}
$$

where

$$
S_{y_{i+}^{(g)}}^2 = \sum_i (Y_{i+}^{(g)} - \overline{Y}_{++}^{(g)})^2/m_g, \quad S_{y_{i+}^{(g)}, z_{i+}^{(g)}} = \sum_i (Y_{i+}^{(g)} - \overline{Y}_{++}^{(g)})
$$
$$
\times (Z_{i+}^{(g)} - \overline{Z}_{++}^{(g)})/m_g, \quad \text{and} \quad \overline{Z}_{++}^{(g)} = \sum_i Z_{i+}^{(g)}/m_g.
$$

However, using this approach may produce an inaccurate estimate of the sample size if the chosen value Δ_0 of interest is quite different from the underlying true value Δ in the pilot study. This is because the cell probabilities $\pi_{rc}^{(g)}$'s themselves can also be functions of the underlying value of Δ (for example, see Exercise 6.14). Furthermore, because all the parameter estimates are subject to sampling variation, we may wish to calculate a range of the required sample sizes corresponding to various combinations of plausible parameter values especially when the underlying parameter values are needed to determine from a pilot study. These may provide clinicians with a general crude picture regarding how large the minimum required sample size subject to their budget constraints would be needed.

6.5.2.2 Using the ratio of proportions

When calculating the minimum required sample size for testing noninferiority based on the PR, we consider use of the test statistic (6.14). Given the ratio $k = n_0/n_1$ of sample allocation, we can re-express the asymptotic variance $Var(\log(\hat{\gamma}^{(RE)}))$ as a function of $\underline{E}_1, \underline{E}_2, \gamma$ and k,

$$V_{LPR}^{(RE)}(\underline{E}_1, \underline{E}_2, \gamma, k)/n_1, \tag{6.38}$$

where $\underline{E}_g$ ($g = 1, 0$) denotes the column vector consisting of $E_{rc}^{(g)}$'s, and

$$\begin{aligned}
V_{LPR}^{(RE)}(\underline{E}_1, \underline{E}_2, \gamma, k) = &\{[\sum_r r^2 E_{r+}^{(1)} - (\sum_r r E_{r+}^{(1)})^2 \\
&+ 2\gamma(\sum_r \sum_c rc E_{rc}^{(1)} - (\sum_r r E_{r+}^{(1)})(\sum_c c E_{+c}^{(1)})) + \gamma^2(\sum_c c^2 E_{+c}^{(1)} \\
&- (\sum_c c E_{+c}^{(1)})^2] + [\sum_r r^2 E_{r+}^{(0)} - (\sum_r r E_{r+}^{(0)})^2 + 2\gamma(\sum_r \sum_c rc E_{rc}^{(0)} \\
&- (\sum_r r E_{r+}^{(0)})(\sum_c c E_{+c}^{(0)})) + \gamma^2(\sum_c c^2 E_{+c}^{(0)} - (\sum_c c E_{+c}^{(0)})^2)]/k\}/ \\
&[\gamma^2(\sum_c c E_{+c}^{(0)} - \sum_c c E_{+c}^{(1)})^2].
\end{aligned}$$

Based on the test procedure (6.14) and $V_{LPR}^{(RE)}(\underline{E}_1, \underline{E}_2, \gamma, k)$ (6.38), we obtain an estimate of the minimum required number of patients n_1 from the experimental treatment for a desired power $(1 - \beta)$ of detecting noninferiority with a given specified value γ_0 ($> 1 - \gamma_l$) at a nominal α-level as

$$n_1 = Ceil\{(Z_\alpha + Z_\beta)^2 V_{LPR}^{(RE)}(\underline{E}_1, \underline{E}_2, \gamma_0, k)/(\log(\gamma_0) - \log(1 - \gamma_l))^2\}. \tag{6.39}$$

Note that one can easily see that the sample size calculation formula n_1 (6.39) reduces to that (2.35) when there is only a single measurement per patient (i.e. $J = 1$) under the monotonicity assumption. Note also that in application of (6.39), assigning the value for the individual parameter $E_{rs}^{(g)}$ is difficult. For a given γ_0 of interest, we may provide an approximate value of $V_{LPR}^{(RE)}(\underline{E}_1, \underline{E}_2, \gamma_0, k)$ from a pilot study via the following formula:

$$\{[S_{x_{i+}^{(1)}}^2 + 2\gamma_0 S_{x_{i+}^{(1)}, x_{i+}^{(1)*}} + (\gamma_0)^2 S_{x_{i+}^{(1)*}}^2] + [S_{x_{i+}^{(0)}}^2 + 2\gamma_0 S_{x_{i+}^{(0)}, x_{i+}^{(0)*}} + (\gamma_0)^2 S_{x_{l+}^{(0)*}}^2]/k\}/$$

$$[\gamma_0^2 (\overline{X}_{++}^{(0)*} - \overline{X}_{++}^{(1)*})^2], \tag{6.40}$$

where

$$S_{x_{i+}^{(g)}}^2 = \sum_i (X_{i+}^{(g)} - \overline{X}_{++}^{(g)})^2/m_g, \quad S_{x_{i+}^{(g)}, x_{i+}^{(g)*}} = \sum_i (X_{i+}^{(g)} - \overline{X}_{++}^{(g)})$$

$$\times (X_{i+}^{(g)*} - \overline{X}_{++}^{(g)*})/m_g, \quad S_{x_{i+}^{(g)*}}^2 = \sum_i (X_{i+}^{(g)*} - \overline{X}_{++}^{(g)*})^2/m_g,$$

$$\overline{X}_{++}^{(g)} = \sum_i X_{i+}^{(g)}/m_g, \quad \text{and} \quad \overline{X}_{++}^{(g)*} = \sum_i X_{i+}^{(g)*}/m_g.$$

As for testing noninferiority based on the PD, however, using this approach can produce an inaccurate estimate of the minimum required sample size if the chosen value γ_0 of interest is quite different from the underlying value γ in the pilot study. Thus, it is advisable to determine the final estimate of the minimum required sample size based on a range of n_1 (6.39) corresponding to various combinations of possible parameter values in practice.

6.5.3   Sample size calculation for testing equivalence

When determining the minimum required number of patients in testing equivalence, we need to make an additional approximation of the power function to derive the closed-form sample size calculation formulae. When the equivalence margins are pre-determined to be not small or the non-null parameter value of interest is chosen in the neighborhood of the null value, as noted in Section 2.5.3, using these closed-form sample size calculation formulae tends to underestimate the minimum required number of patients for a desired power at a nominal α-level. Thus, we should apply the trial-and-error adjustment procedure to correct this possible underestimation in these particular cases.

6.5.3.1   Using the difference in proportions

Note that using the normal approximation, we can easily show that the power function for testing $H_0 : \Delta \leq -\varepsilon_l$ or $\Delta \geq \varepsilon_u$ at the α-level based on the test procedure (6.15) for a given Δ_0 (where $-\varepsilon_l < \Delta_0 < \varepsilon_u$) is given by

$$\phi_{PD}(\Delta_0) = \Phi(\frac{\tanh^{-1}(\varepsilon_u) - \tanh^{-1}(\Delta_0)}{\sqrt{Var(\tanh^{-1}(\hat{\Delta}^{(RE)}))}} - Z_\alpha)$$

$$- \Phi(\frac{-\tanh^{-1}(\varepsilon_l) - \tanh^{-1}(\Delta_0)}{\sqrt{Var(\tanh^{-1}(\hat{\Delta}^{(RE)}))}} + Z_\alpha), \quad (6.41)$$

where $\Phi(X)$ is the cumulative standard normal distribution. Following the same arguments as those for a single measurement per patient (see Section 2.5.3.2), we may obtain an estimate of the minimum required number n_1 of patients from the experimental treatment for a desired power $(1 - \beta)$ of detecting equivalence with a specified value $-\varepsilon_l < \Delta_0 < \varepsilon_u$ at a nominal α-level as

$$n_1 = Ceil\{((Z_\alpha + Z_\beta)^2 V_{PD}^{(RE)}(\underline{\pi}_1, \underline{\pi}_2, \Delta_0, k)/[(1 - \Delta_0^2)^2])/$$
$$(\tanh^{-1}(\varepsilon_l) + \tanh^{-1}(\Delta_0))^2\} \quad \text{for} \; -\varepsilon_l < \Delta_0 < 0, \quad (6.42)$$

$$n_1 = Ceil\{((Z_\alpha + Z_\beta)^2 V_{PD}^{(RE)}(\underline{\pi}_1, \underline{\pi}_2, \Delta_0, k)/[(1 - \Delta_0^2)^2])/$$
$$(\tanh^{-1}(\varepsilon_u) - \tanh^{-1}(\Delta_0))^2\} \quad \text{for} \; 0 < \Delta_0 < \varepsilon_u, \quad (6.43)$$

and

$$n_1 = Ceil\{((Z_\alpha + Z_{\beta/2})^2 V_{PD}^{(RE)}(\underline{\pi}_1, \underline{\pi}_2, \Delta_0, k))/(\tanh^{-1}(\varepsilon_u))^2\}$$
$$\text{for} \; \Delta_0 = 0 \; \text{and} \; \varepsilon_l = \varepsilon_u. \quad (6.44)$$

When the pre-determined equivalence margins ε_l and ε_u are not small or when the chosen value $\Delta_0(\neq 0)$ is in the neighborhood of 0, using n_1 (6.42) or n_1 (6.43) tends to underestimate the minimum required number of patients from the experimental treatment resulting from an inaccurate approximation of power (Section 2.5.3.2). If this occurs, we may use n_1 (6.42) or n_1 (6.43) as the initial estimate and apply trial-and-error procedure to find the minimum integer n_1 such that the power function $\phi_{PD}(\Delta_0)$ (6.41) is greater than or equal to the desired power $1 - \beta$.

6.5.3.2   Using the ratio of proportions

When we test equivalence based on the PR used to measure the relative treatment efficacy, the power function of the test procedure (6.16) is given by

$$\phi_{PR}(\gamma_0) = \Phi(\frac{\log(1 + \gamma_u) - \log(\gamma_0)}{\sqrt{Var(\log(\hat{\gamma}^{(RE)}))}} - Z_\alpha)$$
$$- \Phi(\frac{\log(1 - \gamma_l) - \log(\gamma_0)}{\sqrt{Var(\log(\hat{\gamma}^{(RE)}))}} + Z_\alpha), \qquad (6.45)$$

where $1 - \gamma_l < \gamma_0 < 1 + \gamma_u$. Using the test procedure (6.16) and $V_{LPR}^{(RE)}(\underline{E}_1, \underline{E}_2, \gamma, k)$ (6.38), we obtain an estimate of the minimum required number n_1 of patients from the experimental treatment for a desired power $(1 - \beta)$ of detecting equivalence with a given specified value $1 - \gamma_l < \gamma_0 < 1 + \gamma_u$ at a nominal α-level as given by

$$n_1 = Ceil\{(Z_\alpha + Z_\beta)^2 V_{LPR}^{(RE)}(\underline{E}_1, \underline{E}_2, \gamma_0, k)/$$
$$(\log(\gamma_0) - \log(1 - \gamma_l))^2\} \quad \text{for } 1 - \gamma_l < \gamma_0 < 1, \qquad (6.46)$$

$$n_1 = Ceil\{(Z_\alpha + Z_\beta)^2 V_{LPR}^{(RE)}(\underline{E}_1, \underline{E}_2, \gamma_0, k)/$$
$$(\log(\gamma_0) - \log(1 + \gamma_u))^2\} \quad \text{for } 1 < \gamma_0 < 1 + \gamma_u, \qquad (6.47)$$

and

$$n_1 = Ceil\{(Z_\alpha + Z_{\beta/2})^2 V_{LPR}^{(RE)}(\underline{E}_1, \underline{E}_2, \gamma_0, k)/(\log(1 + \gamma_u))^2\}$$
$$\text{for } \gamma_0 = 1 \text{ and } \log(1 + \gamma_u) = -\log(1 - \gamma_l). \qquad (6.48)$$

When the pre-determined equivalence margins γ_l and γ_u are not small (say, $\gamma_l = 0.50$ and thereby, $\gamma_u = 1$ for a symmetric equivalence region on the log scale) or when the chosen value $\gamma_0(\neq 1)$ is in the neighborhood of 1, as noted previously, using n_1 (6.46) or n_1 (6.47) tends to underestimate the minimum required number of patients from the experimental treatment. Thus, we may use these resulting estimates as an initial estimate and apply the trial-and-error procedure to find the minimum integer n_1 such that the power function $\phi_{PR}(\gamma_0)$ (6.45) is greater than or equal to the desired power of $(1 - \beta)$.

Exercises

6.1 For a randomly selected patient i assigned to treatment $g = 1$,

(a) show that under model (6.1), the expectation (Lui, 2007c)

$$E(Y_{i+}^{(1)}) = E(p_{i+}^{(1)}) + \Delta_C E(Z_{i+}^{(1)}|C)P(C) + \Delta_A E(Z_{i+}^{(1)}|A)P(A)$$
$$+ \Delta_N E(Z_{i+}^{(1)}|N)P(N),$$

where $P(S)$ denotes the proportion of subpopulation S ($= C$, A, N) in the sampling population. Similarly, for a randomly selected patient i' assigned to treatment $g = 0$,

(b) show that the expectation

$$E(Y_{i'+}^{(0)}) = E(p_{i'+}^{(0)}) + \Delta_C E(Z_{i'+}^{(0)}|C)P(C) + \Delta_A E(Z_{i'+}^{(0)}|A)P(A)$$
$$+ \Delta_N E(Z_{i'+}^{(0)}|N)P(N).$$

Since we randomly assign patients to one of the two treatments, we may assume $E(p_{i+}^{(1)}) = E(p_{i'+}^{(0)})$. Furthermore, as noted in the context, we make the strong exclusion restriction assumption of treatment-receipt for always-takers and never-takers, and hence we have $E(Z_{i+}^{(1)}|A) = E(Z_{i'+}^{(0)}|A)$ and $E(Z_{i+}^{(1)}|N) = E(Z_{i'+}^{(0)}|N)$. Thus, we have $E(Y_{i+}^{(1)}) - E(Y_{i'+}^{(0)}) = \Delta_C[E(Z_{i+}^{(1)}|C) - E(Z_{i'+}^{(0)}|C)]P(C)$. Furthermore, for any two randomly selected patients i and i' from the experimental treatment and the standard treatment (placebo), respectively,

(c) show that the expectations $E(Z_{i+}^{(1)}) - E(Z_{i'+}^{(0)}) = [E(Z_{i+}^{(1)}|C) - E(Z_{i'+}^{(0)}|C)]P(C)$. Therefore, we obtain $E(Y_{i+}^{(1)}) - E(Y_{i'+}^{(0)}) = \Delta_C(E(Z_{i+}^{(1)}) - E(Z_{i'+}^{(0)}))$.

(d) Define $\overline{\overline{Y}}_{++}^{(g)} = \sum_i Y_{i+}^{(g)}/(n_g J)$ and $\overline{\overline{Z}}_{++}^{(g)} = \sum_i Z_{i+}^{(g)}/(n_g J)$. Show that $E(\overline{\overline{Y}}_{++}^{(1)} - \overline{\overline{Y}}_{++}^{(0)}) = \Delta_C(E(\overline{\overline{Z}}_{++}^{(1)}) - E(\overline{\overline{Z}}_{++}^{(0)}))$. (hint: $E(Y_{i+}^{(1)}) = E(\sum_j E(Y_{ij}^{(1)}|S)))$.

6.2 Show that an estimated variance for $\overline{\overline{Y}}_{++}^{(g)}$ (for $g = 1, 0$) is given by

$$\hat{Var}(\overline{\overline{Y}}_{++}^{(g)}) = [\sum_r (r/J)^2 \hat{\pi}_{r+}^{(g)} - (\sum_r (r/J)\hat{\pi}_{r+}^{(g)})^2]/n_g.$$

6.3 To account for the possible variation of the relative experimental treatment to the standard treatment between different patients and various courses, we may assume the risk additive model for the underlying probability structure of a positive response on patient i $(i = 1, 2, \ldots, n_g)$ assigned to treatment g $(g = 1, 0)$ at course j: $P(Y_{ij}^{(g)} = 1 | p_{ij}^{(g)}, z_{ij}^{(g)}) = p_{ij}^{(g)} + \Delta_{ij} z_{ij}^{(g)}$, where $p_{ij}^{(g)}$ denotes the underlying basic probability of a positive response when patient i is assumed to receive the standard treatment (or placebo) at course j; Δ_{ij} represents the excess effect due to the experimental treatment over the standard treatment (or placebo) on patient i at course j, and for patient $i \in S$ $(S = C, A, N)$, we denote the conditional expectation $E(\Delta_{ij}|S)$ by Δ_S. We further assume that $E(\Delta_{ij} Z_{ij}^{(g)} | S) = E(\Delta_{ij}|S) E(Z_{ij}^{(g)}|S)$. Show that Equation (6.2) holds.

6.4 When there is only a single measurement per patient (i.e. $J = 1$), show that test statistics (6.4) and (6.5) reduce to test statistics (2.3) and (2.4), respectively.

6.5 Using the delta method, show that an estimated asymptotic variance $\hat{Var}(\hat{\Delta}^{(RE)})$ for $\hat{\Delta}^{(RE)}$ (6.7) is given by

$$\sum_g \{\sum_r r^2 \hat{\pi}_{r+}^{(g)} - (\sum_r r \hat{\pi}_{r+}^{(g)})^2 - 2\hat{\Delta}^{(RE)}(\sum_r \sum_c rc \hat{\pi}_{rc}^{(g)}$$
$$- (\sum_r r \hat{\pi}_{r+}^{(g)})(\sum_c c \hat{\pi}_{+c}^{(g)})) + \hat{\Delta}^{(RE)^2}(\sum_c c^2 \hat{\pi}_{+c}^{(g)}$$
$$- (\sum_c c \hat{\pi}_{+c}^{(g)})^2)\} / [n_g (\sum_c c \hat{\pi}_{+c}^{(1)} - \sum_c c \hat{\pi}_{+c}^{(0)})^2].$$

6.6 Show that test statistic (6.9) reduces to test statistic (2.7) for testing noninferiority when there is only a single one measurement taken from each patient under the monotonicity assumption.

6.7 (a) Show that under model (6.10) and the strong exclusion restriction assumption for the treatment-receipt among always-takers and never-takers, we have $E(X_{i+}^{(1)}) - E(X_{i'+}^{(0)}) = \gamma_C (E(X_{i'+}^{(0)*}) - E(X_{i+}^{(1)*}))$. (hint: For a randomly selected patient i assigned to treatment g, show that we have the expectation

$$E(X_{i+}^{(g)}) = \gamma_C [\sum_j E(p_{ij}^{(g)}|C) E(Z_{ij}^{(g)}|C)] P(C)$$
$$+ \gamma_A [\sum_j E(p_{ij}^{(g)}|A) E(Z_{ij}^{(g)}|A)] P(A)$$
$$+ \gamma_N [\sum_j E(p_{ij}^{(g)}|N) E(Z_{ij}^{(g)}|N)] P(N).)$$

(b) Furthermore, under model (6.10), show that the expectations

$$E(X_{i+}^{(g)*}) = E(p_{i+}^{(g)}) - \{[\sum_j E(p_{ij}^{(g)}|C)E(Z_{ij}^{(g)}|C)]P(C)$$
$$+ [\sum_j E(p_{ij}^{(g)}|A)E(Z_{ij}^{(g)}|A)]P(A)$$
$$+ [\sum_j E(p_{ij}^{(g)}|N)E(Z_{ij}^{(g)}|N)]P(N)\}.$$

6.8 Using the delta method, we can show that the asymptotic variance for $\hat{\gamma}^{(RE)}$ (6.12) is given by

$$Var(\hat{\gamma}^{(RE)}) = \sum_g \{\sum_r r^2 E_{r+}^{(g)} - (\sum_r r\pi_{r+}^{(g)})^2$$
$$+ 2\gamma(\sum_r \sum_s rs E_{rs}^{(g)} - (\sum_r r E_{r+}^{(g)})(\sum_s s E_{+s}^{(g)}))$$
$$+ \gamma^2(\sum_s s^2 E_{+s}^{(g)} - (\sum_s s E_{+s}^{(g)})^2)\}/$$
$$[n_g(\sum_s s E_{+s}^{(0)} - \sum_s s E_{+s}^{(1)})^2].)$$

6.9 Show that when $J = 1$, test statistic (6.14) reduces to the test statistic (2.11) for a single measurement per patient. (hint: When $J = 1$, the term $\sum_r \sum_c rc E_{rc}^{(g)}$ is, by definition, equal to 0, and so is $\sum_r \sum_c rc \hat{E}_{rc}^{(g)}$ in $\hat{Var}(\hat{\gamma}^{(RE)})$ (6.13)).

6.10 Show that the expectation $E(T_{PD}^{(RE)}) = 0$, where $T_{PD}^{(RE)} = (\overline{Y}_{++}^{(1)} - \overline{Y}_{++}^{(0)}) - \Delta(\overline{Z}_{++}^{(1)} - \overline{Z}_{++}^{(0)})$, where $\overline{Y}_{++}^{(g)} = \sum_i Y_{i+}^{(g)}/n_g$ and $\overline{Z}_{++}^{(g)} = \sum_i Z_{i+}^{(g)}/n_g$.

6.11 Show that the variance $Var(T_{PD}^{(RE)})$ is equal to

$$\sum_g [\sum_r r^2 \pi_{r+}^{(g)} - (\sum_r r\pi_{r+}^{(g)})^2]/n_g + \Delta^2 \sum_g [\sum_s s^2 \pi_{+s}^{(g)}$$
$$- (\sum_s s\pi_{+s}^{(g)})^2]/n_g - 2\Delta \sum_g [\sum_r \sum_s rs\pi_{rs}^{(g)}$$
$$- (\sum_r r\pi_{r+}^{(g)})(\sum_s s\pi_{+s}^{(g)})]/n_g.$$

6.12 Show that $(T_{PD}^{(RE)})^2/Var(T_{PD}^{(RE)}) \le Z_{\alpha/2}^2$, where $T_{PD}^{(RE)} = (\overline{Y}_{++}^{(1)} - \overline{Y}_{++}^{(0)}) - \Delta(\overline{Z}_{++}^{(1)} - \overline{Z}_{++}^{(0)})$, where $\overline{Y}_{++}^{(g)} = \sum_i Y_{i+}^{(g)}/n_g$ and $\overline{Z}_{++}^{(g)} = \sum_i Z_{i+}^{(g)}/n_g$ and $Var(T_{PD}^{(RE)})$ is given in (6.19), if and only if Δ satisfied the quadratic equation $A^{(RE)}\Delta^2 - 2\Delta B^{(RE)} + C^{(RE)} \le 0$ defined in (6.20). Thus, if $A^{(RE)} > 0$ and $(B^{(RE)})^2 - A^{(RE)}C^{(RE)} > 0$, an asymptotic $100\,(1 - \alpha)\,\%$ confidence interval for Δ would be given by (6.21).

6.13 Under the assumed model (6.23), show that when $\rho_S = 0$, we have
$P(Z_{ij}^{(g)} = 1|S) = P(Z_{ij-1}^{(g)} = 1|S) = \cdots = P(Z_{i1}^{(g)} = 1|S)$.

6.14 By definition, we have $P(Z_{i1}^{(g)} = 1|A) = 1$ and $P(Z_{i1}^{(g)} = 1|N) = 0$ for $g = 1, 0$; as well as we have $P(Z_{i1}^{(1)} = 1|C) = 1$ and $P(Z_{i1}^{(0)} = 1|C) = 0$. Thus, under the assumed model (6.23), show that

(a) we have

$$
P(Z_{i2}^{(g)} = 1|A, Y_{i1}^{(g)}) = (1 - \rho_A) + \rho_A Y_{i1}^{(g)},
$$
$$
P(Z_{i2}^{(g)} = 1|N, Y_{i1}^{(g)}) = \rho_N(1 - Y_{i1}^{(g)}) \quad \text{(for } g = 1, 0),
$$
$$
P(Z_{i2}^{(1)} = 1|C, Y_{i1}^{(1)}) = (1 - \rho_C) + \rho_C Y_{i1}^{(1)}, \text{ and}
$$
$$
P(Z_{i2}^{(0)} = 1|C, Y_{i1}^{(0)}) = \rho_C(1 - Y_{i1}^{(0)}).
$$

Under models (6.1) and (6.23), derive the following conditional probability mass functions;

(b) for a randomly selected patient $i \in A$, we have

$$
P(Y_{i+}^{(g)} = 2|A) = [E(p_{i1}^{(g)}|A) + \Delta_A][E(p_{i2}^{(g)}|A) + \Delta_A],
$$
$$
P(Y_{i+}^{(g)} = 1|A) = [E(p_{i1}^{(g)}|A) + \Delta_A][1 - (E(p_{i2}^{(g)}|A) + \Delta_A)]
$$
$$
+ [1 - (E(p_{i1}^{(g)}|A) + \Delta_A)]E(p_{i2}^{(g)}|A)
$$
$$
+ [1 - (E(p_{i1}^{(g)}|A) + \Delta_A)](1 - \rho_A)\Delta_A, \text{ and}
$$
$$
P(Y_{i+}^{(g)} = 0|A) = [1 - (E(p_{i1}^{(g)}|A) + \Delta_A)][1 - E(p_{i2}^{(g)}|A)]
$$
$$
- [1 - (E(p_{i1}^{(g)}|A) + \Delta_A)](1 - \rho_A)\Delta_A;
$$

(c) for a randomly selected patient $i \in N$, we have

$$
P(Y_{i+}^{(g)} = 2|N) = E(p_{i1}^{(g)}|N)E(p_{i2}^{(g)}|N),
$$
$$
P(Y_{i+}^{(g)} = 1|N) = E(p_{i1}^{(g)}|N)[1 - E(p_{i2}^{(g)}|N)]
$$
$$
+ [1 - E(p_{i1}^{(g)}|N)]E(p_{i2}^{(g)}|N)
$$
$$
+ [1 - E(p_{i1}^{(g)}|N)]\rho_N\Delta_N, \text{ and}
$$
$$
P(Y_{i+}^{(g)} = 0|N) = [1 - E(p_{i1}^{(g)}|N)][1 - E(p_{i2}^{(g)}|A)]
$$
$$
- [1 - E(p_{i1}^{(g)}|N)]\rho_N\Delta_N;
$$

(d) for a randomly selected patient $i \in C$ assigned to the experimental treatment $(g = 1)$, we have

$$P(Y_{i+}^{(1)} = 2|C) = [E(p_{i1}^{(1)}|C) + \Delta_C][E(p_{i2}^{(1)}|C) + \Delta_C],$$
$$P(Y_{i+}^{(1)} = 1|C) = [E(p_{i1}^{(1)}|C) + \Delta_C][1 - (E(p_{i2}^{(1)}|C) + \Delta_C)]$$
$$+ [1 - (E(p_{i1}^{(1)}|C) + \Delta_C)]E(p_{i2}^{(1)}|C)$$
$$+ [1 - (E(p_{i1}^{(1)}|C) + \Delta_C)](1 - \rho_C)\Delta_C, \text{ and}$$
$$P(Y_{i+}^{(1)} = 0|C) = [1 - (E(p_{i1}^{(1)}|C) + \Delta_C)][1 - E(p_{i2}^{(1)}|C)]$$
$$- [1 - (E(p_{i1}^{(1)}|C) + \Delta_C)](1 - \rho_C)\Delta_C;$$

(e) for a randomly selected patient $i \in C$ assigned to the standard treatment or placebo $(g = 0)$, we have

$$P(Y_{i+}^{(0)} = 2|C) = E(p_{i1}^{(0)}|C)E(p_{i2}^{(0)}|C),$$
$$P(Y_{i+}^{(0)} = 1|C) = E(p_{i1}^{(0)}|C)[1 - E(p_{i2}^{(0)}|C)]$$
$$+ [1 - E(p_{i1}^{(0)}|C)]E(p_{i2}^{(0)}|C)$$
$$+ [1 - E(p_{i1}^{(0)}|C)]\rho_C\Delta_C, \text{ and}$$
$$P(Y_{i+}^{(0)} = 0|C) = [1 - E(p_{i1}^{(0)}|C)][1 - E(p_{i2}^{(0)}|C)]$$
$$- [1 - E(p_{i1}^{(0)}|C)]\rho_C\Delta_C.$$

(f) On the basis of the above results, for patients i and i' randomly selected from the experimental and standard treatments, respectively, show that we have

$$E(Y_{i+}^{(1)}) - E(Y_{i'+}^{(0)}) = E(E(Y_{i+}^{(1)}|S)) - E(E(Y_{i'+}^{(0)}|S))$$
$$= \Delta_C\{2 - [1 - (E(p_{i1}^{(1)}|C) + \Delta_C)]\rho_C$$
$$- [1 - E(p_{i'1}^{(0)}|C)]\rho_C\}P(C).$$

Furthermore, show that (h) $E(Z_{i+}^{(1)}) - E(Z_{i'+}^{(0)}) = E(E(Z_{i+}^{(1)}|S)) - E(E(Z_{i'+}^{(0)}|S)) = \{2 - [1 - (E(p_{i1}^{(1)}|C) + \Delta_C)]\rho_C - [1 - E(p_{i'1}^{(0)}|C)]\rho_C\}P(C)$. Thus, we have $E(Y_{i+}^{(1)}) - E(Y_{i'+}^{(0)}) = \Delta_C[E(Z_{i+}^{(1)}) - E(Z_{i'+}^{(0)})]$. Note that when $\rho_C = 1$, a substantial number of patients assigned to the experimental treatment can be switched to receive the standard treatment (or placebo) and vice versa. In this case, the difference $E(Z_{i+}^{(1)}) - E(Z_{i'+}^{(0)})(= \{E(p_{i1}^{(1)}|C) + \Delta_C + E(p_{i'1}^{(0)}|C)\}P(C))$ can be very small when the underlying probability $E(p_{i1}^{(1)}|C) (= E(p_{i'1}^{(0)}|C))$ and $P(C)$ are small. Thus, there is a nonnegligible probability that the estimate of $E(Z_{i+}^{(1)}) - E(Z_{i'+}^{(0)})$ can be 0 or even negative. As noted in the concern of estimation for the PR when its denominator is close to 0 under perfect compliance (Lui, 2004), hypothesis testing procedures and interval estimators discussed here on the basis of $\hat{\Delta}_C^{(RE)}$ for the treatment efficacy can perform poorly in this extreme case. In practice, however, ρ_C is likely to be small especially for a double-blind RCT.

6.15 Show that the randomization-based variance $V_{RB}(t_{PR}^{(RE)})$ (Cochran, 1977) for statistic $t_{PR}^{(RE)}$ is given in (6.28).

6.16 Under models (6.10) and (6.23), derive the following conditional expectations:

(a)
$$E(X_{i+}^{(1)}|C) = \gamma_C\{E(p_{i1}^{(1)}|C) + E(p_{i2}^{(1)}|C)$$
$$- \rho_C[1 - \gamma_C E(p_{i1}^{(1)}|C)]E(p_{i2}^{(1)}|C)\},$$
$$E(X_{i'+}^{(0)}|C) = \gamma_C E(p_{i'2}^{(0)}|C)[1 - E(p_{i'1}^{(0)}|C)]\rho_C,$$

and hence

$$E(X_{i+}^{(1)}|C) - E(X_{i'+}^{(0)}|C) = \gamma_C\{E(p_{i1}^{(1)}|C) + E(p_{i2}^{(1)}|C)$$
$$- \rho_C[1 - \gamma_C E(p_{i1}^{(1)}|C)]E(p_{i2}^{(1)}|C)$$
$$- \rho_C[1 - E(p_{i'1}^{(0)}|C)]E(p_{i'2}^{(0)}|C)\}.$$

Similarly, show that (b)

$$E(X_{i+}^{(1)*}|C) = E(p_{i2}^{(1)}|C)[1 - \gamma_C E(p_{i1}^{(1)}|C)]\rho_C,$$
$$E(X_{i'+}^{(0)*}|C) = E(p_{i'1}^{(0)}|C) + E(p_{i'2}^{(0)}|C)\{1 - [1 - E(p_{i'1}^{(0)}|C)]\rho_C\},$$

and hence

$$E(X_{i'+}^{(0)*}|C) - E(X_{i+}^{(1)*}|C) = E(p_{i'1}^{(0)}|C) + E(p_{i'2}^{(0)}|C)$$
$$- \rho_C[1 - E(p_{i'1}^{(0)}|C)]E(p_{i'2}^{(0)}|C)$$
$$- \rho_C[1 - \gamma_C E(p_{i1}^{(1)}|C)]E(p_{i2}^{(1)}|C).$$

We can further show that (c)

$$E(X_{i+}^{(g)}|A) = \gamma_A\{E(p_{i1}^{(g)}|A) + E(p_{i2}^{(g)}|A)$$
$$- \rho_A[1 - \gamma_A E(p_{i1}^{(g)}|A)]E(p_{i2}^{(g)}|A)\};$$
$$E(X_{i+}^{(g)}|N) = \gamma_N E(p_{i2}^{(g)}|N)[1 - E(p_{i1}^{(g)}|N)]\rho_N;$$
$$E(X_{i+}^{(g)^*}|A) = E(p_{i2}^{(g)}|A)[1 - \gamma_A E(p_{i1}^{(g)}|A)]\rho_A; \text{ and}$$
$$E(X_{i+}^{(g)^*}|N) = E(p_{i1}^{(g)}|N) + E(p_{i2}^{(g)}|N)\{1 - [1 - E(p_{i1}^{(g)}|N)]\rho_N\}.$$

On the basis of the above results, we can show that

$$\gamma_C = [E(X_{i+}^{(1)}) - E(X_{i'+}^{(0)})]/[E(X_{i'+}^{(0)^*}) - E(X_{i+}^{(1)^*})] \quad (6.11).$$

6.17 Show that the sample size calculation formula n_1 (6.33) reduces to the sample size formula (2.31) for testing superiority when there is only a single measurement per patient.

References

Agresti, A. (1990). *Categorical Data Analysis*. New York: John Wiley & Sons, Inc.

Anbar, D. (1983). The relative efficiency of Zelen's prerandomization design for clinical trials. *Biometrics*, **39**, 711–718.

Angrist, J.D., Imbens, G.W. and Rubin, D.B. (1996). Identification of causal effects using instrumental variables. *Journal of the American Statistical Association*, **91**, 444–456.

Baker, S. G. and Kramer, B. (2005). Simple maximum likelihood estimates of efficacy in randomized trials and before-and-after studies, with implications for meta-analysis. *Statistical methods in Medical Research*, **14**, 349–367.

Baker, S. G. and Lindeman, K. S. (1994). The paired availability design: a proposal for evaluating epidural analgesia during labor. *Statistics in Medicine*, **13**, 2269–2278.

Bang, H. and Davis, C. E. (2007). On estimating treatment effects under non-compliance in randomized clinical trials: are intent-to-treat or instrumental variables analyses perfect solutions? *Statistics in Medicine*, **26**, 954–964.

Barnard, J., Frangakis, C.E., Hill, J.E., and Rubin, D.B. (2003). Principal stratification approach to broken randomized experiments: a case study of school choice voucher in New York City. *Journal of the American Statistical Association*, **98**, 299–311.

Binary Data Analysis of Randomized Clinical Trials with Noncompliance, First Edition. Kung-Jong Lui.
© 2011 John Wiley & Sons, Ltd. Published 2011 by John Wiley & Sons, Ltd.

Barnett, H. J. M. and NASCET collaborators. (1991). Beneficial effect of carotid endarterectomy in symptomatic patients with high-grade carotid stenosis. *New England Journal of Medicine*, **325**, 445–453.

Begg, C. B. (2000). Ruminations on the intent-to-treat principle. Controlled Clinical Trials *(Commentary)*, **21**, 241–243.

Bellamy, S. L., Lin, J. Y. and Ten Have, D. R. (2007). An introduction to causal modeling in clinical trials. *Clinical Trials*, **4**, 58–73.

Bernhard, G. and Compagnone, D. (1989). Binary data in prerandomized designs, *Biometrical Journal*, **31**, 19–33.

Bishop, Y. M. M., Fienberg, S. E. and Holland, P. W. (1975). *Discrete Multivariate Analysis, Theory and Practice*. Cambridge, MA: MIT Press.

Blackwelder, W. C. and Chang, M. A. (1984). Sample size graphs for 'proving the null hypothesis'. *Controlled Clinical Trials*, **5**, 97–105.

Bristol, D.R. (1993). Probabilities and sample sizes for the two one-sided test procedures. *Communications in Statistics, Theory and Methods*, **22**, 1953–1961.

Brunner, E. and Neumann, N. (1985). On the mathematical basis of Zelen's prerandomized designs. *Methods of Information in Medicine*, **24**, 120–130.

Casella, G. and Berger, R. L. (1990). *Statistical Inference*. Belmont, California: Duxbury.

Chen, J.J., Tsong, Y., and Kang, S.-H. (2000). Tests for equivalence or noninferiority between two proportions. *Drug Information Journal*, **34**, 569–578.

Clarke, P.S. and Windmeijer, F. (2010). Identification of causal effects on binary outcomes using structural mean models. *Biostatistics*, doi:10.1093/biostatistics/kxq024, in press.

Cochran, W. G. (1977). *Sampling Techniques*, 3rd edition. New York: John Wiley & Sons, Inc.

Cornfield, J.A. (1956). Statistical problem arising from retrospective studies, In J. Neyman (ed.), *Proceedings of the Third Berkeley Symposium on Mathematical Statistics and Probability*. Vol. 4. Berkeley, CA: University of California Press, 136–148.

Coronary Drug Project Research Group (1980). Influence of adherence to treatment and response of cholesterol on mortality in the Coronary Drug Project. *New England Journal of Medicine*, **303**, 1038–1041.

Cox, D. R. (1958). *The Planning of Experiments*. New York: John Wiley & Sons, Inc.

Cuzick, J., Edwards, R. and Segnan, N. (1997). Adjusting for non-compliance and contamination in randomized clinical trials. *Statistics in Medicine*, **16**, 1017–1029.

Dexter, P., Wolinsky, F., Gramelspacher, G., *et al.* (1998). Effectiveness of computer-generated reminders for increasing discussions about advance directives and completion of advance directives. *Annals of Internal Medicine*, **128**, 102–110.

DiMatteo, M.R., Giordani, P.J., Lepper, H.S., and Groghan, T.W. (2002). Patient adherence and medical treatment outcomes. *Medical Care*, **40**, 794–811.

Donner, A. and Klar, N. (2000). *Design and Analysis of Cluster Randomization Trials in Health Research*. London: Arnold.

Dunnett, C.W. and Gent, M. (1977). Significance testing to establish equivalence between treatments, with special reference to data in the form of 2 x 2 tables. *Biometrics*, **33**, 593–602.

Edwardes, M.D. (1995). A confidence interval for $Pr(X<Y)-Pr(X>Y)$ estimated from simple cluster samples. *Biometrics*, **5**, 571–578.

FDA (1997). *Guidance for Industry. Evaluating Clinical Studies of Antimicrobials in the Division of Anti-infective Drug Products*, FDA, 17 Feb., p. 87.

Fischer-Lapp, K. and Goetghebeur, E. (1998). Practical properties of some structural mean analyses of the effect of compliance in randomized trials, *Controlled Clinical Trials*, **20**, 531–546.

Fisher, R. A. (1924). On a distribution yielding the error functions of several well known statistics. *Proceedings of International Congress of Mathematics*, **2**, 805–813.

Fleiss, J. L. (1981). *Statistical Methods for Rates and Proportions*. 2nd ed. New York: John Wiley & Sons, Inc.

Fleiss, J.L., Levin, B. and Paik, M.C. (2003). *Statistical Methods for Rates and Proportions*, 3rd ed. New York: John Wiley & Sons, Inc.

Frangakis, C. E. and Baker, S. G. (2001). Compliance subsampling designs for comparative research: estimation and optimal planning. *Biometrics*, **57**, 899–908.

Frangakis, C. E. and Rubin, D. B. (1999). Addressing complications of intention-to-treat analysis in the combined presence of all-or-none treatment-noncompliance and subsequent missing outcomes. *Biometrika*, **86**, 365–379.

Frangakis, C.E. and Rubin, D. B. (2002). Principal stratification in causal inference. *Biometrics*, **58**, 21–29.

Frangakis, C.E., Rubin, D.B. and Zhou, X.-H. (2002). Clustered encouragement designs with individual noncompliance: Bayesian inference with randomization, and application to advance directive forms. *Biostatistics*, **3**, 147–164.

Garrett, A.D. (2003). Therapeutic equivalence: fallacies and falsification. Statistics in Medicine, **22**, 741–762.

Goetghebeur, E. and Molenberghs, G. (1996). Causal inference in a placebo-controlled clinical trial with binary outcome and ordered compliance. *Journal of the American Statistical Association*, **91**, 928–934.

Goetghebeur, E., Molenberghs, G. and Katz, J. (1998). Estimating the causal effect of compliance on binary outcome in randomized controlled trials, *Statistics in Medicine*, **17**, 341–355.

Goetghebeur, E. and Vansteelandt, S. (2005). Structural mean models for compliance analysis in randomized clinical trials and the impact of errors on measures of exposure. *Statistical Methods in Medical Research*, **14**, 397–415.

Greenland, S. and Robins, J. M. (1985). Estimation of a common effect parameter from sparse follow-up data. *Biometrics*, **41**, 55–68.

Hauck, W.W. and Anderson, S. (1984). A new statistical procedure for testing equivalence in two group comparative bioavailability trials. *Journal of Pharmacokinetics and Biopharmaceutics*, **12**, 83–91.

Hauck, W.W. and Anderson, S. (1986). A proposal for interpreting and reporting negative studies. *Statistics in Medicine*, **5**, 203–209.

Heitjan, D.F. (1999). Causal inference in a clinical trial: a comparative example. *Controlled Clinical Trials*, **20**, 309–318.

Hernan, M. and Robins, J.M. (2006). Instruments for causal inference: an epidemiologist's dream? *Epidemiology*, **17**, 360–372.

Hirano, K, Imbens, G.W., Rubin, D.B. and Zhou, X.-H. (2000). Assessing the effect of an influenza vaccine in an encouragement design. *Biostatistics*, **1**, 69–88.

Holland, P. (1986). Statistics and causal inference. *Journal of the American Statistical Association*, **81**, 945–970.

Hosmer, D. W. and Lemeshow, S. (1989). *Applied Logistic Regression*. New York: John Wiley & Sons, Inc.

Ialongo, N.S., Werthamer, L., Kellam, S.G., Brown, C.H., Wang, S. and Lin, Y. (1999). Proximal impact of two first-grade preventive interventions on the early risk behaviors for later substance abuse, depression and antisocial behavior. *American Journal of Community Psychology*, **27**, 599–642.

Jacobson, J.M., Spritzler, J., Fox, L. *et al.* (1999). Thalidomide for the treatment of esophageal aphthour ulcers in patients with human immunodeficiency virus infection, *Journal of Infectious Diseases*, **180**, 61–67.

Jo, B. (2002). Statistical power in randomized intervention studies with noncompliance. *Psychological Methods*, **7**, 178–193.

Jo, B., Asparouhov, T. and Muthén, B.O. (2008). Intention-to-treat analysis in cluster Randomized trials with noncompliance. *Statistics in Medicine*, **27**, 5565–5577.

Jo, B., Asparouhov, T., Muthén, B.O., Ialongo, N.S., and Brown, C.H. (2008). Cluster randomized trials with treatment noncompliance. *Psychological Methods*, **13**, 1–18.

Johnson, N.L. and Kotz, S. (1970). *Continuous Univariate Distribution: I Distribution in Statistics*. New York: John Wiley & Sons, Inc.

Katz, D., Baptista, J., Azen, S.P. and Pike, M.C. (1978). Obtaining confidence intervals for the risk ratio in cohort studies. *Biometrics*, **34**, 469–479.

Lachin, J.M. (2000). Statistical Considerations in the intent-to-treat principle. *Controlled Clinical Trials*, **21**, 167–189.

Last, J.M. (1988). *A Dictionary of Epidemiology*, 2nd edn. Oxford: Oxford University Press.

Laupacis, A., Sackett, D. L., and Roberts, R. S. (1988). An assessment of clinically useful measures of the consequences of treatment. *New England Journal of Medicine*, **318**, 1728–1733.

Li, F. and Frangakis, C. E. (2005). Designs in partially controlled studies: messages from a review. *Statistical Methods in Medical Research*, **14**, 417–431.

Light, R.J. and Margolin, B. H. (1971). An analysis of variance categorical data. *Journal of the American Statistical Association*, **66**, 534–544.

Lipsitz, S.R. Dear, K.B.G, Laird, N.M. and Molenberghs, G. (1998). Tests for homogeneity of the risk difference when data are sparse. *Biometrics*, **54**, 148–160.

Little, R.J.A. and Yau, L.H.Y. (1998). Statistical techniques for analyzing data from prevention trials: Treatment of no-shows using Rubin's causal model. *Psychological Methods*, **3**, 147–159.

Little, R.J.A. and Rubin, D.B. (2002). *Statistical Analysis with Missing Data*, 2nd edition. New York: John Wiley & Sons, Inc.

Liu, J.P. and Chow, S.C. (1992). Sample size determination for the two one-sided tests procedure in bioequivalence. *Journal of Pharmacokinetics and Biopharmaceutics*, **20**, 101–104.

Liu, J.P. and Chow, S.C. (1993). On assessment of bioequivalence of drugs with negligible plasma levels. *Biometrical Journal*, **35**, 109–123.

Liu, J.P. and Weng, C. S. (1995). Bias of two one-sided tests procedures in assessment of bioequivalence. *Statistics in Medicine*, **14**, 853–861.

Loey, T., Vansteelandt, S. and Goetghebeur, E. (2001). Accounting for correlation and compliance in cluster randomized trials. *Statistics in Medicine*, **20**, 3753–3767.

Lui, K.-J. (1991). Sample sizes for repeated measurements in dichotomous data, *Statistics in Medicine*, **10**, 463–472.

Lui, K.-J. (1994). The effect of retaining probability variation on sample size calculations for normal variates. *Biometrics*, **50**, 297–300.

Lui, K.-J. (1997a). Sample size determination for repeated measurements in bioequivalence test. *Journal of Pharmacokinetics and Biopharmaceutics*, **25**, 507–513.

Lui, K-J. (1997b). Exact equivalence test for risk ratio and its sample size determination under inverse sampling. *Statistics in Medicine*, **16**, 1777–1786.

Lui, K.-J. (2000a). Notes on life table analysis in correlated observations. *Biometrical Journal*, **42**, 93–110.

Lui, K.-J. (2000b). A note on the log-rank test in life table analysis with correlated observations. *Biometrical Journal*, **42**, 457–470.

Lui, K.-J. (2001). A test procedure of equivalence in ordinal data with matched-pairs. *Biometrical Journal*, **43**, 977–983.

Lui, K.-J. (2002). Notes on estimation of the general odds ratio and the general risk difference for paired-sample data. *Biometrical Journal*, **44**, 957–968.

Lui, K.-J. (2004). *Statistical Estimation Epidemiological Risk*. New York: John Wiley & Sons, Inc.

Lui, K.-J. (2005). Interval estimation of the proportion ratio under multiple matching. *Statistics in Medicine*, **24**, 1275–1285.

Lui, K.-J. (2006a). A note on hypothesis test in binary data under the single-consent randomized design. *Drug Information Journal*, **40**, 219–227.

Lui, K.-J. (2006b). Interval estimation of risk difference in simple compliance randomized trials. *Journal of Modern Applied Statistical Methods*, **5**, 395–407.

Lui, K.-J. (2006c). Risk Ratio Analysis. In: Chow SC, editor. *Encyclopedia of Biopharmaceutical Statistics*, Taylor and Francis Group, Dekker, New York. DOI 10.1081/E-EBS-120041874.

Lui, K.-J. (2007a). Interval estimation of risk ratio in the simple compliance randomized Trial. *Contemporary Clinical Trials*, **28**, 120–129.

Lui, K.-J. (2007b). Estimation of proportion ratio in non-compliance randomized trials with repeated measurements in binary data. *Statistical Methodology*, **5**, 129–141.

Lui, K.-J. (2007c). Correction for non-compliance of repeated binary outcomes in randomized clinical trials: Randomized analysis approach. *Statistics in Medicine* (Letter to the Editor), **21**, 4679–4685.

Lui, K.-J. (2007d). Notes on test equality in stratified noncompliance randomized trials. *Drug Information Journal*, **41**, 607–618.

Lui, K.-J. (2007e). Testing homogeneity of the risk ratio in stratified noncompliance randomized trials. *Contemporary Clinical Trials*, **28**, 614–625.

Lui, K.-J. (2007f). Sample size calculation for non-compliance trials with repeated measurements in binary data. *Computational Statistics and Data Analysis*, **51**, 3832–3843.

Lui, K.-J. (2007g). Interval estimation of the risk difference in non-compliance randomized trials with repeated binary measurements. *Statistics in Medicine* **26**, 3140–3156.

Lui, K-J. (2008a). Estimation of the risk difference under a noncompliance randomized clinical trial with missing outcomes. *Journal of Biopharmaceutical Statistics*, **18**, 273–292.

Lui, K.-J. (2008b). Notes on interval estimation of risk difference in stratified noncompliance randomized trials: A Monte Carlo evaluation. *Computational Statistics and Data Analysis*, **52**, 4091–4103.

Lui, K.-J. (2009). On estimating treatment effects under non-compliance in randomized clinical trials: Are intent-to-treat or instrumental variables analyses perfect solutions? *Statistics in Medicine* (Letter to the Editors), **28**, 531–534.

Lui, K.-J. and Chang, K.-C. (2007). Five interval estimators for proportion ratio under a stratified randomized clinical trial with noncompliance. *Biometrical Journal*, **49**, 613–626.

Lui, K.-J. and Chang, K.-C. (2008a). Test equality and sample size calculation based on risk difference in a randomized clinical trial with noncompliance and missing outcomes. *Biometrical Journal*, **50**, 224–236.

Lui, K.-J. and Chang, K.-C. (2008b). Sample size determination for assessing equivalence based on proportion ratio under a randomized trial with non-compliance and missing outcomes. *Statistics in Medicine*, **27**, 47–67.

Lui, K.-J. and Chang, K.-C. (2008c). Testing homogeneity of risk difference in stratified trials with noncompliance. *Computational Statistics and Data Analysis*, **53**, 209–221.

Lui, K.-J. and Chang, K.-C. (2009a). Estimation of risk ratio in a noncompliance randomized clinical trial with trichotomous dose levels. *Statistical Methodology*, **6**, 164–176.

Lui, K.-J. and Chang, K.-C. (2009b). Interval estimation of odds ratio in a stratified randomized clinical trial with noncompliance. *Computational Statistics and Data Analysis*, **53**, 2754–2766.

Lui, K.-J. and Chang, K.-C. (2009c). Test homogeneity of odds ratio in a randomized clinical trial with noncompliance. *Journal of Biopharmaceutical Statistics*, **19**, 916–932.

Lui, K.-J. and Chang, K.-C. (2010). Notes on odds ratio estimation for a randomized clinical trial with noncompliance and missing outcomes. *Journal of Applied Statistics*, **37**, 2057–2071.

Lui, K.-J. and Chang, K.-C. (2011a). Sample size determination for testing equality in a cluster randomized trial with noncompliance, *Journal of Biopharmaceutical Statistics*, **21**, 1–17.

Lui, K.-J. and Chang, K.-C. (2011b). Test non-inferiority and sample size determination based on the odds ratio under a cluster randomized trial with noncompliance. *Journal of Biopharmaceutical Statistics*, **21**, 94–110.

Lui, K.-J. and Cumberland, W. G. (2001). Sample size determination for equivalence test using rate ratio of sensitivity and specificity in paired sample data. *Controlled Clinical Trials*, **22**, 373–389.

Lui, K.-J. and Cumberland, W. G. (2008). Notes on estimation of proportion ratio under a non-compliance randomized trial with missing outcomes. *Computational Statistics and Data Analysis*, **52**, 4325–4345.

Lui, K.-J., Cumberland, W. G., Mayer, J.A. and Eckhardt, L. (1999). Interval estimation for the intraclass correlation in Dirichlet-multinomial data. *Psychometrika*, **64**, 355–369.

Lui, K.-J. and Kelly, C. (2000a). A revisit on tests for homogeneity of the risk difference. *Biometrics*, **56**, 309–315.

Lui, K.-J. and Kelly, C. (2000b). Tests for homogeneity of the risk ratio in a series of 2x2 tables. *Statistics in Medicine*, **19**, 2919–2932.

Lui, K.-J. and Lin, C.-D. (2003). Interval estimation of treatment effects in double consent randomized design. *Statistica Sinica*, **13**, 179–187.

Lui, K.-J. and Zhou, X.-H. (2004). Testing non-inferiority (and equivalence) between two diagnostic procedures in paired-sample ordinal data. *Statistics in Medicine*, **23**, 545–559.

McDonald, C.J., Hui, S.L., and Tierney, W. M. (1992). Effects of computer reminders for influenza vaccination on morbidity during influenza epidemics. *M .D. Computing*, **9**, 304–312.

McHugh, R. (1984). Validity and treatment dilution in Zelen's single consent design. *Statistics in Medicine*, **3**, 215–218.

Mark, S. D. and Robins, J. M. (1993). A method for the analysis of randomized trials with compliance information: An application to the multiple risk factor intervention trial. *Controlled Clinical Trials*, **14**, 79–97.

Matsui, S. (2005). Stratified analysis in randomized trials with noncompliance. *Biometrics*, **61**, 816–823.

Matsuyama, Y. (2002). Correcting for noncompliance of repeated binary outcomes in randomized clinical trials: randomized analysis approach. *Statistics in Medicine*, **21**, 675–687.

Matts, J. P. and McHugh, R. B. (1987). Randomization and efficiency in Zelen's single consent design. *Biometrics*, **43**, 885–894.

Matts, J. P. and McHugh, R. B. (1993). Precision estimation in Zelen's single-consent Design. *Biometrical Journal*, **35**, 65–72.

Mealli, F. and Rubin, D.B. (2002). Assumptions when analyzing randomized experiments with noncompliance and missing outcomes. *Health Services and Outcomes Research Methodology*, **3**, 225–232.

Mealli, F., Imbens, G.W., Ferro, S., and Biggeri, A. (2004). Analyzing a randomized trial on breast self-examination with noncompliance and missing outcomes. *Biostatistics*, **5**, 207–222.

Multiple Risk Factor Intervention Trial Research Group. (1982). Multiple risk factor intervention trial: Risk factor changes and mortality results. *Journal of the American Medical Association*, **248**, 1465–1477.

Nagelkerke, N., Fidler, V., Bernsen, R. and Borgdorff, M. (2000). Estimating treatment effects in randomized clinical trials in the presence of non-compliance. *Statistics in Medicine*, **19**, 1849–1864.

Obuchowski, N. A. (1997). Testing for equivalence of diagnostic tests. *American Journal of Roentgenology*, **168**, 13–17.

Ohno, R., Miyawaki, S., Hatake, K., *et al.* (1997). Human urinary macrophage colony-stimulating factors reduces the incidence and duration of febrile neutropenia and shortens the period required to finish three courses of intensive consolidation therapy in acute myeloid leukemia: a double-blind controlled study. *Journal of Clinical Oncology*, **15**, 2954–2965.

O'Malley, J. A. and Normand, S.-L. T. (2005). Likelihood methods for treatment noncompliance and subsequent nonresponse in randomized trials. *Biometrics*, **61**, 325–334.

Piantadosi, S. (1997). *Clinical Trials: a Methodological Perspective.* New York: John Wiley & Sons, Inc.

Rae, G. (1988). The equivalence of multiple rater kappa statistics and intraclass correlation coefficients. *Educational and Psychological Measurement*, **48**, 367–374.

Robins, J. M. (1994). Correcting for non-compliance in randomized trials using structural nested mean models. *Communications in Statistics, Theory and Methods*, **23**, 2379–2412.

Robins, J. M. (1998). Correction for non-compliance in equivalence trials. *Statistics in Medicine*, **17**, 269–302.

Robins, J. M. and Rotnitzky, A. (2004). Estimation of treatment effects in randomised trials with non-compliance and a dichotomous outcome using structural mean models. *Biometrika*, **91**, 763–783.

Rousson, V. and Seifert, B. (2008). A mixed approach for proving non-inferiority in clinical trials with binary endpoints. *Biometrical Journal*, **50**, 190–204.

Rubin, D. B. (1974). Estimating causal effects of treatments in randomized and nonrandomized studies. *Journal of Educational Psychology*, **66**, 688–701.

Rubin, D. B. (1977). Assignment to a treatment group on the basis of a covariate. *Journal of Educational Statistics*, **2**, 1–26.

Rubin, D. B. (1978). Bayesian inference for causal effects: the role of randomization. *Annals of Statistics*, **6**, 34–58.

SAS Institute, Inc. (1990). *SAS Language, Reference Version 6*, 1st edn. Cary, North Carolina: SAS Institute.

Sato, T. (1995). A further look at the Cochran-Mantel-Haenszel risk difference. *Controlled Clinical Trials*, **16**, 359–361.

Sato, T. (2000). Sample size calculations with compliance information. *Statistics in Medicine* 2000, **19**, 2689–2697.

Sato, T. (2001). A method for the analysis of repeated binary outcomes in randomized clinical trials with non-compliance. *Statistics in Medicine*, **20**, 2761–2774.

Schuirmann, D. J. (1987). A comparison of the two one-sided tests procedure and the power approach for assessing the equivalence of average bioavailability. *Journal of Pharmacokinetics and Biopharmaceutics*, **15**, 657–680.

Senn, S. (2000). Consensus and controversy in pharmaceutical statistics (with discussion). *Journal of the Royal Statistical Society*, Series D, **49**, 135–176.

Sheps, M. C. (1958). Shall we count the living or the dead? *New England Journal of Medicine*, **259**, 1210–1214.

Sheps, M. C. (1959). An examination of some methods of comparing several rates or proportions. *Biometrics*, **15**, 87–97.

Sinclair, J.C. and Bracken, M.B. (1994). Clinically useful measures of effect in binary analyses of randomized trials. *Journal of Clinical Epidemiology*, **47**, 881–889.

Sjölander, A. (2008). A note on 'The method of handling non-compliance in clinical trial suggested by Sato/Matsuyama.' *Statistics in Medicine* (Letter to the Editor), **27**, 3920–3924.

Skalski, J. R. (1992). Sample size calculations for normal variates under binomial censoring. *Biometrics*, **48**, 877–882.

Sommer, A., Tarwotjo, I., Djunaedi, E., *et al.* (1986). Impact of vitamin A supplementation on childhood mortality: a randomized controlled community trial. *Lancet*, **i**, 1169–1173.

Sommer, A. and Zeger, S. L. (1991). On estimating efficacy from clinical trials. *Statistics in Medicine*, **10**, 45–52.

Tabár, L., Fagerberg, G., Day, N.E., and Holmberg, L. (1987). 'What is the optimum interval between mammographic screening examinations?' – An analysis based on the latest results of the Swedish two-county breast cancer screening trial. *British Journal of Cancer*, **55**, 547–551.

Ten Have, T.R., Elliott, M.R., Joffe, M., Zanutto, E., and Datto, C. (2004). Causal models for randomized physician encouragement trials in treating in primary care depression. *Journal of the American Statistical Association*, **99**, 16–25.

Ten Have, T.R., Joffe, M. and Cary, M. (2003). Causal logistic models for non- compliance under randomized treatment with univariate binary response. *Statistics in Medicine*, **22**, 1255–1283.

Tu, D. (1998). On the use of the ratio or the odds ratio of cure rates in establishing therapeutic equivalence of non-systemic drugs with binary clinical endpoints, *Journal of Biopharmaceutical Statistics*, **8**, 263–282.

Tu, D. (2003). Odds ratio, In: Chow SC, Editor. *Encyclopedia of Biopharmaceutical Statistics*. New York: Dekker; Taylor & Francis Group.

Vansteelandt, S. and Goetghebeur, E. (2003). Causal inference with generalized structural mean models. *Journal of Royal Statistical Society B*, **65**, 817–835.

Walter, S.D. (2000). Choice of effect measure for epidemiological data. *Journal of Clinical epidemiology*, **53**, 931–939.

Walter, S.D., Guyatt, G. Montori, V.M., Cook, R. and Prasad, K. (2006). A new preference-based analysis for randomized trials can estimate treatment acceptability and effect in compliant patients. *Journal of Clinical Epidemiology*, **59**, 685–696.

Wang, H., Chow, S.-C. and Li, G. (2002). On sample size calculation based on odds ratio in clinical trials. *Journal of Biopharmaceutical Statistics*, **12**, 471–483.

Weng, C.S. and Liu, J. P. (1994). Some pitfalls in sample size estimation for anti-infective study. *Proceedings of Biopharmaceutic Section of American Statistical Association*, 56–60.

Westlake, W. J. (1974). The use of balanced incomplete block designs in comparative bioavailability trials, *Biometrics*, **30**, 319–327.

Westlake, W. J. (1979). Statistical aspects of comparative bioavailability trials. *Biometrics*, **35**, 273–280.

Yau, L.H.Y. and Little, R.J. (2001). Inference for complier-average causal effect from longitudinal data subject to noncompliance and missing data, with application to a job training assessment for the unemployed. *Journal of the American Statistical Association*, **96**, 1232–1244.

Zelen, M. (1979). A new design for randomized clinical trials. *The New England Journal of Medicine*, **300**, 1242–1245.

Zelen, M. (1982). Strategy and alternate designs in cancer clinical trials. *Cancer Treatment Reports*, **66**, 1095–1100.

Zelen, M. (1986). Response, *Journal of Chronic Disease*, **39**, 247–249.

Zelen, M. (1990). Randomized consent designs for clinical trials: an update. *Statistics in Medicine*, **9**, 645–656.

Zhou, X. H. and Li, S.-M. (2006). ITT analysis of randomized encouragement design studies with missing data. *Statistics in Medicine* 2006; **25**, 2737–2761.

Index

STATISTICS IN PRACTICE

Human and Biological Sciences

Berger – Selection Bias and Covariate Imbalances in Randomized Clinical Trials

Berger and Wong – An Introduction to Optimal Designs for Social and Biomedical Research

Brown and Prescott – Applied Mixed Models in Medicine, Second Edition

Carstensen – Comparing Clinical Measurement Methods

Chevret (Ed) – Statistical Methods for Dose-Finding Experiments

Ellenberg, Fleming and DeMets – Data Monitoring Committees in Clinical Trials: A Practical Perspective

Hauschke, Steinijans & Pigeot – Bioequivalence Studies in Drug Development: Methods and Applications

Källén – Understanding Biostatistics

Lawson, Browne and Vidal Rodeiro – Disease Mapping with WinBUGS and MLwiN

Lesaffre, Feine, Leroux & Declerck - Statistical and Methodological Aspects of Oral Health Research

Lui – Statistical Estimation of Epidemiological Risk

Marubini and Valsecchi - Analysing Survival Data from Clinical Trials and Observation Studies

Molenberghs and Kenward – Missing Data in Clinical Studies

O'Hagan, Buck, Daneshkhah, Eiser, Garthwaite, Jenkinson, Oakley & Rakow – Uncertain Judgements: Eliciting Expert's Probabilities

Parmigiani – Modeling in Medical Decision Making: A Bayesian Approach

Pintilie – Competing Risks: A Practical Perspective

Senn - Cross-over Trials in Clinical Research, Second Edition

Senn - Statistical Issues in Drug Development, Second Edition

Spiegelhalter, Abrams and Myles – Bayesian Approaches to Clinical Trials and Health-Care Evaluation

Walters – Quality of Life Outcomes in Clinical Trials and Health-Care Evaluation

Whitehead - Design and Analysis of Sequential Clinical Trials, Revised Second Edition

Whitehead – Meta-Analysis of Controlled Clinical Trials

Willan and Briggs – Statistical Analysis of Cost Effectiveness Data

Winkel and Zhang – Statistical Development of Quality in Medicine

Earth and Environmental Sciences

Buck, Cavanagh and Litton – Bayesian Approach to Interpreting Archaeological Data

Chandler and Scott – Statistical Methods for Trend Detection and Analysis in the Environmental Sciences

Glasbey and Horgan – Image Analysis in the Biological Sciences

Haas – Improving Natural Resource Management: Ecological and Political Models

Helsel – Nondetects and Data Analysis: Statistics for Censored Environmental Data

Illian, Penttinen, Stoyan, H and Stoyan D–Statistical Analysis and Modelling of Spatial Point Patterns

McBride – Using Statistical Methods for Water Quality Management

Webster and Oliver – Geostatistics for Environmental Scientists, Second Edition

Wymer (Ed) – Statistical Framework for Recreational Water Quality Criteria and Monitoring

Industry, Commerce and Finance

Aitken – Statistics and the Evaluation of Evidence for Forensic Scientists, Second Edition

Balding – Weight-of-evidence for Forensic DNA Profiles

Brandimarte – Numerical Methods in Finance and Economics: A MATLAB-Based Introduction, Second Edition

Brandimarte and Zotteri – Introduction to Distribution Logistics

Chan – Simulation Techniques in Financial Risk Management

Coleman, Greenfield, Stewardson and Montgomery (Eds) – Statistical Practice in Business and Industry

Frisen (Ed) – Financial Surveillance

Fung and Hu – Statistical DNA Forensics

Gusti Ngurah Agung - Time Series Data Analysis Using EViews

Kenett (Eds) - Operational Risk Management: A Practical Approach to Intelligent Data Analysis

Jank and Shmueli (Ed.) – Statistical Methods in e-Commerce Research

Lehtonen and Pahkinen - Practical Methods for Design and Analysis of Complex Surveys, Second Edition

Ohser and Mücklich - Statistical Analysis of Microstructures in Materials Science

Pourret, Naim & Marcot (Eds) – Bayesian Networks: A Practical Guide to Applications

Taroni, Aitken, Garbolino and Biedermann - Bayesian Networks and Probabilistic Inference in Forensic Science

Taroni, Bozza, Biedermann, Garbolino and Aitken – Data Analysis in Forensic Science